THE REAL MEAL REVOLUTION
SUPER FOOD FOR SUPERCHILDREN

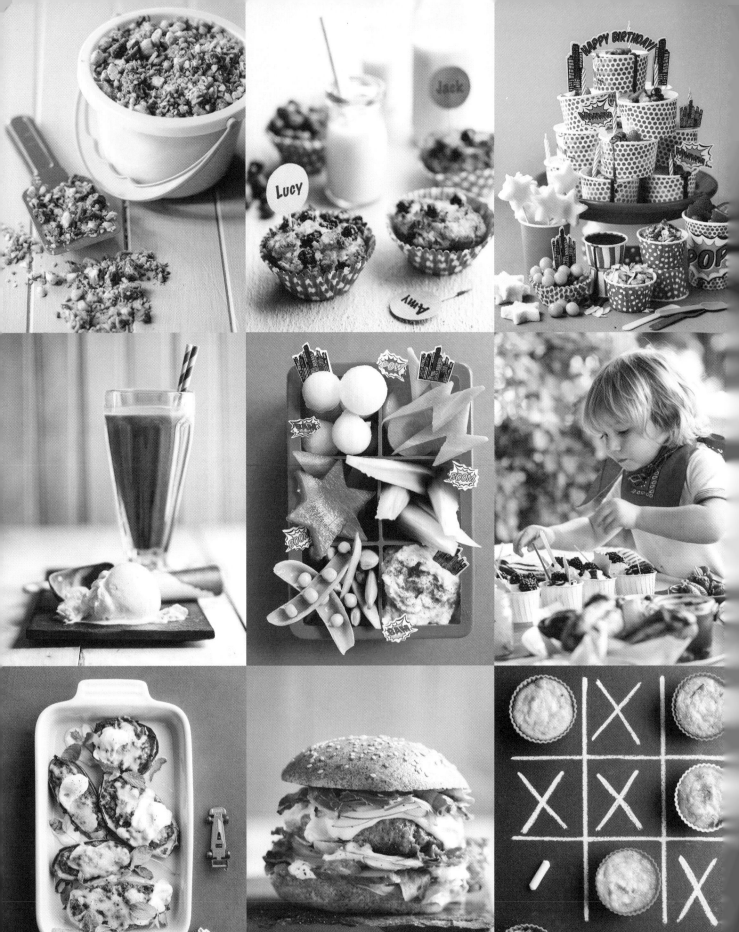

THE REAL MEAL REVOLUTION
SUPER FOOD FOR SUPERCHILDREN

PROFESSOR TIM NOAKES

JONNO PROUDFOOT

BRIDGET SURTEES

ROBINSON

CONT

KA-BOOM

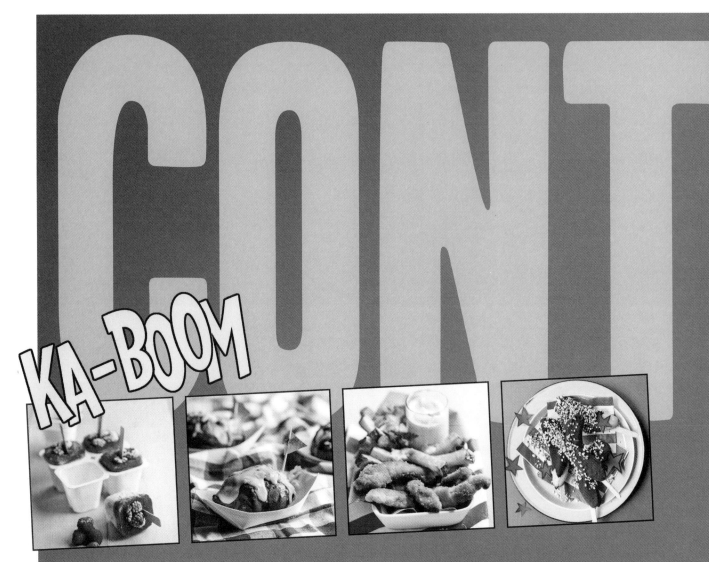

POW!

ENTS

BLAM!

"I find it ironic that if you **TELL YOUR DOCTOR THAT YOU PLAN TO EAT LOW CARB DURING PREGNANCY,** THEY'LL SAY IT'S UNSAFE. But if you say you plan to eat a diet based on **FRESH VEGETABLES, MEAT, FISH, EGGS, DAIRY, NUTS, SEEDS, AND A LITTLE FRUIT,** they'll encourage you to stay the course."

– Lily Nichols, author of *Real Food For Gestational Diabetes*

"**WE CREATED THIS OBESOGENIC ENVIRONMENT; IT DID NOT HAPPEN TO US.** We told people to avoid real food and to eat processed food. We passed legislation to ensure trans fats and sweeteners into our food chain. **WE ALLOWED OUR CHILDREN TO BE GIVEN TOYS, CARTOON CHARACTERS AND JUNK FOOD BY 'STRANGERS'.**"

– Dr Zoe Harcombe, author of *The Obesity Epidemic: What caused it? How can we stop it?*

PROLOGUE
BY PROF TIM NOAKES

I was born in 1949, one of the Baby Boomers, the child of parents who had survived the prolonged stress and deprivations of the Second World War in Liverpool, England. The war taught my parents' generation life lessons it would never forget. The first was frugality; waste and excess were considered equally sinful.

The second was the nutritional value of the foods like meat, eggs, cheese and butter that had been severely rationed during the war. So during my childhood, first in Harare, Zimbabwe and then in Cape Town, my parents made sure I was provided with the nutrition they believed to be optimum. This meant there was always plenty of eggs, meat, fish and dairy, not to forget organ meats like liver, kidneys and my special favourite, sheep's brains. My parents also grew their own vegetables and in time we acquired a cow that provided us with raw milk and butter. I now suspect that my height (1.88m) has much to do with the nutritionally dense foods that my parents provided me in my critical first 18 years.

When it came to sweets, sugary drinks and ice creams, those were strictly rationed treats. I recall the special moment on Sundays when my father would drive my sister and me to the local Dairy Den ice-cream parlour to purchase an especially decadent ice cream in a cone, the centre of which contained a chocolate bar! The feeling of illicit pleasure that the treat produced remains with me today. I remember too the precise birthday party at which I first overindulged in sweets and chocolates and, as a result, felt ill for several days.

I now know that one outstanding result of our parental generation's nutritional practices was that in our adolescence almost all my generation were lean. In my high-school class in Cape Town there was only one boy who would today be classified as obese. So rare was the condition that we considered it probable that he had an uncommon disease, perhaps cancer. Not only were we boys lean, but so too were the adolescent girls in our sister schools. Watching the films of the 1960s confirms that the vast majority were lean at any age during that period.

But today when I speak at high schools I notice that the situation is quite different. It is uncommon to meet many children who are as lean as we were. And the number who are already unhealthily heavy in their teens is frightening.

Five years ago, before I had myself undergone the dietary transformation that saw me lose 20kg of excess body fat, and before we had written *The Real Meal Revolution*, I assumed that the obesity I see in today's younger generation is, just like the weight gain I had experienced in my middle age, completely unavoidable. I had come to believe that this obesity is simply a natural consequence of our errant human biology over which we, as individuals, have little or no control.

I assumed this because my own overweight state had happened insidiously over 20 years during which I had religiously followed the dietary advice of my clever teachers at medical school. Beginning in 1977 these experts admonished us that the dietary practices of our parents' generation were abysmally in error. They warned us that if we continued eating all that protein, and especially too much saturated fat, we would most assuredly die from a heart attack at a young age. Or if we survived that, then cancer would get us.

So compelling did I find this messaging that as a novice and impressionable (but now properly "educated") young professional, I was amongst the very first South African doctors fully to commit to the novel 1977 United States Dietary Goals for Americans (USDGA). Very soon I replaced the delicious whole foods of my youth with the tasteless cereals and grains that I was assured would ensure a longer and healthier life.

Only much later did I realise that once I had made this change my running began to deteriorate almost immediately, and I started to put on weight – at first just a few kilograms. For the first time in my life I had increasing difficulty controlling my weight – because, I now know in retrospect, for the first time in my life I had lost control of my hunger. Over the next 20 years I discovered that the only way I could prevent weight gain whilst eating cereals and grains was to run extraordinarily long distances each week. As I loved running this was fortunately not a hardship. But all that running was completely unnecessary; I could have controlled my weight effortlessly had I simply reverted to the foods I had eaten as a child.

My real wake-up call came in 2010 when I realised that, despite eating the diet the experts assured me was "healthy" and despite running so much,

I still managed to develop Type 2 diabetes mellitus. Since I had done everything "right" according to expert opinion, I could draw only one conclusion – the "experts" must be wrong. But why?

One result of my Damascene conversion was our book *The Real Meal Revolution*, in which we warned that the dietary advice I had embraced too readily was the direct and immediate cause of the obesity and diabetes epidemics that began in 1980. We also told why many of us need to restrict the amount of dietary carbohydrate we ingest if we want to be healthy; why we should avoid eating processed foods; and why a long healthy life begins with eating real, unadulterated foods.

With this first sequel to *The Real Meal Revolution* we turn our attention to our children (and grandchildren). For if we are to reverse the current obesity/ diabetes epidemic in the next decade and optimise their health, we must begin by changing the eating patterns of our children and grandchildren – one child at a time, one meal at a time.

THE POWER-UP GUIDE

Welcome to *Super Food for Superchildren*, about the awesome nutrition your kids deserve, the delicious recipes you can cook to give it to them, and the fascinating story behind the science of it all. Here's a breakdown of the book:

Part I: How To Raise Superchildren is our quick and easy introduction – the summarised take of the Real Meal Revolution's approach to children's nutrition. Especially for busy parents with not much time on their hands, it gets to the point and cuts through all the misinformation and confusion out there. Read this right away so you know what it's all about.

Part II: Nutritional Information And Recipes By Age Group provides specific nutritional advice and delicious kid-friendly recipes for five separate dietary stages of childhood – or, if you'd prefer, five food-providing stages of parenthood. The stages are:

> **Marvellous Mums – pregnancy-6 months.** Nutrition for mum who's in turn providing nutrition for baby, first in utero then while breastfeeding.
> **Wonder Weaning – 6-12 months.** The often tricky always messy transition from breast milk (or formula) to solids.
> **Terrific Toddlers – 1-3 years.** The playgroup years, when junior's eating repertoire expands, though his table manners may still need work.
> **Incredible Kids – 3-13 years.** Time to put on the big-boy pants, go to nursery school (then junior school) – and eat meals with the family.
> **Tremendous Teens – 13 years +.** Advice and recipes to make adolescence, high school and hormonal imbalances that much easier to handle.

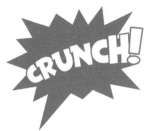

Note: even if your children are teenagers make sure you start at Incredible Kids, as this section includes the bulk of the (family-friendly) recipes.

Part III: The Kids' Nutrition Revolution is Tim Noakes's review of the evidence that supports the advice in this book. Effectively a compendium of the science of children's nutrition, it is riveting, enlightening and sometimes a little frightening. When Prof Noakes began his research he was, as ever, out to challenge the "conventional wisdom" not supported by the science. He has let the peer-reviewed empirical evidence guide him, and the results have been both predictable in some senses and surprising in others. Either way, the children's food industry does not come out of it well – another reason why we believe parents need to educate themselves on how best to feed their families.

NEED TO KNOW

The meals throughout this book have been created according to a clear brief:

- They contain no added sugar, no refined carbohydrates and no overly processed ingredients. They are as low as possible in total sugars, as well as high-gluten grains, specifically wheat, barley and rye.
- They are as practical as possible to shop for and make, so that cooking for your children becomes an enjoyable and thus sustainable experience.
- They are delicious and appealing to kids!

When cooking from our recipes, please bear these notes in mind:

- More than half the recipes are found in the Incredible Kids section, subdivided into Breakfasts, Lunches, Packed Lunches, Dinners, Snacks & Treats, and Party Food. These are meals suitable for all children old enough to eat with the family, teenagers and adults, with the exception of anyone following strict low-carb diets. The Teen section recipes, which are healthy variations on typical teenager convenience food, are similarly suitable.
- Cooking times are approximate; they may vary according to your oven, your equipment, your toddler's propensity for needing emergency entertainment halfway through the preparation, and any number of factors. Use them as a guide. Likewise, the portion sizes are also guides. There's a big size difference between a 4-year-old and a 12-year-old, for instance, so use your common sense (a good parenting rule in general). In fact, feel free to mix and match and adjust ingredients and recipe quantities as necessary.
- More important than getting the times or ingredients exactly right: read through the recipe before you begin so that you understand the process and method from the start.

A NOTE ON GENDERS
We have alternated genders from chapter to chapter when referring to your baby or child. For nutrition purposes, consider the advice for boys and girls as interchangeable unless specified.

THE RECIPES LEGEND

Quick and easy
For rustling up something in a flash

One-pot wonder
Convenient cooking with less washing up (though not necessarily quick)

Freezer friendly
Ideal for convenient freezer storage (usually up to 3 months)

Family friendly
Suitable for the whole family

Family fun
Great for getting the kids involved in the cooking process

Gourmet meal
Not just kid-friendly – perfect for a dinner party

Treat alert
Meals that are a little higher in total sugars or carbs – try to limit your kids to one treat meal a week

THE LISTS

These lists are for children above the age of three who are healthy and at a healthy weight.

GREEN

The green list is made up of foods that can be eaten freely every day to appetite

Fruit & vegetables

All green leafy vegetables (spinach, cabbage, lettuce etc.)

- Asparagus
- Artichoke hearts
- Aubergine
- Avocado
- Broccoli
- Brussels sprouts
- Butternut squash
- Cabbage
- Cauliflower
- Celery
- Courgettes
- Leeks
- Mushrooms
- Olives
- Onions
- Peppers
- Pumpkin
- Radishes
- Sauerkraut
- Spring onions
- Sweet potato
- Tomatoes

Proteins

- Eggs
- All meats, poultry and game (offal is encouraged)
- Naturally cured meat products like bacon, salami, biltong, jerky
- All fish and shellfish

Dairy

- Cottage cheese, cream, cream cheese, full-fat and Greek yogurt (homemade is best; shop-bought second; added starches, sugars and preservatives last resort), sour cream/crème fraîche
- Hard cheeses like Parmesan and pecorino
- Soft cheeses like mozzarella, feta, ricotta
- Firm cheeses like Cheddar, Emmental, Gouda
- Full-fat cheeses like Brie, camembert, gorgonzola, Roquefort
- Double cream

Fats

- Avocado oil (cold-pressed is best)
- Butter or ghee
- Coconut oil
- Macadamia oil (cold-pressed is best)
- Mayonnaise, homemade or preservative-free
- Olive oil (cold-pressed is best) and olives
- Lard, tallow, duck and bacon fat
- Nut oils like groundnut oil (as long as they're not heated)

Nuts & seeds

- All raw nuts
- Homemade nut butters (sugar-free), including peanut butter

All legumes (best prepared soaked or sprouted)

- Alfalfa (sprouts)
- Beans such as green, runner, broad, cannellini, kidney and black-eyed (fresh or dried)
- Chickpeas (sprouts or dried)
- Lentils (sprouts or dried)
- Peanuts (in shells only)
- Peas (fresh, frozen or dried)
- All whole seeds

To drink

- Water – sparkling or still
- Caffeine-free herbal teas and water (with real slices of fruit and herbs)
- Flavoured waters from the recipes on pages 188, 252 and 254
- Homemade broths

Extras

- Vinegars
- Herbs and spices
- Real mustards
- All condiments without preservatives and sugar

ORANGE

The orange list is made up of foods that are safe to eat but should be consumed in moderation; as a result, portion control is important.

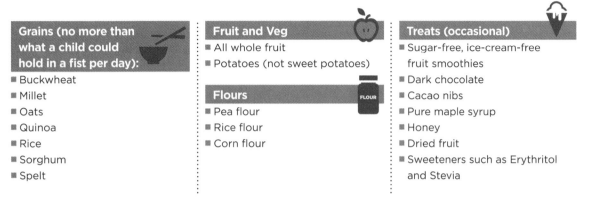

Grains (no more than what a child could hold in a fist per day):
- Buckwheat
- Millet
- Oats
- Quinoa
- Rice
- Sorghum
- Spelt

Fruit and Veg
- All whole fruit
- Potatoes (not sweet potatoes)

Flours
- Pea flour
- Rice flour
- Corn flour

Treats (occasional)
- Sugar-free, ice-cream-free fruit smoothies
- Dark chocolate
- Cacao nibs
- Pure maple syrup
- Honey
- Dried fruit
- Sweeteners such as Erythritol and Stevia

RED

All items on the red list should be avoided wherever practical.

Glutinous foods
- All flours and all breads made from grains containing gluten (wheat flour, rye flour, barley flour)
- All confectionary
- Commercially breaded or battered food such as breaded chicken nuggets or battered fish
- Commercial breakfast cereals like muesli, granola or boxed cereals
- Corn products, for example popcorn, polenta, corn thins, maize meal
- Couscous
- Crackers and cracker breads

Other refined products
- All processed corn products like popcorn, corn thins, maize meal
- All processed rice products

Beverages
- Fruit juices, including homemade
- All soft drinks, including diet drinks
- Energy drinks
- Commercial iced teas
- Flavoured milk and milkshakes

Dairy/dairy-related
- Commercial cheese spreads and other processed portions
- Powdered milk/coffee creamers
- Condensed milk
- Sweetened single cream
- Ice cream and commercial, sweetened frozen yoghurt
- Baked and steamed puddings

Fats
The following oils and fats are unhealthy on their own and as ingredients in other products.
- Industrial seed and vegetable oils, for example:
  - Cottonseed oil
  - Corn oil
  - Rice bran oil
  - Sunflower oil
  - Safflower oil
- Hydrogenated or partially hydrogenated fats, for example:
  - Butter spreads
  - Margarine and shortening

Animal/vegetable protein
- Meats cured with excessive sugar (for example, honey-glazed ham)
- Highly processed sausages and luncheon meats
- Soya

Sweet things
- All confectionery and (non-dark) chocolates (including 'protein', 'energy' or 'breakfast'/'snack' bars)
- Agave anything
- Artificial sweeteners (aspartame, acesulfame K, saccharin, sucralose)
- Cordials
- Canned fruit in syrup
- Fructose
- Jam
- Malt
- Sugar
- Sugared or commercially pickled foods
- Syrup

General
- Any food with added sugar
- Crisps
- Fast food (unless you trust the brand and you know the ingredients)
- Supermarket convenience meals (unless you trust the brand and you know the ingredients)
- Sugary condiments like ketchup, marinades and salad dressings

INTRODUCTION:
HOW TO RAISE SUPERCHILDREN

WHAT'S IT ALL ABOUT?
(THE SHORT VERSION)

Super Food for Superchildren is the follow-up title to *The Real Meal Revolution*. But it is neither a book about Banting nor a guide to losing weight and rejuvenating health. Rather,

Super Food for Superchildren is an

anti-sugar, anti-refined carb, pro-real foods

proclamation to the world

to say that we want to raise
our children so that they

never have to lose weight in the future.

This rather bold intention is the short version. There are many other similarly bold (evidence-based) recommendations and there are dozens of fantastic and delicious recipes along the way. But we'll get there. For now, we wanted to prime you. You're a parent and we know your time is precious. In creating this book, we hope to help you raise superchildren.

WHAT'S IT ALL ABOUT?
(THE SLIGHTLY LONGER VERSION)

When *The Real Meal Revolution* was published in South Africa in November 2013 we were, as the name suggests, intending to start an eating revolution. Tim Noakes, always an advocate of "challenging beliefs", had been vocal in the three years to that point about the ever-increasing evidence that the global obesity epidemic was being fuelled by the Western high-carb low-fat diet. We hoped a book filled with compelling science and delicious low-carb high-fat recipes would change the way South Africans thought about nutrition and health. With luck, we thought, the book might even be published internationally and make a meaningful contribution to the global conversation.

To say the phenomenal success of *The Real Meal Revolution* has exceeded our expectations is more than an understatement. The book has sold like hotcakes. (Or should that be cauli-mash?) It won the Nielsen Booksellers' Choice Awards after topping the South African Bestseller list for most of 2014, and was still in the top 10 as this book went to print two years after publication. As the Real Meal Revolution and Prof Noakes have made regular headlines – often amidst some controversy – the term "Banting", a word that originated in the 19th century, has returned to modern conversation. Suddenly there are Banting support groups, online Banting programmes (including our own), Banting menus, even entire Banting restaurants springing up across the country. Tens of thousands of South Africans are changing their health for the better by changing the way they eat, and *The Real Meal Revolution* is to be published in a further 21 countries around the world.

The success of *The Real Meal Revolution* has surprised us in many ways, and we've had to remind ourselves that this is exactly what we were hoping to achieve: we really *are* trying to start – and maintain – an eating revolution.

So, where to next?

Of course, we want to continue fighting the good (fat) fight, which we are doing online at realmealrevolution.com with great results. But for genuine long-term success – bearing in mind our modest goal is to cure the world of obesity and its related illnesses – we need to fight a smarter fight. We need to prevent rather than cure.

Rather than (just) trying to
turn overweight, unhealthy people
into SLIMMER, HEALTHIER
versions of themselves,
what about
STOPPING THEM becoming overweight
and unhealthy in the first place?

Hence, *Super Food for Superchildren*, a book that we hope will set children everywhere on the path to long-lasting good health. Having seen so many grown-ups rejuvenate themselves so incredibly in the last year-and-a-half – losing dozens of kilograms; feeling alive with energy after years of sickness;

running and cycling faster than they have for a decade or more – our goal is to prevent future generations from ever having to go to all that trouble. Rather, let them be happy and healthy from the start so they can grow into the superchildren they deserve to be.

Jonno, Kate and the can of cola

"The moment the underlying message of *Super Food for Superchildren* struck me came not long after production on the book had begun, when my wife, Kate, and I went for the 13-week scan on our first child. When our little girl, in utero and fast asleep, refused to perform for the ultrasonographer, she suggested that Kate drink a can of cola to get things going. Interesting advice coming from a doctor, we thought, but she insisted it was the only way we would get our baby to move into the correct position for the scan.

Kate drank only a few sips, and the reaction was mind-blowing. Within minutes our girl was going ballistic, bouncing off the walls, putting on the performance of her little lifetime. As fantastic as it was to see my active future child, I couldn't stop thinking: carbonated water mixed with sugar, a bit of caffeine and some additives can do *that*?

My take-home message was:

An unborn baby gets a similar rush when its mother takes A FEW SIPS OF A FIZZY DRINK to a grown-up taking CLASS-A DRUGS.

It struck me just how sensitive a foetus can be to what her mother eats and drinks. And how sensitive our babies and children must be to what they eat and drink. Something needs to be done!"

– JONNO PROUDFOOT

The philosophy of *Super Food for Superchildren*

Global nutrition is in a transitional phase. After decades of expanding waistlines and diminishing health, we're finally coming around to the fact that low-fat high-carb eating has been a profound and hugely costly mistake, one that has negatively affected the lives of tens of millions of people. As documented in *The Real Meal Revolution* and elsewhere (and summarised on p20), the rationale that led us to demonise fat was disastrous from start to end: the early studies were inherently flawed and contradictory, the arguments that won the day were driven by personality rather than fact, and the guidelines that were implemented around the world as a result were ultimately sustained by the vice grip of commercial farming and food manufacturing. Accurate science was a mere bystander.

Today, anyone who has delved into the questionable history of it all simply has to be sceptical of "prevailing wisdoms" and the advice that is peddled from so many competing platforms. When a study suggests that something *may* cause something else, should we believe it? But who sponsored the study? What's the agenda behind it? Is the science accurate and unadulterated or has it been distorted – for any number of reasons?

In short, how do we know what advice to follow? And specifically, in the case of this book, how do we approach our children's nutrition when nutrition in general is so divided by different lines of thinking and conflicts of interest?

Good questions. Particularly when the politics of modern parenting are added to the debate. From a scientific perspective, there's an expanse of murky moral ground to cross when compiling data on pregnant women, infants and young children. It's simply very difficult to perform studies that draw accurate causative (rather than associative) conclusions. And from a social perspective, specific parenting decisions and child behaviours can be divisive and controversial amongst even the closest of family and friends. Just ask a dinner table of parents which is better: natural birth or Caesarean section, breastfeeding or formula feeding, intensive hands-on mothering or nannies and babysitters to ease the load? Good luck with the conversation that follows...

In our opinion, the answers to these and other questions are not about which option is "better", but about making informed decisions so you can apply the known science as accurately as possible to your specific situation.

Bearing all this in mind,

here's what you'll get from *Super Food for Superchildren*: the best science available on children's nutrition from as objective a viewpoint as possible, married to a practical way of implementing it successfully (along with amazing recipes!).

As a scientist who has run hundreds of studies himself during his career yet is not affiliated to the children's food industry in any way, Tim Noakes is in the ideal position to offer an accurate overview of the available science that isn't clouded by subjective interests – because there *is* scientific consensus on a great deal of the most relevant aspects of children's nutrition. And you, as the parent, need to know what that consensus is and how food-industry marketing (and other parties) may try to mask these facts from you.

Meanwhile, Bridget Surtees specialises in low-carb nutrition for children and offers workable evidence-based advice. Importantly, whatever we recommend is underscored by the practicalities of parenthood.

Of the expanded team of six copy contributors to the book, three have children already and four were expecting during the course of production. So we're *very* aware that well-intentioned dietary advice and scientifically formulated eating plans for a pregnant woman can go out the window when all you want to eat is chocolate milk for lunch and cheesecake for dinner. We know that after you've slaved over a nutritious, carefully balanced meal for your two-year-old, there's a chance he'll take one bite, turn up his nose and demand ice cream for yum-yum. We believe that a less-stressed parent makes for a happier and healthier child, and that a mother's (and father's) wellbeing may be the most important factor in raising a happy, healthy child.

So, in *Super Food for Superchildren* we will be very clear when the science is unambiguous, and we will strongly recommend that you follow it in such cases whenever possible. Elsewhere, the evidence may be less definitive and we'll suggest the path that we might take in that instance. Whenever possible, we will offer alternatives, and we'll always be practical about it.

In general,

this is a wake-up call to today's parents.
We're advising a radical shift away
from the nutrition orthodoxy that has produced
OVERWEIGHT, UNHEALTHY CHILDREN
at alarming rates in the last three decades.

But while we're advocating important fundamental nutritional positions – see from p22 – our guiding position is one of education for both you, the parents, and your children. Don't be tied to the conventional wisdom of your past because you're comfortable with it or "because what was good enough for me must be good enough for my child". Make decisions that are as informed as possible, and that will benefit your children in the long run.

What exactly is a "treat"?

Before you think we're being overly diplomatic, let's make something clear right now: we are committedly anti-sugar. There is no way of interpreting the science differently. Sugar lines the path to adult obesity, metabolic syndrome, diabetes and a host of other health problems we'll get to, and it offers no nutritional benefits. None of the recipes in this book includes added sugar, and the strongest, most emphatic advice in this is book is: *don't serve sugar to your children*. Right on its tail is: *don't serve refined carbohydrates to your children*.

One of the perceived problems with this advice is it can seem a bit mean and Grinch-like. What about the joy of eating an ice cream or slurping down a strawberry milkshake? After all, good parenting isn't just about responsible nutrition; it's also about bringing happiness into your child's life. Right?

This is where we would like your mindset to change. Just because you, the parent, may have a sweet tooth and find the decadent joys of a death-by-chocolate cake one of the finer things in life, that doesn't mean your child has to. In other words, *your* high-sugar, high-carb treat doesn't have to be *his*. You're not treating your child by offering him future bad health, and if he's brought up on a diet low in sugar (and refined carbs) and thus has avoided an affinity for particularly sweet things, then there's a much higher chance he won't get the same joy as you do out of that chocolate cake anyway.

He can, however, still take great pleasure in many foods and you can still spoil him on special occasions. (See from p226 for 40 pages of recipes dedicated to snacks, treats and party foods.) All you have to do is redefine *in your own mind* what a treat is – because your child is a blank slate to start; he doesn't know what a treat is until you show him. So try not to think of treats as bargaining tools or everyday things. An ice cream with the family on Sundays? That's a treat. Processed sugar explosions every day after meals shouldn't be. A handful of biltong or a bowl of strawberries can be. Or a meal that he loves but takes you a little longer to prepare. Or perhaps it's not food: if you're down to the last resort of parenting – bribery – then maybe it's a toy or a movie or a trip to the beach. Just steer clear of "treating" your kids with sugar.

The sooner you realise that
a chocolate or a box of biscuits
IS NOT A TREAT,
the healthier your child is likely to be
throughout his or her entire life.

THE REAL MEAL RECAP

Before outlining the nutritional gist of *Super Food for Superchildren*, we need to briefly review the ground covered in *The Real Meal Revolution*. The summarised message from that book goes something like this.

Once upon a time we were generally slim and free from chronic diseases. As modern medicine advanced and we learnt how to combat infectious diseases, we started living longer. (At the beginning of the 20th century global average lifespan was 31 years, by mid-century it was 48 years, and today it's over 70 years.[1]) Other non-infectious conditions became more prominent, and heart disease and stroke, in particular – now the leading causes of death around the world[2] – captured the imagination of the western world. In looking to identify why heart disease was becoming so prevalant, an American researcher by the name of Ancel Keys came to prominence in the 1950s. It was, he theorised, caused by elevated blood-cholesterol concentrations, which were caused by too much dietary fat, particularly saturated fat. The cause of heart disease, therefore, was a diet high in fat. This was the diet-heart hypothesis.

As there are only three macronutrients for humans to consume – protein, fat and carbohydrates – and because proteins are essential for our survival and occur in so many foods, the recommendations that ultimately emerged from Keys's work were straightforward: eat more carbohydrates, eat fewer fats and ensure that the fats you do eat are not saturated and of animal origin.

Keys's methods and conclusions were criticised by his contemporaries. He had used basic association studies (rather than causative studies) and critically flawed science to reach his conclusions; in some cases he made the errors to be expected of pioneering research in a field; in others he simply interpreted the data to satisfy his fixed preconceptions. Nevertheless, Keys was a forceful personality and he and his allies slowly came to dominate the debate. Despite convincing arguments against his work from many quarters, it was accepted in 1977 as the basis for the United States Dietary Goals for Americans, which was translated into US government policy in 1980. Americans would henceforth be advised to remove as much fat from their diet as possible, and replace it with carbohydrates. This was a government policy that was expected to produce far-reaching health improvements comparable to those that arose from the famous Surgeon General's Advisory Committee on Smoking and Health of 1964.

But the very opposite has happened.

Instead, an American-led global obesity epidemic has emerged over the last 35 years, spreading from country to country and bringing with it a disastrous rise in a host of related chronic diseases. According to the World Health Organization, global obesity rates have more than doubled since 1980. As of 2014, 1.9 billion adults were overweight, of whom 600 million were obese.[3] A full two-thirds of American adults are overweight or obese, and half of them "have one or more preventable, chronic diseases that are related to poor quality dietary patterns and physical inactivity".[4] The rest of the world is similarly beset.

There are many problems with the diet-heart hypothesis, which have been regularly confirmed in these intervening years. For one, the argument that saturated fat raises blood-cholesterol concentrations which alone directly cause heart disease is at best a gross oversimplification and at worst just plain wrong. And two, carbohydrates are both entirely unnecessary for our nutritional needs (unlike proteins *and* fats) and actively bad for us, especially for those of us with insulin resistance, when consumed in bulk. The sugars and starches within carbohydrates are broken down to glucose during the digestion process, which is then absorbed into the body's cells with the help of the hormone insulin. Eat too many carbohydrates – your limit depends on your insulin tolerance – and your glucose concentration levels start spiking to the point that your body can't process the glucose so rather stores it as fat. The more elevated your insulin and glucose levels remain, the harder and harder it becomes to process those carbs, and a steady cycle of weight gain and deteriorating health ensues.

So, nutritious, delicious, satiating fats have been unfairly demonised while unsatisfying, fat-inducing, health-ruining carbs have been left to run rampant.

There is, however, good news. *The Real Meal Revolution* has by no means been a lone voice in the fight to overhaul global eating guidelines, with its low-carb high-fat message. New books, studies, articles and dietary guidelines appear by the week to endorse our position with sensible science, well-argued hypotheses and responsibly sourced evidence.

Having featured Ancel Keys himself on its cover in January 1961, *Time* magazine ran a single coverline in June 2014 that advised "Eat Butter". Below it appeared the teaser "Scientists labelled fat the enemy. Why they were wrong" and a picture of an enormous curl of butter.

Again in 2014, the food journalist Nina Teicholz released her comprehensive demolition of the low-fat orthodoxy, *The Big Fat Surprise*, which quickly became a *New York Times* bestseller. Researched over nine years, and critically reviewed by *The Economist*, *The Financial Times*, *The Wall Street Journal*, *The British Medical Journal*, *The Times of London* and others, it makes the inarguable case *for* fat and *against* carbs. (We highly recommend it.)

Even the US's Dietary Guidelines Advisory Committee – the descendant of the very committee that first adapted the diet-heart approach back in 1977 – has started acknowledging the errors of its past. Its latest five-yearly guidelines, released in February 2015, have softened its stance on daily fat limits and completely dropped its long-standing recommendation to restrict consumption of dietary cholesterol. Though we're not entirely in agreement with everything the committee has to say – it's a slowly righting ship – this is real progress. Most pertinently, fat is no longer its prime villain; that position is now, correctly in our opinion, taken by sugar. [5]

THE BASICS OF
SUPER FOOD FOR SUPERCHILDREN

The history of nutrition as described in *The Real Meal Revolution*, and much of the advice that comes from it, underscores all of *Super Food for Superchildren*. But the differing nutritional requirements of children set the two books apart. As mentioned already, we are not necessarily advocating strict Banting (i.e., extremely low-carb eating) for kids here, and we are, for example, less wary of starch-heavy vegetables than in *The Real Meal Revolution*. Any source of good nutrition is recommended as long as there are no negative long-term effects. Besides, we don't want to push our message *too* hard. As it stands, what we're advising is a far cry from the received cereal-box wisdom out there, and will require a major shift in thinking for many parents. We are sensitive to this.

Beyond the major and minor differences in dietary guidelines, the modern take on children's nutrition comes with its very own murky past, one that stretches back to the 1920s and '30s when the company that would become Gerber's Baby Foods "successfully medicalised motherhood", as Prof Noakes explains in detail later (see p312). It was then that commercial baby food manufacturers in the US began establishing their hold on the psyche of the modern parent. Commercially prepared baby foods were not just more convenient than homemade foods, the message went; they were better. But it was a message without any meaningful evidence to back it up; it was simply a clever marketing spiel that was peddled first to dieticians through sponsored advertising in scientific publications and then to mothers with effective, targeted advertising in the mainstream.

Today, nothing much seems to have changed. Fast-forward to the modern family kitchen and we find it stocked with "easily digestible" baby foods that are worryingly low in nutrition (and high in additives) designed for infants who are desperate for energy-rich brain food. And for older children we have "fortified" cereals that are apparently enhanced with certain vitamins and minerals, and yet are invariably overloaded with sugar and based on the worst kind of refined carbs, such as wheat. Our kids are literally becoming addicted to an unhealthy, destructive way of eating.

Combined with the general advice to drink skim milk, eat low-fat everything and stock up on unnecessary carbs whenever convenient, the dietary pitfalls for a well-intentioned parent seem insurmountable. But they aren't.

We'll start with the three golden rules of *Super Food for Superchildren*:

No added sugar!

No refined carbs!

Keep it real!

GOLDEN RULE 1: NO ADDED SUGAR!

If it took you a while to get your head around the fact that eating fat doesn't make you fat, then you may want to take a second to understand the various definitions of sugar.

In biochemical terms, *sugars* are the building blocks of carbohydrates, and the ones you hear of regularly are glucose (avoid), fructose (doubly avoid!) and lactose (found in dairy; be wary).

In (informal) medical terms, *blood sugar* refers to the amount of glucose in the bloodstream (low and stable levels are good; spikes or constant elevations are not good). We'll refer to this as *blood-glucose concentration* from here.

And in culinary terms, *sugar* is the sweet stuff that people around the world pour on their cereal in the morning – more easily specified as table sugar or sucrose – and it's what we're talking about in this book, except where specified.

For our purposes, *added sugar* includes table sugar that might go into a cup of tea or on top of a bowl of cereal or into a meal you cook at home, *plus* it includes the sucrose (or high fructose corn syrup) that gets added into commercial foods and drinks such as ready-made meals, sauces, sweets and soft drinks.

How bad is sugar?
To put it in perspective, think of it as
COCAINE FOR YOUR KID.

It's been known for decades now that high sugar consumption causes dental problems and may be a possible cause of obesity. If you grew up in the '80s, for example, your parents might have restricted your table sugar intake to avoid costly visits to the dentist. That was a valid precaution.

But sugar, it has now been conclusively proven, is far more insidious than mere caries and cavities. Because it is genuinely addictive – you can binge on it, crave it and get withdrawal symptoms from it – it's not necessarily the immediate effects that most concern us. Rather, it's the path it leads you down – the one that ends up with metabolic syndrome, obesity, diabetes and all their related chronic problems, from strokes and heart disease to kidney disease, blindness and nerve damage, not to mention the variety of cancers it has been linked to. Dental cavities are thus not in themselves the primary problem; they are, however, an early indicator that there are major problems on the way.

The World Health Organization, American Heart Association and other authorities generally recommend a daily allowance of around 3 to 8 teaspoons of sugar a day for children, depending on age. It sounds harsh, but we believe you should be veering towards the lower end of the spectrum – at best!

When we say "no added sugar", we're advising – in the strongest terms we can – that you never add table sugar to your child's food, and that you do your best not to offer him food that is prepared with added sugar. Of course you can't (and shouldn't) be monitoring every spoonful that passes his lips, and there will probably be birthday cakes at school and sweets at parties and granny giving him muffins for breakfast when you're not looking – and all that is fine. But if you implement the No Added Sugar rule the rest of the time, it will make an unimaginable difference to his health and wellbeing in the longer term. If you must add a small amount of sugar to his diet, we suggest honey (see p143).

In summary, sugar makes you eat the wrong things (including more sugar), and the less your child is exposed to it in his earlier years, the less likely he is to develop a sweet tooth (actually sugar addiction) in his later years.

When you realise that OBESITY is a DISORDER OF THE BRAIN,
suddenly sugar's true danger is crystallised.

See from p306 for more on sugar.

Where's the sugar?
Once you start analysing the ingredients of popular children's foods and drinks, it's frightening to see how much sugar is out there. Soft drinks, cereals and sauces are some of the worst offenders, and we recommend you avoid the commercial variations in their entirety. Consider, for example, that a 330ml can of Coca-Cola (in the UK) contains 35g, or nearly 9 teaspoons, of sugar.

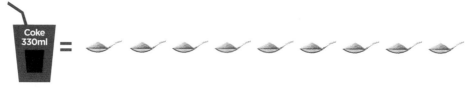

This translates to nearly 14 teaspoons for a 500ml bottle.

Or, imagine it's a hot summer's day; the kids are running around in the garden and you've got a 2-litre bottle in the fridge. If they get through all of it in the course of the day they will have consumed *53 teaspoons of sugar*.

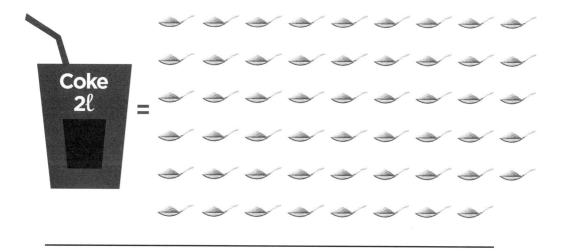

HOW MUCH SUGAR ARE YOUR KIDS DRINKING?

The amount of sugar in soft drinks is astounding. One standard can of Coke or Fanta, or a large glass of fruit juice, quite easily maxes a child's entire daily recommended allowance of sugar, according to *all* the major guidelines. Here are six popular drinks, rated by sugar per typical serving. (NB: the amount of sugar in a glass of water is 0g.) [6]

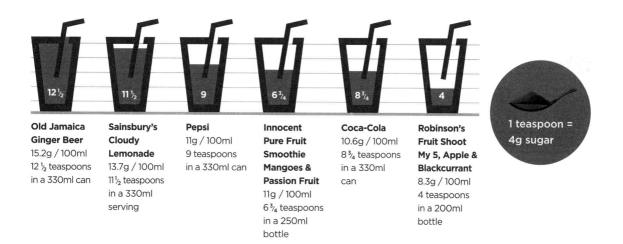

Old Jamaica Ginger Beer
15.2g / 100ml
12½ teaspoons in a 330ml can

Sainsbury's Cloudy Lemonade
13.7g / 100ml
11½ teaspoons in a 330ml serving

Pepsi
11g / 100ml
9 teaspoons in a 330ml can

Innocent Pure Fruit Smoothie Mangoes & Passion Fruit
11g / 100ml
6¾ teaspoons in a 250ml bottle

Coca-Cola
10.6g / 100ml
8¾ teaspoons in a 330ml can

Robinson's Fruit Shoot My 5, Apple & Blackcurrant
8.3g / 100ml
4 teaspoons in a 200ml bottle

1 teaspoon = 4g sugar

HOW MUCH SUGAR ARE YOUR KIDS EATING FOR BREAKFAST?

The amount of sugar in popular cereals is possibly more disconcerting than that in drinks because cereals are seen as everyday staples, and even healthy. Ignore for a moment the refined carbs that form the bulk of the cereal (see Golden Rule 2, opposite), and there are a number in which added sugar makes up a full *third* of the content. Our graphic shows the amount of sugar per 100g serving of six popular cereals, excluding anything your kid may add on top. Note that some cereal manufacturers try to convince buyers that a serving equates to 30g, an unlikely amount to satisfy a hungry 10-year-old. [7]

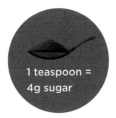

1 teaspoon = 4g sugar

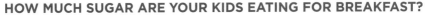

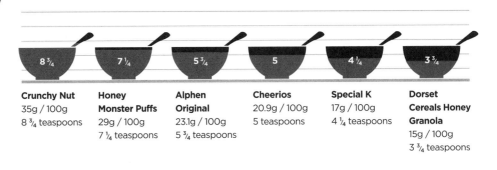

Crunchy Nut	Honey Monster Puffs	Alphen Original	Cheerios	Special K	Dorset Cereals Honey Granola
35g / 100g	29g / 100g	23.1g / 100g	20.9g / 100g	17g / 100g	15g / 100g
8 ¾ teaspoons	7 ¼ teaspoons	5 ¾ teaspoons	5 teaspoons	4 ¼ teaspoons	3 ¾ teaspoons

HOW MUCH SUGAR IS THERE IN POPULAR CONDIMENT SAUCES?

You probably don't consider ketchups, chutneys, mayonnaise or other condiment sauces as principal ingredients in a meal, but consider how much ketchup or mayo a hungry child might add to a burger or plate of chips. We think 50ml (2 shot glasses) is a fair bet, which works out to 4 or 5 teaspoons of added sugar in particularly sugar-laden sauces. [8]

1 teaspoon = 4g sugar

Sainsbury's Chutney Caramelised Onion	HP Sauce	Heinz Tomato Sauce	Sainsbury's Tomato Ketchup	Heinz Salad Cream	Nando's Peri-Peri Sauce
31.3g / 100ml	23.1g / 100ml	22.8g / 100ml	21.6g / 100ml	17g / 100ml	7.7g / 100ml
4 teaspoons / 50ml serving	2 ¾ teaspoons / 50ml serving	2 ¾ teaspoons / 50ml serving	2 ¾ teaspoons / 50ml serving	2 teaspoons / 50ml serving	1 teaspoon / 50ml serving

A note on Type 1 diabetes

While sugar may have no nutritional value, it is medically advised for the treatment of acute hypoglycaemic attacks in Type 1 diabetes sufferers. We would never advise against the use of sugar in these circumstances, though we will point out that a low-carb high-fat diet, as outlined in these pages and (more strictly) in *The Real Meal Revolution*, would benefit children with Type 1 diabetes by better regulating blood-glucose levels and thus decreasing the likelihood of future glycaemic attacks.

GOLDEN RULE 2: NO REFINED CARBS!

Refined carbohydrates are carbs that have been broken down in the food-preparation process to the point that they are more easily digestible. In general, the whiter a carb the more refined it is. Flour, for instance, is created by grinding grain, usually wheat. The process removes the fibrous outer layer of the grain, which contains most of the vitamins and minerals, and leaves you with nice long chains of glucose molecules that are perfect for spiking blood-glucose and thus insulin levels (while contributing little or no nutritional value).

Consider it this way. If your child eats a bowl of luminous rice-based cereal for breakfast he would be consuming a scary amount of added sugar in the process (see previous page). But all the actual rice he's eating rapidly breaks down to sugar, too. *So he's effectively just eaten an entire bowl of sugar.*

As we've detailed above, this is the path to future obesity and ill health, so steer clear of all refined carbs. You can start by being highly, highly sceptical of any commercially available cereal. The average breakfast cereal is exactly *not* what you should be giving your kid first thing in the morning.

What about carbs in general?

Though we are less concerned about the consumption of complex carbohydrates – carrots, butternut, beetroot and the like – bear in mind a few things. First, even complex carbs break down to sugars, and the restriction of any carbs controls blood-glucose concentrations, which is generally advisable no matter the age. Second, even complex carbs aren't as nutritious as they are sometimes perceived to be, and children need nutrient-dense foods. And third, the evidence seems to be mounting against gluten-containing grains, in general, whether refined or otherwise. They are hard on the gut (particularly in children) and have been linked to chronic digestion difficulties. As a result, we prefer ancient grains such as millet, quinoa and buckwheat whenever possible, rather than wheat, rye and barley.

See from p315 and from p325 for more on white rice cereal for infants, and from p306 and specifically p335 for more on grains.

GOLDEN RULE 3: KEEP IT REAL!

Real, non-processed, whole foods are the basis of healthy eating. This rule transfers directly from *The Real Meal Revolution*, but is even more relevant here because of the all-pervasive influence of convenience foods on children's nutrition. We know how hard it can be to make the effort to cook from scratch for yourself, let alone your children, but we wouldn't make this a golden rule unless it was absolutely critical.

Processed foods aimed at children are filled with all the bad stuff we're trying so hard to avoid, notably sugars, refined carbs and carbs in general. Beyond that there are the colourants that make corn chips luminous orange and ice cream neon pink, and there are the flavourants, stabilisers, glazing agents, colour retention agents, humectants, conditioners, preservatives, thickeners and sweeteners, most of them represented on ingredients lists as codes rather than names, that really shouldn't be passing through your child's body.

If ever we've got the right to pull the guilt card it's now: your kids deserve better than this.

How to shop for real food

Ideally when cooking, you'd use the best ingredients bought fresh every day, but this can be expensive, time-consuming and impractical, especially if you're feeding a family. Here are two shortcuts.

- **Cook in bulk and freeze.** Many of the recipes in this book are designed to work beautifully out of the freezer, so kill two meals with one pot as often as you can: double up recipe quantities and make enough for dinner tonight *and* dinner in a couple of weeks' time. If you can, set aside blocks of cooking time to get several dishes done, for example on a Saturday morning. This is particularly useful for bolognaise, ratatouille and other sauces that you can freeze in portions for quick use. (See the kitchen staples recipes from p290.)
- **Shop smart.** Frequent last-minute trips to the supermarket are sure-fire ways to waste time and money, and are more likely to result in you falling back on convenience meals. Get organised. Give your meals some thought in advance. Make a weekly meal plan and shop for as many of your ingredients as possible in one trip.

Here is our extra smart-shopping advice. Try to:

Shop without your kids. This advice is linked to the point above and not always practical, but it's highly recommended. Kids are easily distracted at the best of times, and if you're doing a big shop there's a good chance they'll find numerous ways to distract you too. When you're trying to just hurry up and get to the till, you start buying the wrong (read: convenient, non-real) things.

And speaking of the till, don't forget about the sweet and savoury delights that await you and your wide-eyed, hungry child in temptation aisle... It takes magnificent parenting skills to wait to pay for your groceries next to a wall of chocolates and sweets and not give in to "Can I have a choccie? Can I have a choccie? Can I have a choccie?" Rather avoid the problem in the first place.

Find out about your food. Where does it come from? How was it farmed? Modern supermarkets have done a lot to place us at arm's length from our (vacuum-packed) food, and though they have their place, we encourage the movement back to specialist stores. Whenever you can – and it's easier these days – try to shop at a grocer, butcher and fishmonger so you can talk to them about the food they're selling. Of course, this isn't always practical for busy parents, in which case try to frequent supermarkets with specialist departments. If there's a butcher to actually mince your mince in front of you, or a fishmonger to fillet your fish fresh, it makes a difference.

Buy local. It's cheaper and more sustainable.

Buy seasonal. Strawberries in summer, plums in autumn. A logical step from buying local; it's once again less expensive and more sustainable – plus the quality is likely to be better.

Buy free-range and organic. Particularly eggs and chicken. They're healthier and genuinely taste much better (proper organic eggs are amazing!), so if you can stretch your budget, please do.

Buy grass-fed meat. Not grain-fed. Watch out for meats and sausages that are processed, sugar-cured or contain grains, colourants and dodgy preservatives.

Buy fresh fish. Ensure they are sustainably caught and that the cold-chain has been maintained.

Buy full-cream dairy. Milk, yoghurt and cheeses are all far healthier this way (and better tasting, we think). And the best dairy is from grass-fed cows.

Grow your own food! Carrots, spinach, beetroot, cabbage, lettuce and many herbs grow like weeds. Plant a garden or use pots and get your kids involved. Teach them about real food, responsibility and sustainability.

Educate yourself and your children. And realise that knowledge moves on, so keep learning.

THE SILVER RULES

The Kids' Nutrition Revolution by Tim Noakes, starting on p303, is packed with the latest science on children's nutrition. Every parent should read it to stay as informed as possible (so please do). For quick reference here are key points that we feel deserve mention up front, with page references for further reading.

Breast is indeed best. The breastfeeding versus formula-feeding debate can be emotional and controversial, for reasons that go well beyond nutrition. But the science and global guidelines on breastfeeding leave no room for doubt: breast milk provides superior nutrition to baby formulas. From a purely nutritional point of view, we strongly advise that parents feed breast milk exclusively until 4-6 months and then in combination with foods until age 2 or even beyond.

From a physiological point of view, we believe that the majority of mothers should be able to breastfeed successfully. That said, we know that breastfeeding *can* be problematic for some mothers, and in time can become logistically difficult for mothers who work. So although we strongly recommend breastfeeding, of course there are non-dietary considerations to bear in mind.

See from p42 and p311, and specifically p319.

Wean onto real foods, whether purées or not. The history of commercial baby-food manufacturing is doubtful at best and, as ever, we believe real foods trump what you get out of a jar. Today there is a strong movement to return to baby-led weaning, which bypasses the now-traditional purées stage of weaning and encourages a direct transition from breast milk to easily edible whole foods (in combination with breast milk). We can see the appeal of it, though we have certain reservations; as a result, we suggest a combination of non-commercial purées and baby-led weaning as a good compromise. Either way, it's the type and quality of food that weaning babies eat, rather than the form in which they are offered, that is vital for both short- and long-term health.

See from p68 and p340.

Don't go vegetarian before age 2. And be wary of vegetarianism in later years. The first two years of a child's life are vital for brain development in particular, and certain proteins, fats, minerals (notably iron and zinc) and vitamins are essential in this time. The evidence is clear that babies weaned onto nutrient-dense foods such as meat and eggs are at an advantage over those weaned on to less nutrient-rich foods, so we strongly advise against grain-based formulas and vegetarian diets at this point. In fact, we recommend that pregnant women and children in general avoid vegetarian (and certainly vegan) diets.

See from p328.

Be wary of dairy. We strongly recommend (full-cream) dairy for children because it offers plenty of nutritional benefits. But it does appear to have certain negative health effects in some children (and adults) who are unable to digest lactose, the sugar found in milk. As a result, we advise that you monitor your child's dairy intake as a potential cause of bloating, diarrhoea, cramps or other digestive issues.

See p144.

Be especially wary of grains. *No refined carbs* is our second golden rule, but we're not convinced by grains in general, whether "whole grain" or not. Coeliac disease, a reaction to eating the gluten found in wheat, barley and rye, is relatively well known, while non-coeliac gluten sensitivity is becoming an increasingly recognised problem. We suggest avoiding gluten-rich grains if possible, in favour of non-gluten varieties such as oats, buckwheat, millet and quinoa.

See from p306 and specifically from p335.

Keep an eye on your kids. Related to the previous point, and the book in general, this may seem a parenting basic but it's perhaps overlooked: be aware of your child's relationship with food. How and what does he like to eat and how does he react to certain foods? Ideally he will be eating a wonderful fully balanced diet that satisfies his health needs (as well as his taste buds). But that may not always be the case, so keep an eye out for the potential deficiencies that crop up at various stages of development. Most importantly, be aware of the early indicators of insulin resistance, as outlined later.

See p344.

THE SUPERGOAL

This book is not about putting your children on a diet to lose weight; it's about turning them into the healthiest people then can be for the rest of their lives by teaching them how to eat well. Imagine them all grown up one day without a lust for the foods that ruin health in adulthood (soft drinks, sweets, junk food, you name it) – not because they've been denied any pleasures of eating, but because they define those pleasures differently.

Our end goal is for children everywhere to eat healthily, to genuinely enjoy what they're eating, and to learn enough about what they're putting into their bodies so that as they tread the path to adulthood they find themselves heading towards good health rather than chronic disease. If we can allow them this opportunity, they'll fly!

MARVELLOUS MUMS

Super food for ages

Pregnancy -6 months

If you're reading this book while pregnant, first things first: congratulations! And secondly, well done for prioritising your child's nutrition at such an early point – because how you look after yourself from now until you've stopped breastfeeding is likely to have a direct effect on the health of your baby, in both the shorter and longer term. (Not forgetting, of course, that you will benefit from looking after yourself, too.) Living with a growing baby inside you is challenging at the best of times, so getting your nutrition right from the start is paramount. But one of the annoying truisms of being pregnant is that *everyone* is an expert – from your mother-in-law to the girl who does your nails – and they all have a bit of secret advice that you *have* to follow. Know what? You'll go mad if you try to listen to everyone. Choose one or two trusted sources of information and stick to them. When it comes to nutrition while pregnant and breastfeeding, we've got you covered. For our purposes, there are effectively four stages: the three trimesters of pregnancy, plus the breastfeeding stage that comes after birth.

WHAT'S GROWING ON?

What's growing on is you're having a baby! It's an epic story in the making, and you've got the lead role. No doubt you'll have read up on the development process elsewhere already – from poppy seed to sesame seed to blueberry to melon to watermelon, and all that comes with it – so we'll stick to the nutrition basics (which don't involve progressive fruit-size comparisons).

Naturally, what you put in your body affects your baby. It's not so much that you're eating for two (you're not); it's that you're eating with two people in mind. Good nutrition is vital.

To start, let's answer a common question from Real Meal mums:

SHOULD I BE BANTING WHILE PREGNANT OR BREASTFEEDING?

As we've discussed already in the Introduction and return to elsewhere in the book, there's nothing quite like pregnancy and child-rearing to create controversy and differences of opinion. Add high-carb low-fat versus high-fat low-carb eating to the equation and the stakes are raised. So let's be clear about this: we don't necessarily advise that pregnant or breastfeeding women should be following a fully ketogenic Banting diet. In other words, we're not recommending that you exclude carbohydrates from your daily intake to such a degree that your body's energy source switches completely from glucose to ketone bodies. (The scientific evidence on a fully ketogenic diet during pregnancy is insufficient to make definitive calls, though we suspect it would be perfectly fine.)

We do, however, strongly advocate a healthy high-fat low-carb diet that follows the Real Meal principles. This means steering clear of sugar, refined carbohydrates and processed foods, and eating your fill of iron-rich proteins, fresh vegetables and healthy fats, as well as some fruit and dairy. (Pretty much what we recommend throughout this book.)

Our advice does, however, come with a healthy dose of practicality. Pregnancy is (often) not easy. Your hormones may rage, your body may do strange and scary things, and your cravings may at times consume you. Realise that this is normal, and try to walk a sensible line as much as you can when it comes to your diet (and other things!). Pregnancy is not a time to diet to lose weight (except in very specific circumstances); but, equally, it isn't an excuse to binge on junk food, pack on unnecessary pounds and risk gestational diabetes or other problems. Do your best to follow sound nutritional principles as outlined here, and remember that you can still eat delicious, satisfying foods – but don't beat yourself up when you slip.

WHAT TO EAT? WHAT NOT TO EAT?

Foods to embrace during pregnancy

All of the foods listed below are good and healthy throughout pregnancy (and in general), but your different trimesters come with different nutritional requirements. We recommend stocking up as follows.

First Trimester

Leafy greens: The likes of spinach and kale are jammed with folic acid and iron. Iron is an essential mineral that we return to throughout the book, and folic acid is important during the first trimester to prevent neural tube defects in your foetus. Your doctor may have put you on a multivitamin high in folic acid, but don't let that stop you from getting more in your diet.

Meat and eggs: Packed with important proteins, they are Real Meal staples and excellent foods for the first trimester.

Bananas: A fantastic source of vitamin B6, potassium, vitamin C and fibre, and also good for reducing nausea, bananas should be a staple at this stage. That said, don't binge on them.

Second Trimester

Cheese: High in calcium and protein (not to mention deliciousness), cheese is beneficial to you throughout your pregnancy, but is particularly good now. (You may, however, want to be wary of certain cheeses – see p37.)

Eggs: Eggs contain choline, a key nutrient for the brain.

Avocados: Great for brain and tissue growth, a good source of fibre and healthy fat, and a wonderful nausea suppressant thanks to the high vitamin B6 content.

Third Trimester

Salmon: Full of protein and omega-3s, this is another food we can't recommend more highly (and return to in later chapters); essential for your baby's growing brain and visual development.

Artichokes: Packed with fibre and iron and great for soothing indigestion, which can be problematic at this stage. Excellent if you're suffering from heartburn.

Nuts: You may well be feeling permanently full at this stage, in which case nuts make the perfect protein snack. Almonds, pecans and walnuts are also bursting with omega-3s.

SUPERNUTRIENTS FOR YOU AND YOUR SUPERCHILDREN		
NUTRIENT	**BENEFIT**	**GOOD SOURCES**
Calcium	Combats insomnia. Builds baby's bones	Broccoli, sardines, hard cheese
Fibre	Relieves constipation and helps with overall gut health	Artichokes, avocados, (ripe) bananas, spinach
Folic acid	For the prevention of neural tube defects; for example, spina bifida	All dark green leafy vegetables, asparagus, broccoli, Brussels sprouts, avocado, celery, citrus fruit, beans, peas, lentils, sunflower seeds, almonds
Iron	Essential "blood-building" nutrient, and important for baby and placenta growth	Animal protein, cheese, yoghurt
Magnesium	Important for muscle and organ growth	Chicken, fish, dark leafy greens, bananas and yoghurt
Omega-3s	Essential for your baby's brain development. May reduce risks of pre-term labour and allergies after birth	Anchovies, sardines, salmon, fatty fish in general, pecans, walnuts, pumpkin seeds, almonds
Vitamin B6	Essential for the development of your baby's brain and nervous system. Also helps combat morning sickness	Chicken, other animal protein, milk, avocados
Vitamin C	Facilitates iron absorption	Citrus, broccoli, avocados, tomatoes, red peppers, spinach
Vitamin K	Helps blood clotting	Avocados, blueberries, real butter, yellow and orange vegetables

POW!

Foods To Avoid During Pregnancy: Two Separate Approaches

We've covered what you *should* be eating; but what specifically should you *not* be eating (and drinking) when pregnant? Your approach to this question will most likely be a reflection of your personality rather than any hard science on the matter, as this is a topic of contrasting viewpoints but often insufficient evidence to back them up.

Some healthcare professionals will advise that you can eat anything and everything; others may provide you with a long list of foods to be avoided at all costs. Note that contamination of the food and thus food-borne illness, as opposed to an inherent problem with the food itself, is the primary threat from many of them. For example, listeria is a nasty bacterium that can find its way into various foods; pregnant women are more susceptible to it, especially in the third trimester when their immune systems may be compromised, and it can cause serious problems for both mum and baby.

For those who would like to err on the side of caution, this is the extended list of what to avoid and/or how to approach certain foods during pregnancy.

AVOID

 Raw sprouts: Steer clear to avoid the risk of campylobacter or toxoplasma, the result of nasty bacteria and parasites respectively.

Undercooked eggs: The Real Meal team *loves* eggs – as you'll see in the recipes to come throughout this book. Just ensure that you cook your eggs well to avoid the risk of salmonella.

Soft, mould-ripened cheeses: Potential carriers of listeria and other pathogens. Unpasteurised mould-ripened and blue-veined cheeses are traditionally avoided by pregnant women; these include the likes of brie, camembert, chevin, gorgonzola, Danish blue, and their close relations. Note, however, two things:

1 all cheese sold in the UK must be clearly labelled as pasteurised or unpasteurised; most of it is pasteurised, though you may want to be wary of smaller-scale, artisanal manufacturers;

2 cooking unpasteurised cheese eliminates the problem; for example, a blue-cheese sauce properly heated on the stove top.

Raw and undercooked meat and fish: Potential listeria carriers. Eat them cooked through unless you're 100 percent sure of their quality.

Unpasteurised milk and juices: Potential listeria carriers.

Pre-made deli meals and street foods: Potential carriers of listeria and other contaminants. Frankfurters, hot dogs, hams, pâtés, meat spreads, smoked seafood and the like, especially those that sit forlornly in less-than-hygienic surrounds, are risky and best avoided.

WATCH OUT FOR

Alcohol: This shouldn't be a revelation – excess alcohol and pregnancy don't mix. Heavy drinking can seriously harm the development of your foetus, causing everything from abnormal brain development to actual miscarriage. The safest option is to abstain from drinking, though recent research apears to show that a very limited intake is fine.[1]

High-mercury fish: Certain apex-predator fish, such as swordfish, marlin and tuna, can contain high levels of mercury, which may be harmful to the foetus. When you're pregnant or planning to get pregnant, the NHS in England advises you to avoid swordfish, marlin and shark, and to limit the amount of tuna you eat (to four 140g portion per week). Always eat cooked rather than raw shellfish.

Flaxseed, flaxseed oil and soy: Flaxseed and soy have a potentially hazardous effect on pregnancy due to their ability to exert an oestrogen-like effect. The evidence is mixed, but it's best not to overdo them. (Not forgetting that we're not big fans of soy, as it is.)

Caffeine: If you're a caffeine fiend this may be tough... Sadly, you need to cut right back. (And yes, this will be ironic when pregnancy fatigue kicks in.) To avoid the complications of excess caffeine, stick to no more than 300mg/day, which equates to 1-2 cups of coffee. Remember that most tea and chocolate also contains caffeine.

Certain herbs and tinctures

There are wide varieties of herbs and herbal remedies that are considered suspect or have documented adverse affects in pregnant women, including camomile, ginseng, sage, ginko, St John's Wort and tea tree oil. If you use these or others regularly, you may want to research them in more detail.

If you'd prefer a more fundamental approach to eating and drinking during pregnancy, follow these guidelines:

AVOID:
- rubbish food and drink, as per the general Real Meal approach;
- alcohol (or at least limit it substantially);
- unpasteurised dairy products;
- anything that is likely to make you physically sick.

ENSURE YOU:
- wash your fruit and veg well;
- eat food prepared hygienically and preferably fresh;
- properly cook anything you're unsure of;
- know where your food comes from.

This approach entails not eating junk food, not getting drunk, steering clear of imported French cheese that may be unpasteurised, and avoiding food that might necessitate a trip to the A&E; for example, mussels and oysters at a mid-summer buffet. Bearing in mind that keeping stress-free, happy and positive is hugely important while pregnant (and forever, come to think of it), it would be hard to fault your rationale if you followed this route.

And don't forget that Mother Nature also offers her two cents by endowing many mothers-to-be with food aversions and a heightened sense of smell so as to avoid any foods that may pose a danger to the foetus. As with most things, common sense will usually suffice. For example, if the idea of raw fish turns your stomach, then avoid the sashimi. Equally, if you find yourself craving something, listen to your body – just try to differentiate between what your body wants and what your (indulgent) mind *thinks* you want. Are you, for instance, really craving those sugared bonbons with extra sugar, or are you just suffering from fatigue and need an energy boost?

COMMON PREGNANCY COMPLAINTS

Morning sickness: The classic pregnancy downer, morning sickness is probably the best-known side effect of being pregnant (and often the first clue that you are). Think of it as an early warning sign: parenthood isn't a walk in the park. The good news (for most women) is that the nausea and vomiting usually pass after the first trimester. That, however, can be poor comfort when you're a month and a half away from hitting your second trimester and you're finding yourself spending more time with your toilet bowl than your family. So, here are some tips to nuke the nausea.

- Make sure you take your pregnancy multivitamin *after* food. Omega-3 supplements, for example, are usually easier to stomach with food.
- Vitamin B6 is a nausea suppressant; see that you're getting enough of it.
- Both hunger and overeating can lead to nausea and vomiting, so try to eat small amounts frequently to avoid either of them.
- Ginger is a well-known anti-nausea remedy. A bit of fresh ginger and lemon juice in hot water can be a lifesaver, and see the various ginger-laced recipes coming up. (NB: the ginger biscuits on p48). Ginger supplements can also be effective in the fight against nausea, though you may want to chat to a doctor or your gynaecologist about them first.

Fatigue: Fatigue often comes hot on the heels of morning sickness, and it can be the most debilitating of all the pregnancy ailments, especially if you enjoyed your coffee. It's usually worst in the first trimester, before returning again in the third. The best way to combat fatigue? Take naps. Easier said than done if you have the inconvenience of a job and/or other children to worry about, but well worth it, especially if you're struggling with – oh, the irony – insomnia. Otherwise try the obvious solution: get to bed earlier. And the not-so-obvious: exercise. The best energy-boosting foods you can eat are eggs and animal protein because they're packed with iron. If you're short of iron you may well be falling asleep at your desk (and possibly anaemic) – remedy that quickly.

Constipation: Sometimes pregnancy can feel like a practical joke. You're nauseous yet violently hungry, and you're flatulent (oh, the shame) yet surprisingly constipated! And while friends are, for whatever reason, happy to listen to you describe how your latest mid-morning vomiting session interrupted the weekly accounts meeting, they're not so keen to listen to your constipation travails. It can be horribly painful during pregnancy and, worst of all, can lead to piles, which nobody – especially a pregnant woman – needs. Combat the constipation with these tips:

- Make fibre your friend.
- Keep hydrated. Water and vegetable juices will help keep things moving.

(And fibre and water go hand in hand; fibre without water isn't ideal.)

■ Exercise. Get yourself moving to get your insides moving.

Extreme hunger: Despite what your mother may say, you shouldn't actually be eating for two. Make sure you have enough food but be careful not to balloon as a result of extreme hunger. Eat your fill of fibrous foods (especially vegetables) and make sure you include protein in every meal. Hard-boiled eggs are a great appetite satisfier that you can have as a snack any time of day. High-carb foods, particularly refined carbs, are the enemy because they don't satisfy your hunger – but you know that by now, right?

Cravings: Specific food cravings are most common in the first three months of pregnancy. Providing you are getting all the nutrients that you and your growing foetus require, it's okay to have some of the foods you crave, but be very wary of sugar cravings. Watch that indulgent trigger – usually tiredness – which makes you feel like you "deserve" something sweet, and try to keep the focus: you're eating for your baby, so eat what you'd want her to eat. Bear in mind that carb cravings are generally caused by unstable blood-sugar levels and that refined carbs will only make things worse in the long run. In emergencies try berries and fruit instead of cakes and sweets – or turn to the Snacks & Treats recipes from p226 if you're really struggling. In general, try to eat stabilising foods that will sustain your blood-sugar levels.

Insomnia: How can you be permanently exhausted *and* still not be able to sleep properly? Ah, the joys of pregnancy, where counting sheep just makes you hungry, and a glass of hot milk just makes you nauseous. And then, when you *are* feeling sleepy, the future Olympic gymnast inside you wakes up and gets a bout of the hiccups... There's no point in fighting the insomnia. Rather than lying in bed staring at the ceiling, get up, read a book, watch an episode of your favourite TV show – then try sleeping again in 45 minutes. The rest of the time, try the following:

■ Avoid all caffeine-containing foods and drinks (including coffee, tea and chocolate), especially before bedtime;

■ Avoid eating a big meal before bedtime; if necessary have a light snack before lights out so you don't go to bed hungry;

■ Eat foods containing tryptophan, an amino acid that aids sleep; you can find it in red meat, dairy products, nuts, seeds, bananas and shellfish;

■ Consider upping your magnesium (nuts, leafy greens) and calcium (dairy) levels, as these deficiencies have been linked to sleep disorders;

■ Stay well hydrated;

■ Keep exercising, even if it's just an evening walk.

BREASTFEEDING

Once your baby is born, the real fun begins, and breastfeeding is one of the first big challenges. (Don't worry; she'll provide you with various others in the next 18-21 years!)

Make no mistake about it; breastfeeding is the gold standard of nutrition for your child, and it comes with a range of health benefits, as we cover elsewhere (see from p311). From a purely nutritional point of view, you should be aiming to exclusively breastfeed until 6 months, and continue breastfeeding in combination with solid foods for longer – until two years, at least. Yes, we know: that's an intimidating thought, especially if you're a working mum.

Some women find breastfeeding the easiest thing in the world, but many experience a plethora of problems despite their best efforts, ranging from an inability to feed to an embarrassing oversupply of milk. Cracked nipples, mastitis, blocked milk ducts and engorged breasts are some of the more common complaints that can arise, and the whole process can be incredibly painful. For many women, breastfeeding is difficult and can be extremely disheartening, especially to start. But if you can get it right it's worth the effort.

One of the biggest hurdles facing breastfeeding mothers, especially first-timers, is anxiety. Try to stay calm – although that's easier said than done when you have a newborn waking you six times a night and you feel like you don't have a clue… From a technical point of view, incorrect latching is often the cause of unsuccessful feeding; a failure of the baby to latch properly to the nipple and areola is more likely to be the problem rather than an insufficient milk supply or any other physiological problem. Do what you can to get this right. Surround yourself with and take advice from people you trust. If necessary, seek help from a lactation consultant or attend a reputable breastfeeding clinic. For excellent advice on breastfeeding, La Leche League International is well worth investigating; see www.llli.org.

The only proven way to increase your breast milk supply is to have your baby suckle, which should be happening 8-12 times per 24-hour period to start, and regularly after that. If you are successful, it's important to ensure that your own nutritional needs are being met.

- Drink plenty of fluids, including a large glass of water before or after feeds;
- Eat 2 servings of oily fish a week (for omega-3 intake);
- Eat at least 4 servings of vegetables per day;
- Eat 2-3 servings of dairy per day;
- Keep up your intake of healthy fats, including avocados, nuts and olives;
- Keep up your intake of animal protein to ensure you're getting enough iron and zinc;
- Limit your intake of alcohol, caffeine and sweeteners, though you can

welcome back on to the menu the other foods you may have worried about during pregnancy.

■ Consider taking a folic acid supplement, or simply continuing your pregnancy multivitamin.

When it comes to breastfeeding, perseverance is the guiding light. But if you've done everything you can to breastfeed and it's just not working, or if your lifestyle prevents you from breastfeeding for as long as you ideally might, then take heart; there *are* alternatives. Don't fall into the trap of feeling like a bad mother or that you have "failed". You have your whole life to feel parental guilt; don't let it start with breastfeeding!

Alternatives to breastfeeding

Commercial formula: Practical and viable, commercial formulas are the most common alternative to breastfeeding. Even if still breastfeeding, many mums find they are able to supplement their breastfeeds with formula and thus gain relief from a voracious baby. Note, however, that they come with several drawbacks. For one, as stressed already, they simply aren't as nutritionally beneficial as breast milk. And secondly, many commercial formulas use glucose syrup or corn starch as a base carbohydrate source – which, you won't be surprised to hear, we disagree with. Try to avoid these.

The two most common types of commercial formula are:

■ formula based on cow's milk
■ formula based on soy milk

Because infants struggle to process the large protein molecules within cow's milk, which can lead to colic, eczema and other problems, this type of formula is often modified, or hydrolysed, to break up the proteins. Should you be unable to feed your child cow's-milk formula, or choose not to, you may be considering soy. We strongly advise against this at all ages (and standard dietetic teaching advises against this until 6 months at least). Soy formula contains phytoestrogens, which appear to have detrimental effects on infants, including impairing the function of the thyroid gland.[2] More than this, soy in general is not a favoured Real Meal food and there haven't been sufficient studies on soy-based formulas to determine their long-term effects. As a result, if your baby is struggling with a cow's-milk formula, we would recommend you rather try an extensively hydrolysed cow's-milk formula or a whey-based one. Whey, as opposed to casein, is the easier of the two main cow's-milk proteins to digest. Goat's milk infant formulas are relatively new on the market, and may provide a viable alternative to cow's-milk formula, though they are not suitable for a baby with identified cow's-milk allergy. If you are trying something a little different, we recommend consulting a professional on the matter; in other words, a doctor or specialist – not that guy who works at the wellness shop.

Home-enriched formula: Many formulas are sold enriched with probiotics and omega-3s, but you can also do this to standard formula by adding your own. Some experts advise adding 500mg of fish oil per day and a probiotic specifically designed for infants, which will help maintain a healthy gut that breastfed babies experience naturally. Before you start doing this, though, consult a professional to advise which brands to use and how exactly to go about it.

Homemade formula: Homemade formulas are a real can of worms, and we certainly *cannot* recommend them. Their appeal to those sceptical of the baby-food industry is that in creating your own formula from scratch you know exactly what and how much you are giving your baby, and you don't have to worry about the potentially unhealthy and unknowable ingredients in commercial formulas. However, there hasn't been sufficient research conducted to verify the safety of homemade formulas; they may be so low in nutrients as to cause malnutrition and illness and they could potentially harbour dangerous bacteria.

As homemade formulas have become more popular in recent years so they have made headlines around the world. Several Canadian health authorities cautioned against their use in November 2014, and a publisher in Australia decided not to publish a paleo cookbook for babies when health officials found out it included a homemade formula recipe based on chicken livers.

Wet nurses: If there's something more controversial than a homemade baby formula then it must be the suggestion to get a wet nurse instead. But in the absence of your own breast milk, breast milk from another source really is considered the best option – superior to both commercial and homemade formulas. Of the various problems it raises, including ready availability and simply whether you're comfortable with it, the most glaring, especially in a country like South Africa, are the health risks. We strongly advise against this option unless it is from a reputable milk bank, as it can be difficult to be certain that milk obtained via milk-sharing networks and similar organisations is safe.

SUPPLEMENTS

These days parents are widely – and wisely – advised to keep their babies out of the sun for health reasons. The downside is a possible shortage of vitamin D, and as a result breastfed babies in particular may need a vitamin D supplement for their first year.[3] Chat to your paediatrician or health professionalism about this, and any other supplements that have been suggested to you; don't just stock up at the health shop because it seems like a good idea.

ASIAN CHICKEN-AND-GINGER BROTH

Makes 6 portions
Prep time: 30 mins
Cooking time: 30 mins

This recipe may sound a little intricate but it's actually really easy, especially if you keep homemade chicken stock in the freezer. It's light, fresh and wonderfully nourishing. You can add any extra vegetables you'd like, then pour yourself a giant bowl and tuck in.

For the broth:
10cm section fresh ginger, unpeeled
1.5 litres chicken stock
3 chicken legs and thighs
1 tablespoon coriander seeds
4 whole cloves
3 tablespoons fish sauce
1 small handful fresh coriander

For the bowls:
2 cups (200g) bean sprouts
½ onion, sliced paper-thin, soaked in cold water for 30 minutes and drained
3 spring onions, green part only, thinly sliced
2 carrots, peeled and julienned
5cm piece of ginger, peeled and shredded
10-12 sprigs mint
10-12 sprigs Thai basil
12-15 fresh coriander leaves
2 or 3 limes, cut into wedges
2 or 3 chillies, thinly sliced

TO MAKE THE BROTH:
- Halve the ginger lengthways, bruise lightly with the broad side of a chef's knife, and set aside.
- Pour the chicken stock into a pot and add the chicken pieces, spices, ginger, fish sauce and coriander. Bring to a boil over high heat then reduce to a gentle simmer. Cook uncovered for 25-30 minutes, until the chicken is cooked through.
- Remove the chicken from the pot and allow it to cool enough to handle. Meanwhile, keep the broth at a steady simmer.

TO PREPARE THE BOWLS:
- Carefully shred the chicken, and set aside.
- Place a portion of the bean sprouts and shredded chicken at the bottom of each bowl. Top with a mound of the finely sliced onion and carrots in the centre and then sprinkle over some spring onion, ginger and the herbs.
- Strain the broth through muslin cloth or a very fine sieve. Season with some extra fish sauce if desired and fresh lime juice.
- Ladle about 2 cups (500ml) of the hot chicken broth into each bowl, distributing the hot liquid evenly to warm all the ingredients. Serve immediately with fresh lime and a little chopped chilli for spice.

THE GINGER IN THIS DISH WILL HELP EASE THAT NASTY MORNING SICKNESS

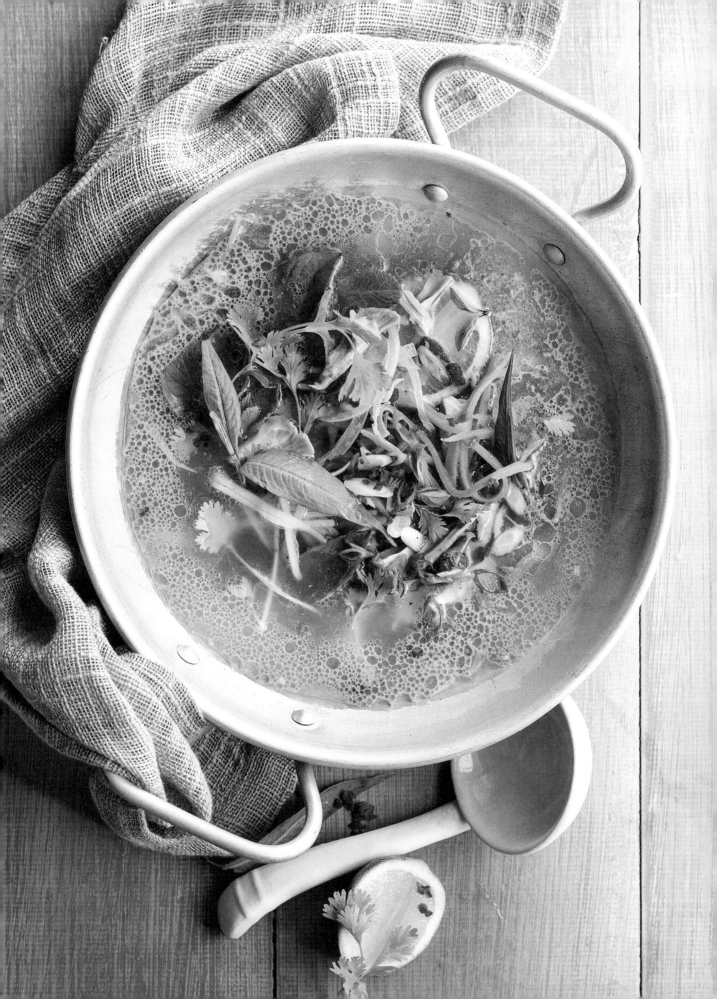

GINGER OAT BISCUITS

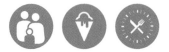

Makes 20 biscuits
Prep time: 20 mins
Cooking time: 25 mins

As we've already mentioned, ginger is a wonderful natural remedy for nausea and morning sickness. In this case, you'll have a snack you can make in advance and call on at a moment's notice – which is sometimes all you have!

1 ½ cups (135g) organic rolled oats
½ cup (55g) chopped almonds
½ cup (40g) desiccated coconut
1 teaspoon ground ginger
½ teaspoon ground cinnamon
¼ teaspoon grated nutmeg
2 ½ tablespoons coconut oil or butter
2 tablespoons raw honey (optional)
1 teaspoon vanilla extract, or
  ½ teaspoon vanilla paste
1-2 tablespoons milk

- Preheat the oven to 150°C.
- In a food processor, combine the oats, chopped almonds, desiccated coconut and spices with the coconut oil or butter, honey and vanilla. Blitz for about 15 seconds.
- Add the milk and blitz again.
- Line two baking sheets with silicone baking paper and roll the dough into 20 small balls.
- Place them onto the baking sheet and flatten down a little. Make sure there's enough room around each biscuit for them to spread.
- Bake for 25 minutes or until golden brown.
- Cool completely before eating.

KEEP AN EMERGENCY SUPPLY OF THESE BISCUITS IN YOUR HANDBAG FOR SURPRISE NAUSEA ATTACKS

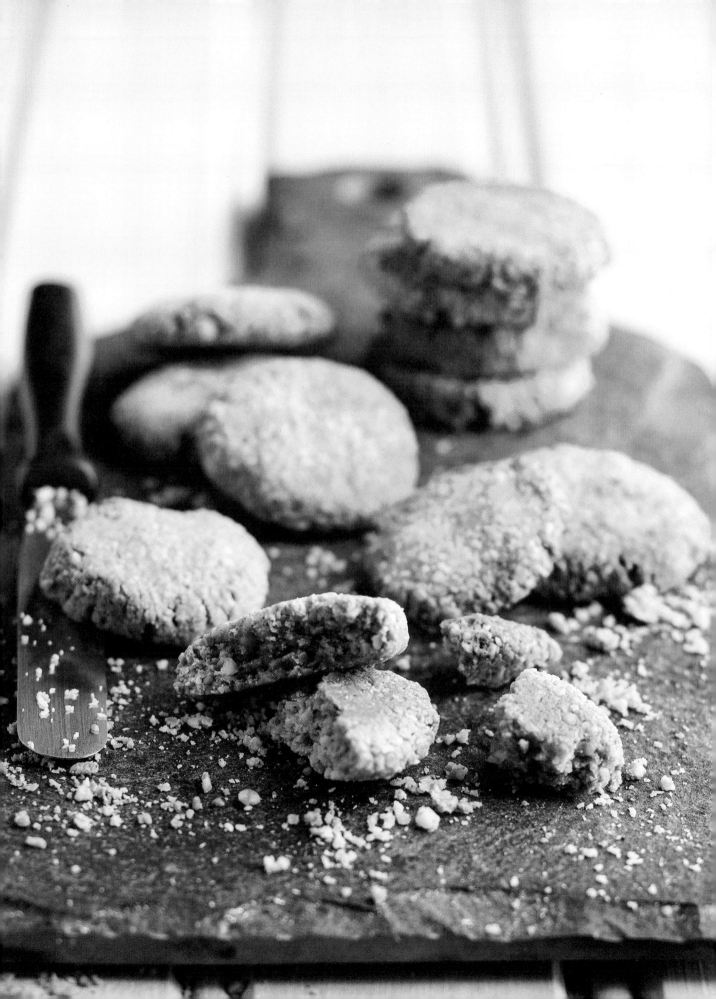

BOILED EGG, BASHED AVO AND BACON BREKKIE

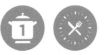

Makes 1 portion
Prep time: 10 mins
Cooking time: 10 mins

If you're prone to those awful mid-morning bouts of nausea, do your best to have a good breakfast early in the day. The healthy fats in this dish will line your stomach and help to keep that morning sickness at bay.

½ avocado
½ tomato, diced
1 tablespoon chopped coriander
1 spring onion, thinly sliced
a squeeze of lemon juice
salt and pepper
3 rashers streaky bacon, cooked until crispy
2 eggs, boiled to your preference
a drizzle of extra virgin olive oil

- Spoon the avocado into a bowl, and mash it using a potato masher or fork until it's soft but not completely smooth. Stir in the tomato, coriander, spring onion and lemon juice. Season with salt and pepper.
- Spread the avo mix onto a plate, top with the crispy bacon and boiled eggs.
- Sprinkle a little fresh coriander over the top and – voilà! – gourmet brekkie is served.

IF THE AVO ADDITIONS ARE TOO MUCH OF A SCHLEP JUST KEEP IT PLAIN – NO HASSLE!

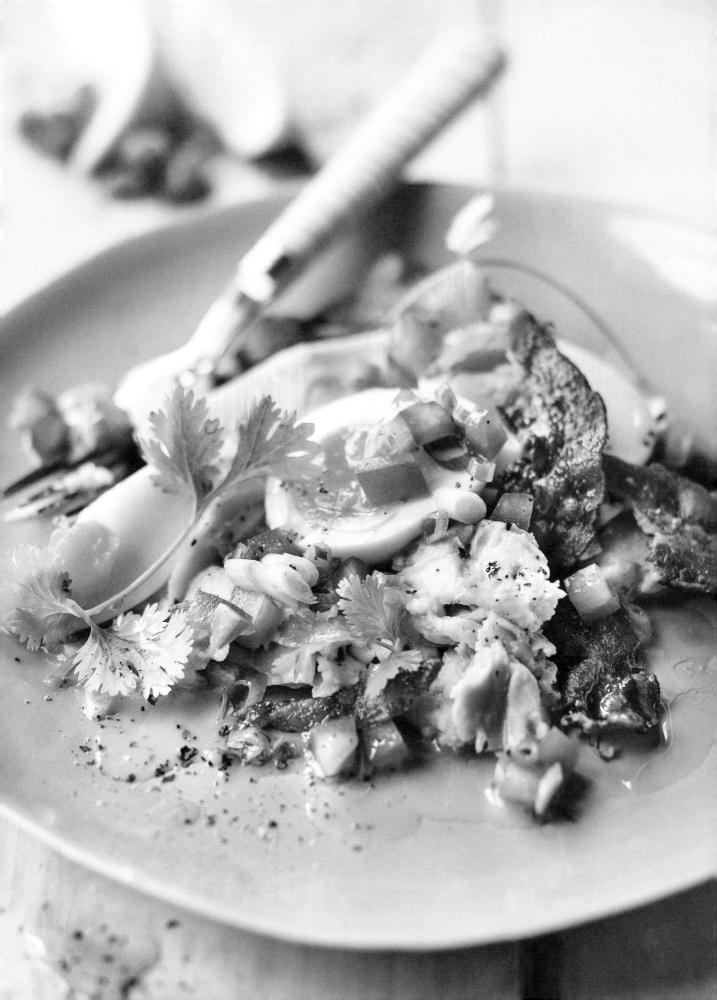

'BABY BAKING' SALAD

Makes 2 portions
Prep time: 20 mins
Cooking time: 20 mins

As you know by now, folic acid is essential for the healthy growth of your baby – if you ever need a boost of the stuff, this salad is the answer. For a hearty lunch, bulk it up with some seared salmon or grilled chicken.

For the dressing:
1 tablespoon raspberry
   or red wine vinegar
4 tablespoons olive oil
1 clove garlic, crushed
1 teaspoon Dijon mustard
salt and pepper

For the salad:
2 handfuls spinach leaves
1 handful fresh kale, shredded
100g broccoli florets, blanched
100g Brussels sprouts, roasted in
   a little olive oil at 200°C for
   35 minutes until crispy
1 small beetroot, peeled and shredded
1 carrot, peeled and shredded
½ stalk celery, finely sliced
1 avocado, peeled and sliced
100g raspberries
100g strawberries, trimmed and
   quartered
100g high-fat creamy feta
50g toasted sunflower seeds

- To make the dressing, whisk together all the ingredients.
- To make the salad, toss all the ingredients together in a salad bowl, except the feta and sunflower seeds; add these on top afterwards.
- Drizzle with the salad dressing and serve.

THIS RECIPE WORKS WELL WITH GOAT'S CHEESE INSTEAD OF FETA, BUT IF YOU'RE WARY OF CHEESE IN GENERAL, JUST LEAVE IT OFF

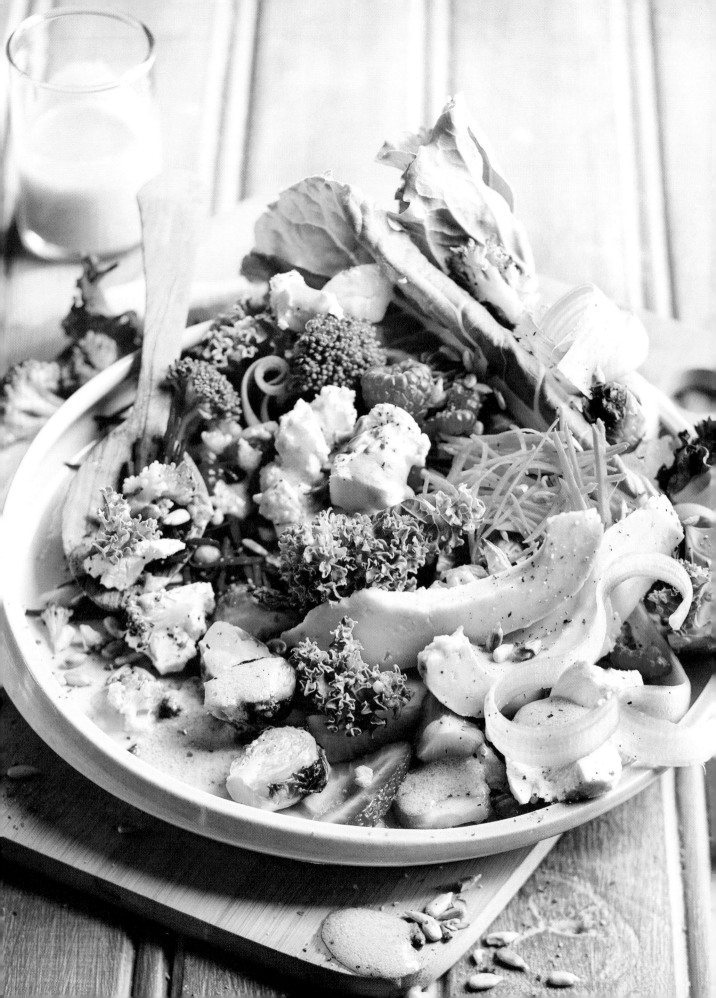

ROASTED ROOT VEGETABLE 'RISOTTO' WITH PARMESAN AND ORANGE ZEST

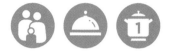

Makes 4 portions
Prep time: 20 mins
Cooking time: 45 mins

Risotto is an ideal vessel for delicious flavours and makes for wonderful comfort food, but in this case we're using cauliflower instead of high-carb rice. The root vegetables are great for a hearty winter dish that will help keep your stomach working and control that pesky gas.

1 large head cauliflower, broken into florets
1 large sweet potato, peeled and cubed
1 large aubergine, cubed or sliced
125g baby carrots, trimmed
200g pumpkin, peeled and diced
5 radishes, quartered
2 sprigs rosemary
2 tablespoons coconut oil melted with 2 tablespoons butter
salt and pepper
3 tablespoons butter
1 large onion, finely chopped
2 cloves garlic, crushed
½ cup (125ml) dry white wine
the zest of 1 orange
1 cup (250ml) cream
½ cup (45g) grated Parmesan
2 tablespoons chopped fresh sage (optional)

- Preheat the oven to 180°C.
- Place the cauliflower in the bowl of a food processor and blitz until it's the consistency of rice. Set aside.
- Spread the vegetables on a roasting tray with the rosemary and drizzle with the melted coconut oil and butter mixture. Season well with salt and pepper.
- Roast in the oven for 45 minutes, until the vegetables are soft and caramelised.
- While the vegetables are roasting, melt the butter on a medium heat in a pot. Add the onion and gently fry until soft. Add the garlic and fry for a further minute.
- Turn up the heat of the pot and add the white wine. Let the wine simmer until it's almost gone. (Don't worry about the alcohol; it will cook off.) Add the orange zest and cream, and simmer for another 5 minutes until it starts to thicken.
- Add the cauliflower, and let everything cook together for 10 minutes.
- Take the pot off the heat and stir in the roasted vegetables, Parmesan and sage. Season well with salt and pepper and serve immediately.

THIS DISH IS SUPERB FOR USING UP LEFTOVERS. TRY VARIOUS CONCOCTIONS, DEPENDING ON WHAT'S IN THE FRIDGE

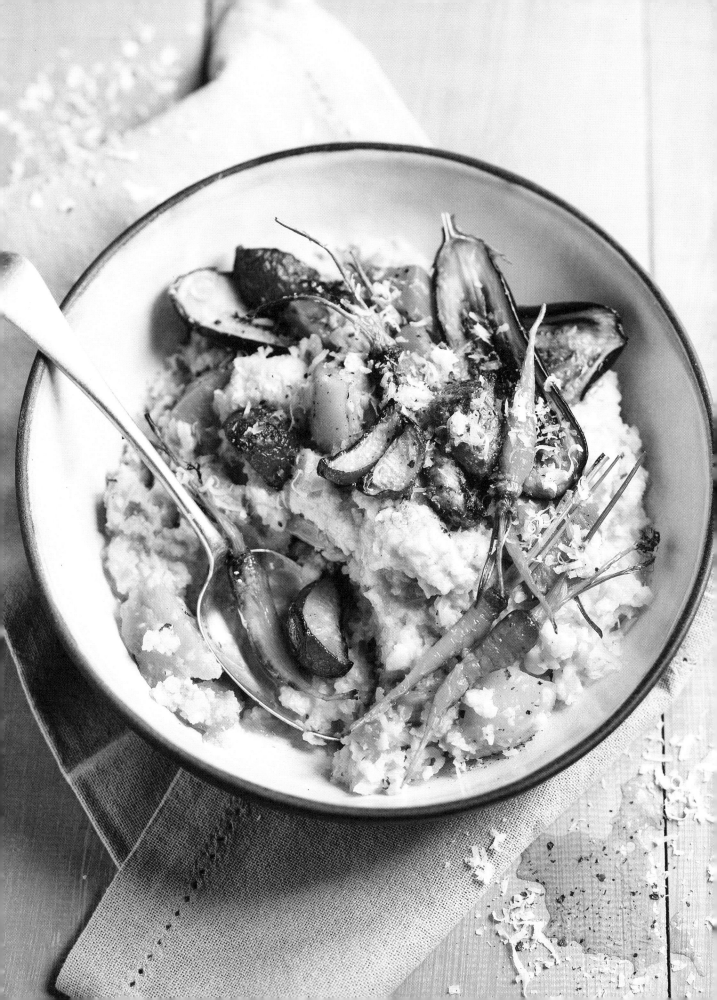

YUMMY CHOCOLATE MILK

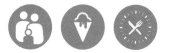

Makes 1 giant glass
Prep time: 2 mins

Never drunk chocolate milk before and now you're craving it by the litre? You're not the first. This recipe, using stevia for sweetness, is far healthier than the commercial stuff and just as satisfying.

2 tablespoons good-quality cocoa
  powder
2 tablespoons boiling water
3 cups (750ml) milk, chilled
½ teaspoon vanilla extract
a little stevia or honey to taste

- Drop the cocoa into a small bowl and stir in the boiling water to cook it a little.
- Pour all the ingredients and the cocoa into a blender and blitz together for 30 seconds.
- Pour into a glass, add a straw and gulp it down!

SIMPLE VANILLA ICE CREAM

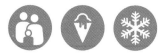

Makes 1 litre
Prep time: 20 mins
Freeze overnight

Pregnant women crave ice cream; it's a cliché because it's true. Problem is, the commercial ones are packed with sugar. Here's a basic ice-cream recipe that works a charm and is easy to make.

10 egg yolks
500ml milk
500ml double cream
1 teaspoon vanilla extract
a little stevia to taste

- Using an electric mixer with the whisk attachment, whisk the egg yolks until they are light and fluffy.
- Pour the milk and cream into a saucepan with the vanilla extract and put it on the stove. Bring the cream mixture to the boil, then take off the heat.
- Add a little of the hot cream mixture to the egg yolks, then pour the egg-yolk mixture into the cream mixture in the saucepan. Stir well to combine.
- If you like a sweet ice cream, add a little sweetener to taste at this stage.
- Return the saucepan to a very low heat. Stirring constantly with a wooden spoon, let the mixture cook until it has thickened enough to coat the back of a spoon. Allow the mixture to cool completely and place in an ice-cream churner to freeze. Eat as needed!

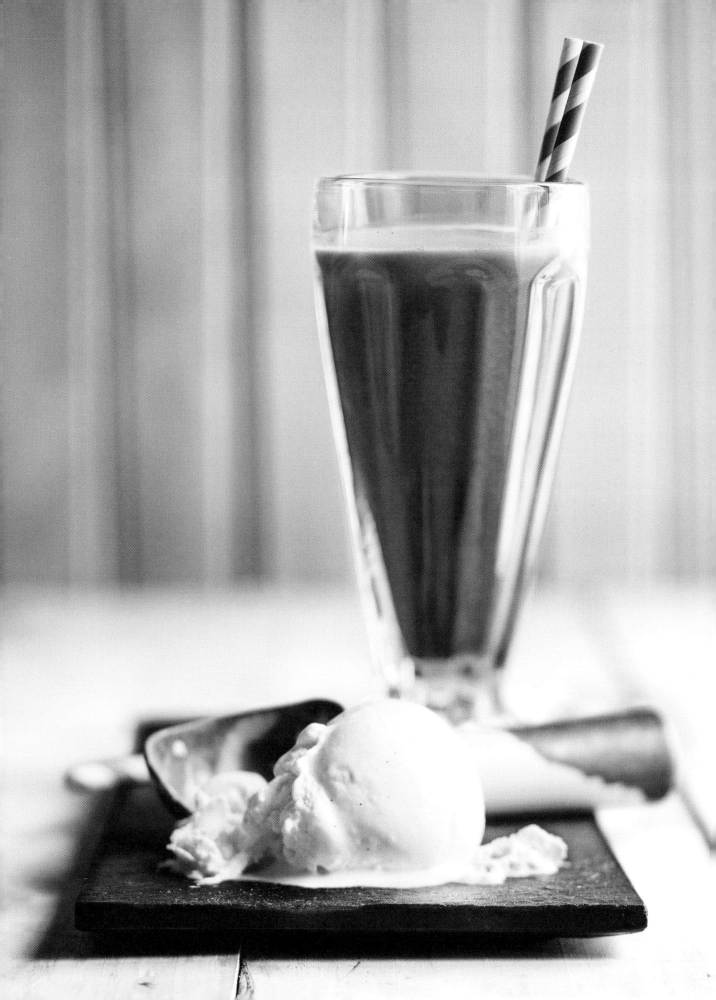

KIWI AND KALE SUPERSMOOTHIE

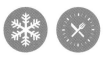

Makes 1 portion
Prep time: 5 mins

Pregnancy can take a toll on your teeth. These smoothies will give you the vitamin-C boost those pearly whites need to keep your smile glowing.

50g kale, with the thick rib removed, washed and chopped
1 green apple, peeled, cored and roughly chopped
1 kiwi fruit, peeled and roughly chopped
¼ avocado, peeled
1 teaspoon grated fresh ginger
6 fresh mint leaves
125ml coconut water
1 cup (105g) ice cubes

- Place all the ingredients, including the ice, in a good-quality blender and blend until smooth. Pour into a glass and drink immediately.

ORANGE, PAPAYA, CARROT AND YOGHURT SMOOTHIE

Makes 1 smoothie
Prep time: 5 mins

The kiwi and kale smoothie is super-healthy, but if you'd prefer something a little less green, you can't go wrong with this recipe.

1 orange, peeled and sliced
½ cup (70g) papaya, peeled and diced
1 carrot, peeled and grated
1 cup (225g) Greek yoghurt
1 cup (105g) ice cubes

- Place all the ingredients, including the ice, in a good-quality blender and blend until smooth. Pour into a glass and drink immediately.

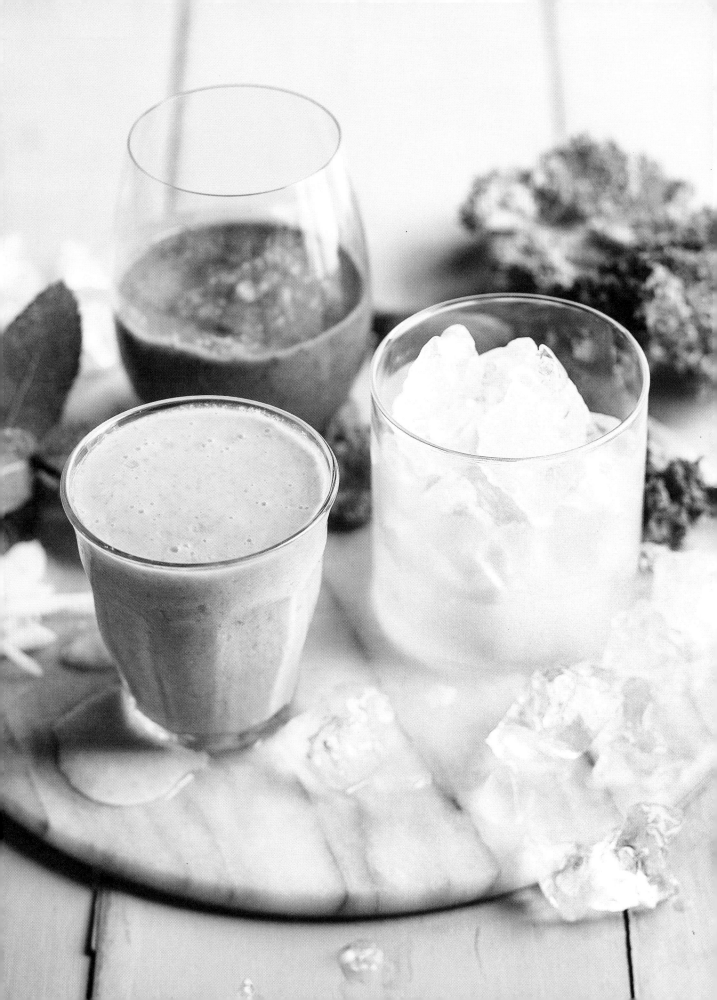

FRESH MEDITERRANEAN-STYLE SARDINES WITH TOMATO AND PEPPERS

Makes 6 portions
Prep time: 25 mins
Cooking time: 45 mins

Pregnancy drains your calcium levels. To keep up with your body and baby's demands you need to refuel regularly. Fresh dairy is an obvious calcium source, but sardines are also fantastic. This recipe will have you eating them all the time.

2 whole red peppers
3 tablespoons butter
1 red onion, thinly sliced
2 garlic cloves, thinly sliced
2 tablespoons tomato paste
¼ cup (65ml) dry white wine
¼ cup (65ml) white wine vinegar
1 x 400g tin whole peeled tomatoes, blended
2 tablespoons fresh flat-leaf parsley, chopped
2 tablespoons drained capers
½ teaspoon dried oregano
salt and pepper
8 whole fresh sardines, scaled, gutted and deboned
4 tablespoons melted butter
fresh dill to garnish
extra virgin olive oil for drizzling
lemon wedges to serve

- Preheat the grill of your oven.
- Grill the peppers, turning occasionally, until they are dark and blistered all over. Transfer them to a bowl and cover them with plastic wrap. Let them sit and sweat for 15 minutes. Peel, seed and slice them into 1cm wide strips and set aside.
- Turn off the grill and preheat the oven to 200°C.
- Melt the butter in a large frying pan over medium heat and gently fry the onion and garlic until soft.
- Increase the heat to medium-high and add the tomato paste, stirring until the paste begins to darken.
- Pour in the wine and vinegar and cook for 2 minutes. (Don't worry about the alcohol; it will cook off.)
- Add the tinned tomato and simmer for 10 minutes.
- Mix in the roast peppers, parsley, capers and oregano, and cook for 5 minutes. Season with salt and pepper and pour into an ovenproof dish.
- Season the sardines inside and out with salt and pepper and brush them with some melted butter. Lay them on top of the tomato mix and bake for about 25 minutes, until the sardines are firm and beginning to brown.
- Garnish with fresh dill and a drizzle of olive oil, and serve with lemon wedges.

SARDINES ARE ALSO AN EXCELLENT SOURCE OF OMEGA-3S, VITAMINS AND MINERALS – A GREAT AND MORE AFFORDABLE ALTERNATIVE TO SALMON

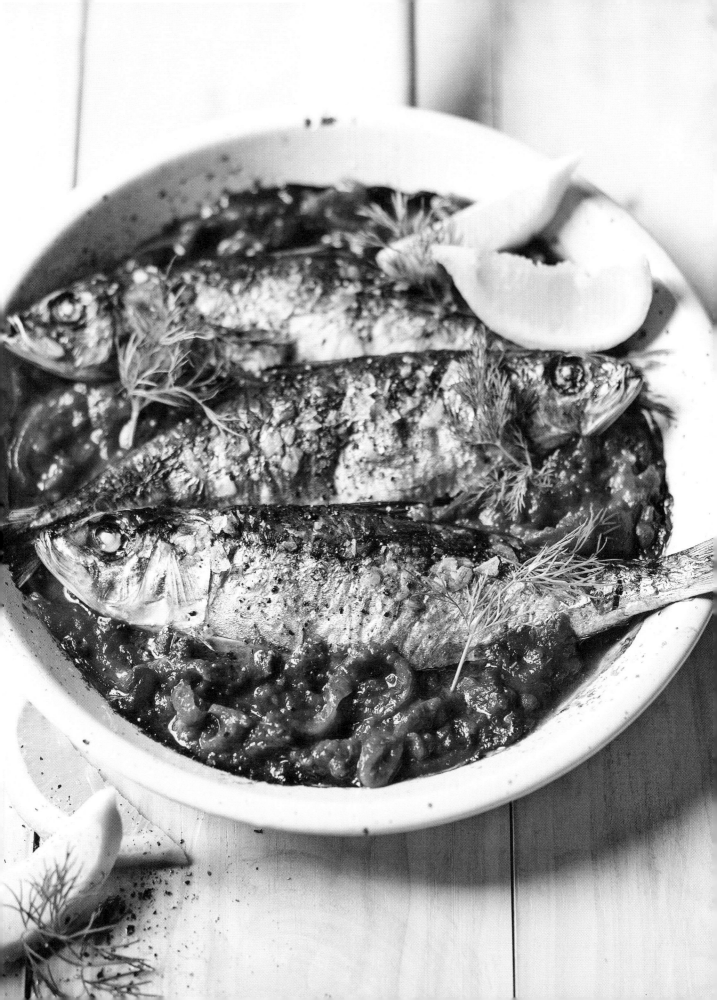

SMOKED TROUT AND ASPARAGUS 'PASTA' WITH COURGETTE NOODLES, CREAM AND MUSTARD

Makes 2 portions
Prep time: 10 mins
Cooking time: 20 mins

Those omega-3s we mentioned in the previous recipe are important to turn that baby of yours into a mini-Einstein (as well as to counteract the effects of your preggie brain). The best source of good omegas is fatty fish, and you can't go wrong with salmon or trout.

180g asparagus, trimmed and halved

400g courgettes, sliced into thin noodles

350ml cream

1 teaspoon Dijon mustard

125g cream cheese

2 tablespoons capers, rinsed, drained and roughly chopped

juice and zest of 1 lemon

2 tablespoons chopped dill

salt and pepper

100g smoked trout

extra virgin olive oil and shavings of Parmesan for garnish

- Fill a small saucepan with water and bring it to the boil. Add a pinch of salt and the asparagus. Cook them for 1-2 minutes, refresh in ice-cold water, and set aside.
- Drop the courgette noodles in the boiling water for 30 seconds, refresh in cold water and drain.
- Pour the cream into a saucepan with the Dijon mustard and bring to the boil. Reduce the heat and simmer until it thickens slightly. This should take about 5 minutes. Stir in the cream cheese, capers, lemon zest and juice and chopped dill. Season with salt and pepper.
- Stir in the asparagus, courgette noodles and the smoked trout. (We've added the trout at this point so that the heat of the sauce gently cooks it, without drying it out.)
- Garnish with a drizzle of olive oil and some Parmesan shavings.

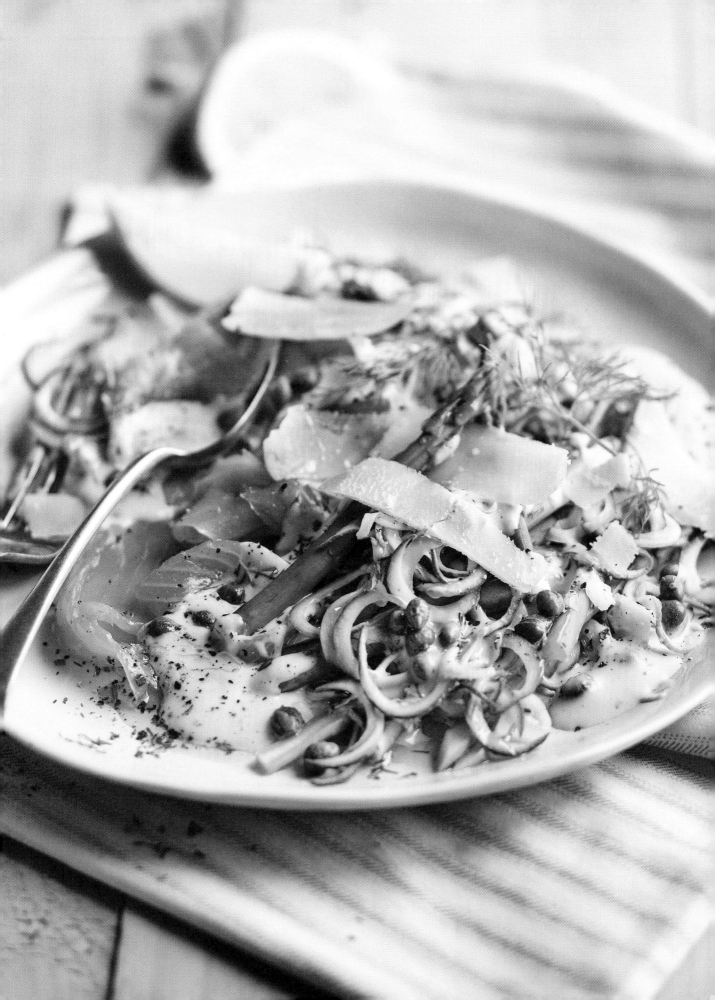

SEARED SALMON ON GARLIC-AND-GINGER MUSHROOMS WITH BOK CHOI AND SESAME

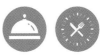

Makes 2 portions
Prep time: 15 mins
Cooking time: 20 mins

Here's another wonderful salmon recipe to boost those omega-3s, and it's sophisticated enough to use for a dinner party if you're entertaining. This time we're using salmon portions and giving it an Asian twist. The ginger should, once again, help with pregnancy-related nausea.

For the sauce:
2 cloves garlic, crushed
1 tablespoon grated ginger
3 tablespoons sake mirin
2 tablespoons tamari soya sauce
1 tablespoon sesame oil
juice of 1 lime

For the fish:
1 tablespoon coconut oil
150g exotic mushrooms, trimmed
100g bok choi, halved lengthways
2 x 200g Norwegian salmon portions

For the garnish:
2 tablespoons toasted sesame seeds
a sprinkle of Japanese 7 spice
  (optional)

- In a bowl, whisk together the sauce ingredients.
- To make the fish, heat the coconut oil in a frying pan and fry the mushrooms on a high heat until they just start to brown. Add 2 tablespoons of the sauce, give the mushrooms a quick stir and remove them from the pan.
- Fry the bok choi for a minute or two in the same pan. Once it has wilted, remove and set aside.
- Add a little more coconut oil if necessary and fry the salmon for about 2 minutes on each side until it is a beautiful golden colour.
- Pour the remaining sauce over the salmon in the pan and cook for a further minute. Add the mushrooms and the bok choi to the pan to heat through.
- Serve with a sprinkle of toasted sesame seeds and a dash of Japanese 7 spice.

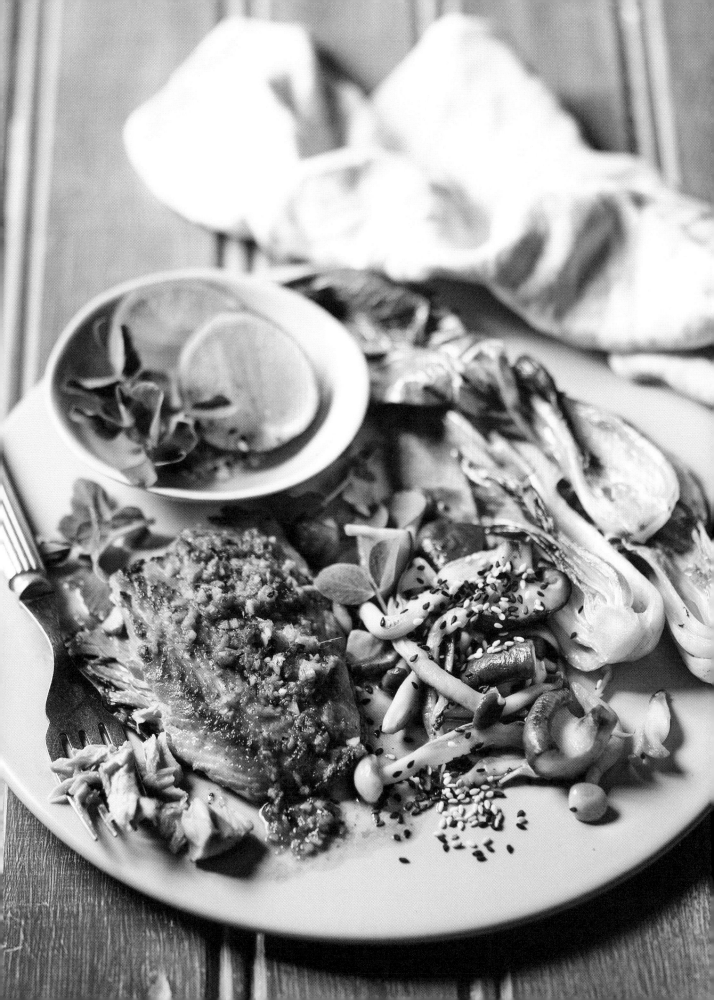

WONDER WEANING

Super food for ages

6-12 *months*

You've made it through childbirth and the exhaustion of the early months, and just when you think you've worked out a great routine with your baby, suddenly everything changes. He's waking for no apparent reason, demanding more milk feeds, never seeming satisfied… Which means he's probably ready for solid food. But where do you start? Which foods come first? How much should your six-month-old be eating? And what about allergies? This is yet another stage of conflicting advice and potentially confounding frustration. Don't panic. Stay away from the internet! And processed baby foods. Break out your steamer and your blender and introduce your child to a delicious, flavour-filled world of potential. You'll need, among other things, persistence, patience, a good handle on textures, and… iron-rich foods.

WHAT'S GROWING ON?

Year one is a time of rapid growth and development. Your baby should double his birth weight by 5 months of age and triple it by 12 months, at which point he'll likely be 25 centimetres longer than he was when you first met him. By 6 months he may be displaying a range of personality traits – he could be active, lazy, stubborn, relaxed, sociable, shy.

At this point he will also likely be running a little low on iron, a need that's no longer being properly satisfied by breast milk or formula. Among other things, iron is important for brain development and for the creation of haemoglobin, which carries oxygen around the body. Without an adequate supply, your baby will be lethargic and can develop anaemia. More than 90 percent of his iron supply – along with his energy, protein and vitamin A needs – will come from food now, and the best source of the iron he needs is meat.[1] This is why the likes of beef, lamb, chicken, pork and small quantities of liver are strongly recommended first foods these days, compared to the vegetable and fruit purées suggested in the past.

HOW DO I KNOW WHEN TO START WEANING?

Your baby's gastrointestinal tract should have developed sufficiently after 4 months to handle solid food, at which stage you could start the weaning process; however, we recommend holding out for another month or two if possible. Breastfeeding exclusively until 6 months is considered ideal, at which point he'll need food to complement his milk (or formula). Wait too long beyond this point and you risk facing growth and developmental problems. [1]

These are the behavioural signs that might indicate it's time to start weaning:
- Your baby's usual milk feeds aren't satisfying him any more.
- He has begun taking an interest in your food (read: he stares you down every time you put something in your mouth).
- He has begun waking during the night, having previously slept through.
- He is able to support his neck and head while sitting.
- He can turn his head away when full.

WHERE DO I START?

Take it easy to begin. There's no rush to get your child eating three meals a day. Start with a teaspoon of puréed food and see how it goes. If you get ½-2 teaspoons down his gullet you've done well. Show him how to do it; eat with him and he'll learn from you. Gradually build it, day by day, to about 2 tablespoons, which you can then consider a meal. Once he's eating 2 tablespoons in a go, you can introduce a second meal in the day. By the time he's 8 months old, he should be on 2-3 meals a day (to complement his continued milk feeds).

A critical factor is food texture. Keep it smooth(ish) initially, and gradually introduce lumps. The sooner you can do this, the better. By the time your baby is 9-10 months old he should be able to handle lumpier food, so as to avoid any fussiness later.[2] Don't worry if he spits out the food to begin with; that's to be expected. If you're struggling with a new food – bearing in mind it might take 8 or 10 attempts before he accepts it, by which time you may be testing your sanity – just move on to the next one. And if you're a type-A personality, it may be wise to get another adult involved as much as possible when feeding because your little angel is going to (and should be allowed to) mess. It's all a learning experience. Remember, as you're cleaning baby-food gunk off the curtains, that patience is a virtue...

A final note when starting out: it may seem blatantly obvious, but chances are you'll be sleep deprived and a little at sea, so we're going to remind you to never leave your child unsupervised when eating.

See the recipe section below for more feeding-specific advice.

ALLERGIES AND HIGH-RISK FOODS

One of the most common fears among parents of young children is the threat of allergic reaction. It's a reasonable one, too, as a reaction could range from a minor runny tummy to life-threatening anaphylactic shock. Naturally the risk is particularly high when weaning, as your baby comes into contact with foods he's never tried before. Unfortunately this is yet another contested realm of the science and art of parenting. When is the right time to introduce a certain food? Is early exposure worse than late exposure? Which side is it safer to err on?

New evidence suggests that withholding high-risk allergenic foods in no way helps prevent allergies in children.[3] In fact, there are theories that suggest that by withholding foods such as eggs, peanuts, shellfish and the like you can actually be *encouraging* allergies to these foods. The hard evidence is still lacking, but the modern consensus – as summarised from national guidelines in the UK, Canada, Australia and New Zealand – is, at least, sensible and practical. Unless a child's family has a history of allergies, eczema or asthma, specifically in the parents (you or your partner) or his siblings (your other children), the risk of reaction is considered slim and you can give foods freely. None of the four countries' guidelines differentiates between allergenic and non-allergenic foods, though they all recommend introducing one food at a time so as to be able to identify a problematic food, and waiting between one and four days before introducing a new one. If you have a particular concern you should consult a professional and consider introducing high-allergenic foods in a controlled environment.

Here's the lowdown on some suspected or previously suspected foods for children under 12 months.

AVOID

Honey: Can cause infant botulism. Do *not* feed your baby honey in year 1.
Cow's milk: Similarly, this should only be introduced as a drink after 12 months of age. Among other things, it is difficult for babies' digestive systems to handle and has a relatively low iron content.

BE WARY

Other dairy products: Cheese, yoghurt and other dairy products can be offered after iron-rich foods have been introduced, before 9 months. As always, make sure it's full cream.
Peanuts: Can cause severe adverse reactions. If there are peanut-allergy sufferers in the family, it may be wise to have him tested in a controlled environment first. Otherwise, peanuts (and real nuts in general) can be offered from six months in ground, chopped and spread form – never whole at this age because of the risk of choking.
Shellfish: As with peanuts, shellfish can be given from 6 months provided there's no history of allergies in the family.

GO FOR IT

Eggs: Don't delay getting eggs into your baby's diet if you can help it. They may be considered a higher-risk allergenic food, but they are the ideal weaning food – indeed, probably the best single weaning food – under normal circumstances, because they are iron- and nutrient-rich. Note, though, that iron absorption is improved when consumed in conjunction with foods rich in vitamin C – so don't forego the fruit and veg. And ensure your eggs are thoroughly cooked through, with no runny bits. (See p80.)

SUPPLEMENTS

If your baby is enjoying a diet high in iron, calcium and veggies, the need for a vitamin supplement should be greatly reduced. But if he's struggling to wean, isn't gaining weight, is unable to eat certain foods or is a vegetarian (not recommended) or vegan (really not recommended), consult your paediatrician about possible supplements.

WHEN DO I STOP BREASTFEEDING OR FORMULA-FEEDING?

This question is an addendum to the often controversial and emotive topic of breastfeeding (which we discuss in detail elsewhere) – so bear this in mind when considering it. From a purely nutritional perspective, the science these days points to breastfeeding to 2 years as the ideal standard to aim for. But there don't seem to be real benefits to formula feeding beyond 12 months; as long as your baby is eating a variety of foods, the advice is to replace it with (full-cream) cow's milk at this point.

Whether breast- or formula feeding, your specific circumstances will dictate what happens, and it may be best to chat to a professional to steer you in the right direction. (See see p42 and p311 for more detail on this topic.)

WHAT'S THE DEAL WITH BABY-LED WEANING?

Baby-led weaning is a responsive feeding technique that is pretty much as it sounds: it's all about letting weaning babies decide what food to put in their mouths instead of their parents spoonfeeding them. Because the (widely accepted) consensus on when to start weaning has been pushed back from 4 to 6 months, the idea is that this extra time allows babies the chance to develop their fine motor skills and digestive ability to the degree that purées are unnecessary. Rather, you provide your child with a variety of foods he can hold and he decides what to put in his mouth (or hair, as the case may be).

Does it make sense? Possibly. Is it a fad? Also possibly. But it does have certain practical advantages. For one, there are no purées to blend and cook and freeze and thaw. Also it is a tactile learning experience that encourages motor-skills development, including the all-important pincer grip. Perhaps most importantly, in the context of our ever-rising infant obesity figures, this type of responsive feeding is believed by its advocates to promote attentiveness and healthier eating habits. By contrast, the logic goes, non-responsive feeding may "override the child's internal hunger and satiety regulatory cues", with the result that weaning babies may learn to eat more than they need. [4]

A major downside with baby-led weaning is that it may test your patience beyond its already stretched limits, especially when you watch your pride and joy grab handfuls of food, throw them across the room and then cry because he's still hungry. Also there is a higher choking risk, it will likely take longer to introduce new foods, and you can't be guaranteed your baby will be getting all the nutrients he needs. Our advice is to mix up the baby- and parent-led weaning. Spend time making the lovely and delicious purées from our recipes (coming up), but also let your child hold and suck on a piece of biltong.

See from p340 for more on baby-led weaning.

Snack ideas and finger foods
- Biltong sticks (low-salt)
- Small pieces of cooked chicken, fish and other soft meats
- Shredded, grated or cut cheese
- Steamed vegetables such as carrot sticks, broccoli, cauliflower, beans and fresh peas
- Dried fruit such as mango or pears (sulphur-free)
- Ripe banana, paw paw and any other very soft and peeled fruit

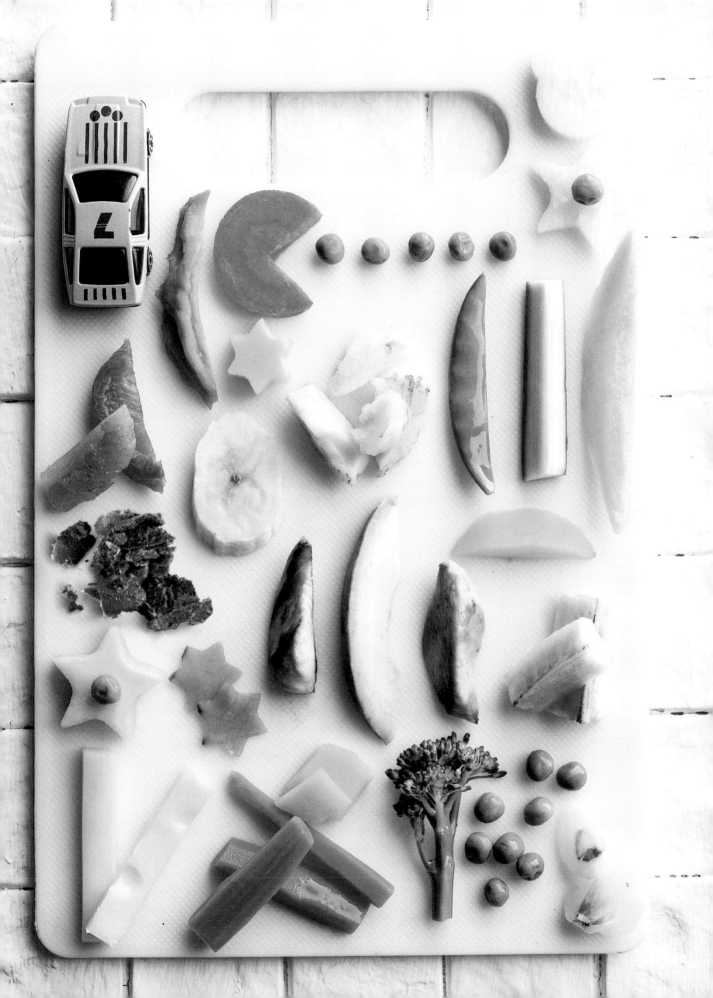

WONDER WEANING: THE KITCHEN BASICS

Cooking for your baby is not quite as mouthwatering a prospect as cooking for diners with teeth who are less likely to mush their food into their hair. Still, if you're going to do it – and, of course, we recommend you do – then it helps to do it properly. Stock your kitchen with the right tools, understand the basic cooking methods and prepare to cook in bulk and freeze. It will make a world of difference.

VITAL EQUIPMENT

Scale: So many baby recipes call for ingredients to be weighed that a scale really is worth getting. A digital scale is a little pricier, but a breeze to use.

Grater: If you aren't into chopping, a grater is invaluable. Make sure it's a good one; not blunt or uncomfortable to use.

Steamer: Dedicated steamers – as opposed to a steaming basket or colander over a pot – are designed specifically for the job, are reasonably priced and are well worth buying because they allow you to cook a few different things at the same time. (See Cooking Methods, overleaf.)

Colander: Useful for draining things, and also as a makeshift or extra steamer.

Strainer/sieve: Also useful to drain things (obviously...), but also brilliant for straining and mashing cooked fruit and vegetables finely to get rid of stubborn lumps. Using a ladle to push cooked food through the sieve works best.

Food processor: One of the most expensive cooking items you can buy, but it's worth it – not only to process food for your baby, but also for chopping, grating and generally making the prep for cooking a breeze. It may be a little daunting at first, with all the various attachments, but once you've got the knack of your food processor you'll never cry from chopping an onion again.

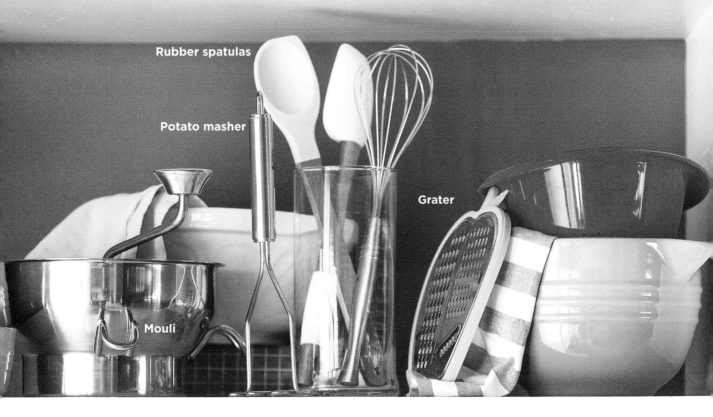

Rubber spatulas

Potato masher

Grater

Mouli

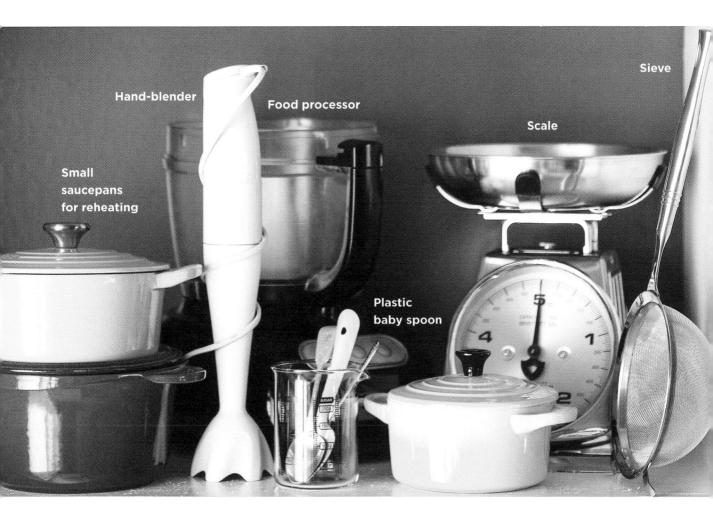

Sieve

Hand-blender

Food processor

Scale

Small
saucepans
for reheating

Plastic
baby spoon

Hand-blender: A frequent life-saver, especially in the first stage of weaning, a hand-blender is small, convenient and easy to clean, and will purée fruit and vegetables to the exact consistency you need. If you're buying new, get a powerful motor; you'll be putting it through its paces.

Mouli: A little old-fashioned, perhaps, but great for creating the right food textures for the phase between food processor and fork. Or try a potato masher.

Rubber spatula: A good rubber spatula (as opposed to an egg-flipper spatula) is invaluable for mixing, stirring and getting everything out of pots and bowls. Make sure it's heat resistant.

Covered ice trays: You're going to need lots of these for all that freezing you'll be doing. The cover prevents spillage or contamination in the freezer.

Sealable bags for freezing: Once your food has frozen in the ice trays, you can pop the cubes out and place them in sealable bags so you can use the trays again. Write the date and type of food on the bags – much easier than cracking open trays of mysterious orange and green blocks.

Small saucepans for reheating: Because you'll be reheating small amounts, small pots make a lot of sense. Large pots are a pain to haul around, you end up losing half the food, and they're more effort to clean. Invest in a couple of good-quality small saucepans for reheating, and you'll be using them daily.

Plastic baby spoon: When your baby is still all gums, a metal spoon can hurt.

COOKING METHODS

Steaming
Steaming food over simmering or boiling water is considered healthier than boiling it. Certain vitamins are water soluble and leach from vegetables into the cooking water when they're boiled. Steaming is a wonderful way to keep the freshness in the food, and is the preferred cooking method for first-stage weaning food to ensure those vitamins don't go missing. Generally it's used for vegetables, white meats and various dumplings.

Boiling
Boiling is usually used for tougher fruit and vegetables. It's a quicker process than steaming and produces a more uniform result; everything

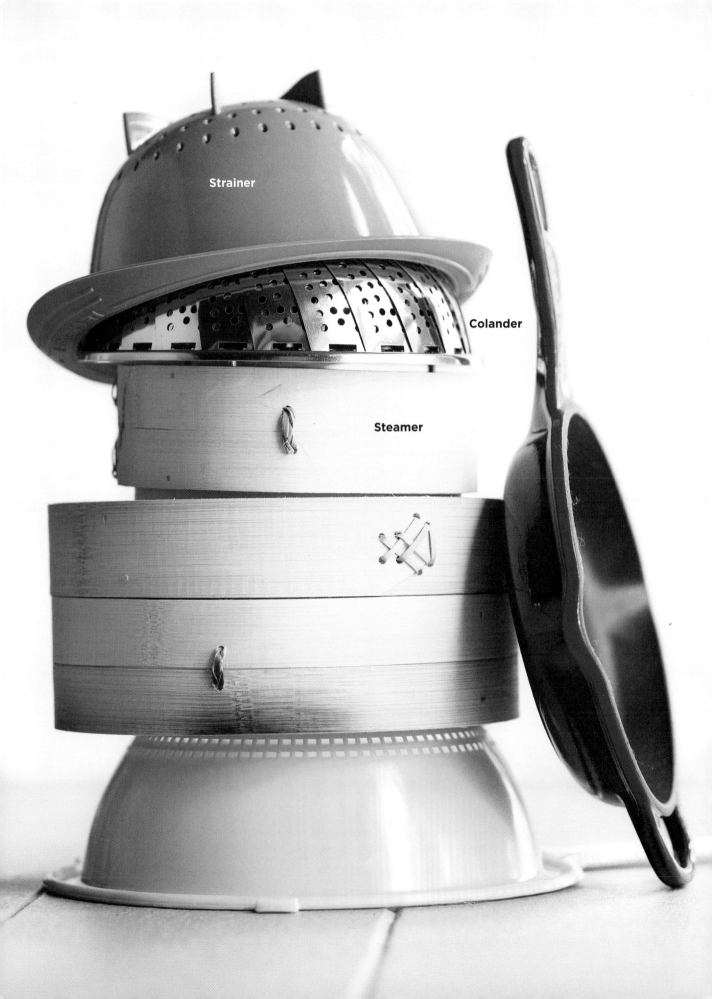

submerged in the water will cook at the same pace. When boiling food for your baby, try to use as little water as possible and keep the lid on. If you incorporate the cooking liquid in your purées, you will lose very little of the vitamins that have made their way into the water.

Baking

Baking is a great way to cook hardy vegetables like potato, sweet potato, aubergine, pumpkin and butternut, especially if you're cooking a family meal. Prick the whole vegetables with a fork, bake for about 45 minutes, then use a spoon to scoop out the soft centre to mash or purée. Remember to remove any seeds.

How to steam vegetables properly

Steaming will likely be the first cooking method you use when weaning, and you're quite possibly going to be mildly exhausted by this stage of motherhood, so it's a good idea to know how to do it well. To start, make sure the vegetables you're steaming have been peeled (if possible) and are the same size; this helps to cook them at the same rate. Then follow these basics.

Steaming in a basket: A steaming basket is basically any heat-resistant container with holes in the bottom. It holds your veggies and allows the steam in through the holes to do the cooking. Fit the basket over a pot that contains at least an inch of boiling water, and loosely cover it with a lid. The lid needs to fit well enough to keep most of the steam in, while allowing enough steam to escape so that there isn't a pressure build-up. Without the lid your veggies will steam unevenly and take forever.

There are many custom-designed steaming baskets available on the market, which are usually adjustable and can fit inside pots of various sizes. They're also designed to stay raised out of the water so you actually steam the food instead of boiling it. If you don't have one, a colander or strainer will do – just be sure it's heat-resistant.

First key point: don't let the the basket get immersed in the water, otherwise the boiling-not-steaming problem strikes.

Second key point: don't forget to turn off the stove when you're done, otherwise the water will boil away and your pot will start to burn. Obvious, you may think, but try steaming veggies on three hours' sleep and with a six-month-old to distract you...

Using a steamer: A dedicated steamer generally makes the process simpler and easier. The water is always at the correct temperature, the vegetables are always above the water, and just enough steam escapes.

A steamer will usually have a few parts and different levels, which allows you to steam different vegetables for different times. The base holds just the right amount of water, and some steamers even have their own element to heat it, so there's less chance of leaving the stove on and burning down the house. The separate element is perhaps unnecessary, but we do recommend you get a stovetop model that allows you to stack two or more baskets at the same time.

Steaming vegetables in a pan: In a bind – if your steamer's on the fritz, for example, and your toddler is using your colander as a helmet – it's possible to steam food using only a pan of water.

You'll need a pot or pan that's big enough to hold all your veggies without them being on top of one another. Add a centimetre or two of water to the pan and, once it's boiling, add the veggies. Because there's so little water, the steam will be doing the cooking. Just be sure to keep an eye on the water level; you may need to keep topping up so that you keep generating steam.

Once again, you'll need a lid to keep most of the steam in. But allow some to escape, especially if you're steaming green veg, because this will help to keep the colour. Since your veggies will be slightly immersed, some of the nutrients and flavour will end up in the water. Save this water and use it as the liquid for blending to incorporate some of the lost nutrients.

Storing and reheating: If you've gone to the effort of making your baby's food (well done!), it's worth storing it and heating it up properly.

The recipes in this section will keep well for 2-3 days in the fridge and up to three months in the freezer. Don't be tempted to refreeze food that you've heated up but not used; the chances of contamination are high. Cooked food should only ever be frozen once, and defrosted food should only be reheated once.

For heating, we recommend using a stovetop rather than the microwave. Place the frozen food from the freezer in a container in the fridge overnight to defrost. (The container will catch the water that will otherwise drip all over your fridge shelf.) The next day, transfer the softened purée into a saucepan or small pot and put it on a low heat. Stir until warmed through and serve. If the consistency is a bit too thick, add a little water or milk and stir it through.

Microwaves can be a lifesaver for an emergency reheat, but they aren't ideal because they heat food unevenly and can create potentially dangerous hot spots in the food. Foods with high fat content, such as meat or eggs, are particularly susceptible to overheating.

Whichever method you use, always check the temperature before serving.

FIRST FOOD: 5-8 MONTHS

In the past, when weaning was recommended from 4 months, first foods were traditionally finely puréed vegetables and fruit (or, worse, processed baby cereals). But starting at 6 months gives your baby's gut more time to develop, and because he's in need of nutrient-rich, energy-dense food containing loads of iron, the best nutritional move is to get straight on to eggs and meat.

But we understand if you're reluctant to let go of the conventional veggie wisdom immediately; it's human nature (like learning that high-fat is good and low-fat isn't all it's cracked up to be). The good news is that veggies are still highly recommended for your baby, they're a little easier to get the right consistency with in purée form, and introducing them now will get him used to their flavours. So we've split the difference, and come up with a mix of vegetable and meat purée recipes.

The idea is to keep things simple and begin with textures and flavours that are most attractive to a growing baby. Start off finer before thickening up the texture. If you need to get him going on a plain butternut purée before he hits the carrot and chicken, then that makes practical sense. You may want to experiment a bit when adding meat to your baby's meals to work out which textures and flavours he likes best. Here are the recommended ways to begin preparing eggs and various meats so that they are soft and palatable.

Eggs

Eggs are a marvellous source of protein. In the past the accepted practice was to introduce egg yolks at first, due to the potentially allergenic egg white, but the science doesn't appear to back this up, so we recommend introducing whole eggs.

If you would still prefer to incorporate yolks only into the meal, then the best method is to boil the whole egg for 9 minutes until hard, then peel away the shell and the egg white, and blend the cooked yolk into the purée you are serving. (See Allergies And High-Risk Foods on p69.)

Scrambled eggs are a good weaning food because they offer lumpier textures. Remember, free-range organic eggs are best.

Chicken

Chicken is the perfect first meat for your baby; it has a mild flavour and is easy to cook. Start with deboned chicken breasts or thighs by chopping them finely and adding them to whatever vegetables you're cooking. Thighs have a little more healthy fat and iron so we recommend them. The chicken will cook in two or three minutes and can be easily blended into whatever you're serving. Try not to overcook it to prevent it becoming stringy and rubbery. Chicken livers are also an excellent weaning food, and we strongly advise incorporating them into your child's diet from 6 months. To prepare them for a dish, simply rinse them in water, then fry in a little butter until no longer pink inside.

Fish

Fish is considered a super food for growing babies and is excellent for brain development, but it's not appealing when overcooked. The skin and all the bones must also be carefully removed. On the plus side, it cooks in minutes.

Start your baby with white fish; it has a gentle flavour and is easy to eat. It can either be chopped and cooked for a minute or two in the pot with your vegetables, and then blended, or you can quickly fry it in a little butter and add it to the veggies afterwards to blend. Move onto oily fish when you feel your baby is ready for a more fishy flavour. Tinned tuna is great in a hurry; opt for tuna in spring water to avoid excess salt. Check the website of your national health authority for advice on recommended weekly servings.

Beef and lamb

Introducing red meat means you're opening up a whole world of new flavours and textures to your baby, but red meat is trickier to get right at the early stages of weaning because it doesn't blend that easily. When starting out, cook it slowly in liquid – i.e. braise it – so that it softens completely, then mix small amounts into your veggies so that the end result is essentially a rich veggie stew. The meat can be blended at the beginning of weaning with vegetables or just shredded later as your baby gets used to different textures. It's best to use shin or shoulder cuts when braising. Lamb and calf livers are also highly recommended, and after a while you can try some mince, too.

Some miscellaneous advice

- Introduce new foods one at a time; if your baby has no reaction you can then combine it with other foods you know he tolerates.
- Avoid adding salt at this stage.
- Introduce your baby to vegetables before fruit, and then the tarter fruits first, to accustom him to less sweet tastes.
- Even in your darkest hour, don't be seduced by the convenience of store-bought rice cereals! If you must use a grain, opt for quinoa, millet or oats.

PUMPKIN OR BUTTERNUT PURÉE & EGG .... Makes 6 portions

Pumpkin and butternut are wonderful first foods because they have a gentle sweetness and a smooth texture when blended. They also combine well with other foods, including butter and even mild spices like nutmeg and cinnamon, and make an excellent base purée. An obvious early addition is egg.

2 cups (250g) pumpkin (or butternut), peeled and diced
1 egg

- Steam the pumpkin for 25-30 minutes with the lid on, until soft. Reserve the liquid.
- Blend the cooked pumpkin in a food processor or using a hand-blender until smooth. Use a little of the reserved cooking liquid to thin it out if necessary.
- If you're adding the egg, boil it for 9 minutes until hard, then blend it into the purée.
- Keep a portion to use now and freeze the rest for later.

CARROT PURÉE & CHICKEN .... Makes 6 portions

Carrots are also slightly sweet and are easy to cook and purée. Start your baby on carrots alone, then try blending in some chicken. You can also mix in some parsnips, which combine very well with carrots, or add a little fresh ginger to introduce new flavours.

2 cups (285g) carrots, peeled and quartered
100g deboned chicken thighs, finely chopped

- Steam the carrots for 15 minutes with the lid on, until soft. If you're adding the chicken, do so now and cook for a further 5 minutes, until no longer pink. Reserve the liquid.
- Blend the cooked carrot and chicken in a food processor or using a hand-blender until smooth. Use a little of the reserved cooking liquid or baby milk to thin it out to the correct consistency. Allow to cool.
- Keep a portion to use now and freeze the rest for later.

GEM SQUASH PURÉE & WHITE FISH .... Makes 6 portions

Gem squash is a quick and easy food, and it purées really well, which makes it a good first food for your baby. It's delicious with a bit of butter or ghee blended through. It's also a great basic with a medley of other veggies, cheese, chicken or white fish.

4 gem squash, halved with the seeds removed
100g skinless, boneless white fish, cut into chunks

- Steam the gem squash, sliced side up, for 15 minutes with the lid on, until soft. If you're adding the fish, do so now and steam for a further 5 minutes. Reserve the liquid.
- Spoon the cooked gem squash and fish into the bowl of a food processor or blend using a hand-blender until smooth. Use a little of the reserved cooking liquid or baby milk to thin it out to the correct consistency. Allow to cool.
- Keep a portion to use now and freeze the rest for later.

APPLE OR PEAR PURÉE & CHICKEN LIVERS .... Makes 6 portions

Apple purée is a delicious and nutritious first baby food. Although apple is sweet, it's unlikely to give your baby an overly sweet tooth. It's high in pectin, which helps to fight constipation, and it's also good for the relief of diarrhoea. When you're ready to introduce your baby to dairy, mix a little apple purée through some full-cream yoghurt as a breakfast option. Pear purée is cooked in the same way and is also a good first food because it's virtually hypoallergenic. Add a little cinnamon for flavour later. Liver is a superb source of iron and is a highly recommended weaning food. By adding it to the sweet-tart flavour of these purées, you will make it much more palatable for your baby.

2 large apples
5 tablespoons water
75g cooked chicken livers

- Peel, core and quarter the apples.
- Place the apples and water in a small saucepan, and heat over a low to medium heat with the lid on.
- Gently cook the apples for about 20 minutes, until they're soft. Give them a stir every few minutes to make sure there is still liquid in the pot and the apple isn't burning.
- Blend using a hand-blender or in a food processor. If you're adding the liver, do so now. Allow the mix to cool.
- Keep a portion to use now and freeze the rest in ice cubes for later use.

BROCCOLI PURÉE & CHEESE .... Makes 6 portions

Broccoli is one of the most nutritious veggies; it's high in vitamin C, beta-carotene, folic acid, iron and potassium. But it comes with a small snag: when cooked, broccoli can be fibrous and cause your baby a little discomfort and gas. The solution is to mix broccoli purée with other vegetables, and also to strain it through a sieve before feeding. To be safe, introduce broccoli a little later on in the weaning process. Once your baby gets used to it, he will love it. A few soft, blanched florets are also great when he starts to feed himself. Cauliflower, beans, fresh peas and asparagus can all be cooked in the same way, but they come with the same warning: they may make your baby a little gassy, so hold back before introducing them and remember that sieve. Both cauliflower and broccoli are delicious with some added butter or ghee and are a great place to start when introducing cheese.

3 cups (525g) broccoli pieces, broken
into florets
a sprinkle of mild cheese, grated

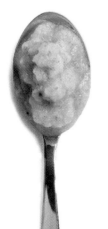

- Steam the broccoli for 5-10 minutes with the lid on, until soft. Reserve the liquid.
- Blend the cooked broccoli in a food processor or using a hand-blender until smooth. Use a little of the reserved cooking liquid or baby milk to thin it out to the correct consistency. Strain it through a sieve to remove any fibrous bits, especially when introducing it into the diet; once your baby is used to it, you can skip this step. If you're adding the cheese, sprinkle it over now. Allow to cool.
- Keep a portion to use now and freeze the rest in ice cubes for later use.

BEETROOT, APPLE AND PARSNIP PURÉE & CHICKEN .... Makes 6 portions

Beetroot is high in calcium, potassium, iron, vitamins A, B6 and C and fibre – another great food to introduce to your baby, and one with an exciting new colour for him to engage with. (Just don't get a fright when that colour is transferred to his nappy later...) For that all-important protein, add some chopped chicken thighs.

250g peeled and sliced parsnips
250ml water or homemade
  vegetable stock
1 cup (150g) grated beetroot
2 apples, peeled, cored and quartered
100g chicken thighs, chopped

- Place the parsnip and water/stock in a small saucepan and simmer for 20 minutes with the lid on, until soft.
- Add the beetroot and apple and simmer for a further 10 minutes, until everything is soft. If you're adding chicken, pop it into the pot for the last 10 minutes of cooking.
- Purée using a blender or hand-blender.
- Keep a portion to use now and freeze the rest in ice cubes for later use.

COURGETTE, POTATO AND BROCCOLI PURÉE & CHEESE .... Makes 6 portions

100g peeled and cubed potato
250ml vegetable stock or water
200g courgettes, washed and sliced
200g broccoli florets
a sprinkle of mild cheese, grated

- Place the potato and water/stock in a saucepan and simmer with the lid on until it softens – about 10-15 minutes.
- Add the courgette and the broccoli and simmer for a further 5-10 minutes, until everything is soft.
- Purée using a blender or hand-blender. Add the cheese if you're using it.
- Keep a portion to use now and freeze the rest in ice cubes for later use.

PUMPKIN, CARROT AND LEEK PURÉE & CHICKEN .... Makes 6 portions

This is another recipe that is perfect with the addition of chopped chicken thighs.

150g peeled and sliced carrot
150g peeled and cubed pumpkin
100g washed and sliced leek (white
  part only)
250ml water or vegetable stock
100g chicken thighs, chopped

- Place the carrot, pumpkin and leeks in a small saucepan and add the water or stock. Simmer for 20 minutes with the lid on, until the vegetables are soft. If you're adding chicken, pop it into the pot for the last 10 minutes of cooking.
- Purée using a blender or hand-blender.
- Keep a portion to use now and freeze the rest in ice cubes for later use.

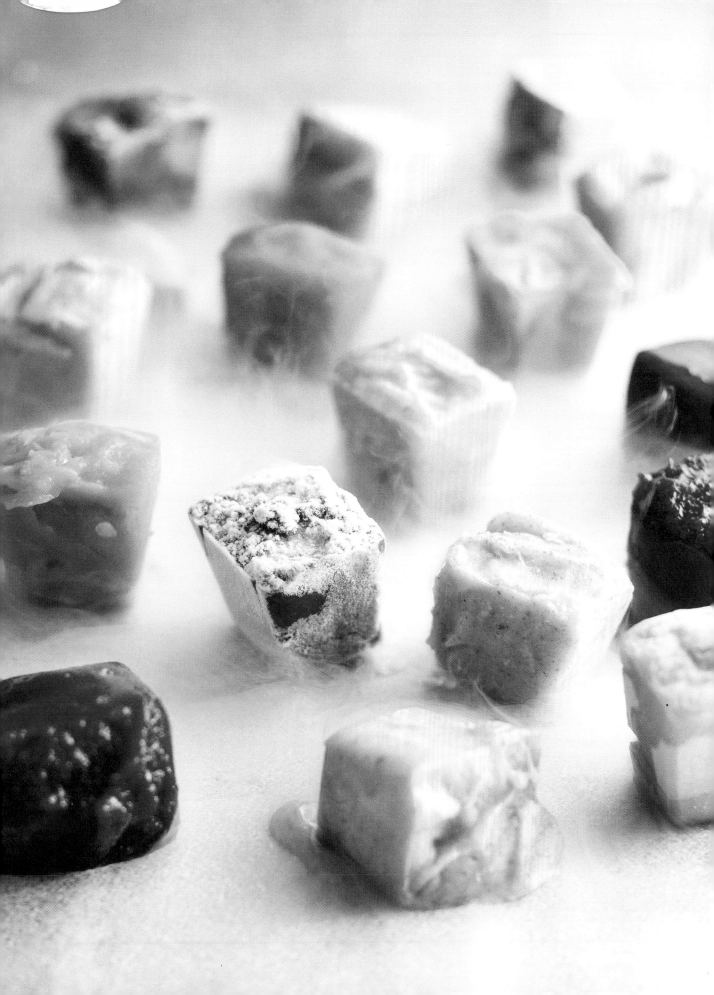

FIRST FOODS: 9-12 MONTHS

Now that you've made it through to the second stage of weaning, your days of puréeing food to a smooth paste should be long gone, especially if you've managed to incorporate some baby-led weaning into meals.

By now, your baby can handle a little more texture; in fact, he needs it so that he can start using his gums in a chewing motion. Start pulsing food in the food processor or use the hand-blender in shorter bursts so that the results aren't perfectly smooth, and slowly move your way through mouliing or mashing food with a fork to chopping it. Fruit can now be raw and grated or mashed. Don't rush the process; let him show you what he's ready for. Just make sure the food is soft throughout, and watch out for choking during feeding.

This is also the time when your baby will want to start feeding himself, so (if you haven't already) start offering finger foods that he can interact with, and perhaps give him his own spoon to experiment with. Try to make this the introduction to every meal. This is an important developmental stage; besides that chewing motion he's working on, he'll also start on the all-important pincer grip, necessary for the holding of crayons and creation of toddler masterpieces in the near future. (See What's The Deal With Baby-led Weaning? on p72.)

As your superchild becomes more aware of colours, mix up the colours on his plate to add to the excitement of eating. (This is where an exciting aeroplane spoon or superhero bowl might start helping, too.) Let him take his time so that he learns to enjoy his dining experience.

By the end of this stage of weaning, your baby should be comfortable eating the food the rest of the family is eating. Lest you forget, though: it's going to get even messier than before – if that's possible...

Adding beans and pulses

Beans and pulses provide another source of protein and are easy to incorporate. They are soft when cooked so blend into vegetables easily, and are gentle on the palate. A few good choices are chickpeas (the tinned ones are fine), broad beans, lentils, butter beans and kidney beans. Soak them overnight in water, drain them and boil them in water until they're soft. Try a little carrot and chickpea with pumpkin, or butter beans and cauliflower with spinach.

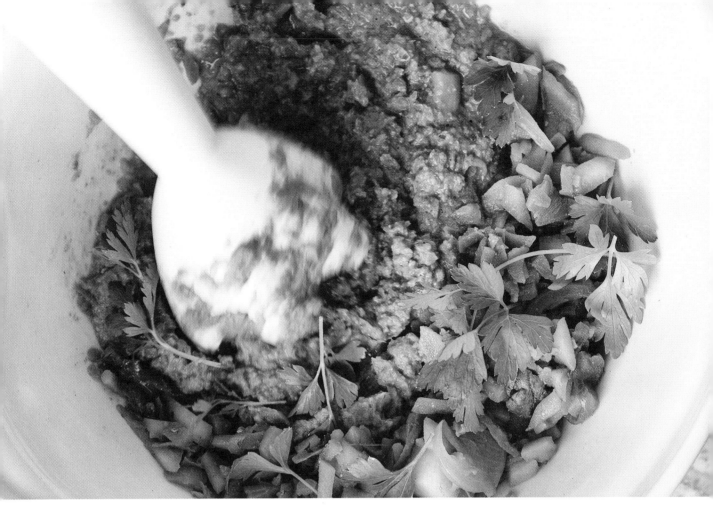

SAUTÉED CHICKEN LIVER, APPLE AND ONION
.... Makes 8 portions

Chicken liver is jam-packed full of goodness and is a cheap and healthy way of feeding kids. The trick is to get your baby used to the taste; after that, you're home free.

2 tablespoons butter or coconut oil
1 onion, peeled and thinly sliced
100g grated carrot
125g cleaned chicken livers (not chopped)
2 apples, peeled, cored and chopped
125ml chicken stock
1 teaspoon chopped parsley

- In a saucepan, melt the butter or coconut oil and fry the onion and carrot together until very soft.
- Add the chicken livers and the apple and fry for 5 minutes.
- Add the chicken stock and the parsley and simmer gently for a further 15 minutes.
- Pour everything into a food processor or use a hand-blender and blend to the desired consistency. As your baby gets used to more lumpy food, this meal is ideal mashed with a potato masher.
- Keep a portion to use now and freeze the rest in ice cubes for later use.

BABY BOLOGNAISE ON CAULI PURÉE .... Makes 6 portions

Bolognaise sauce is real old-fashioned comfort food, and this is a great first recipe for your baby. It freezes like a dream and can be mixed with any number of veggies. It can also be doctored a little and fed to your whole family. Make it in bulk and have it on hand for a quick meal.

For the bolognaise:
2 tablespoons butter
1 large onion, peeled and finely
  chopped
1 clove garlic, crushed
2 medium carrots, peeled and grated
1 stalk celery, finely chopped
200g beef mince
1 teaspoon tomato paste
5 tomatoes, skinned and chopped
200ml chicken stock
1 bay leaf

For the cauli purée:
water, for cooking
450g cauliflower, broken into florets
3 tablespoons butter

TO MAKE THE BOLOGNAISE:

- Melt the butter in a saucepan and gently fry the onion, garlic, carrot and celery until soft.
- Turn the heat up to high and add the beef mince. Fry the mince until it is browned, stirring occasionally and making sure it doesn't make meatballs.
- Turn the heat back down to medium and add the tomato paste, tomatoes, stock and bay leaf. Increase the heat and simmer for 30 minutes. Make the cauliflower purée while the sauce is cooking.
- Remove the bay leaf and blend the sauce in a mouli or blender to an appropriate consistency.
- Keep a portion to use now and freeze the rest for later use.

TO MAKE THE CAULI PURÉE:

- Bring a pot of water to the boil and add the cauliflower. Cook for 8 minutes until the cauliflower is soft. Drain it well.
- Add the butter and purée using a hand-blender until smooth.
- Keep a portion to use now and freeze the rest for later use.
- Serve the bolognaise spooned onto the cauli purée.

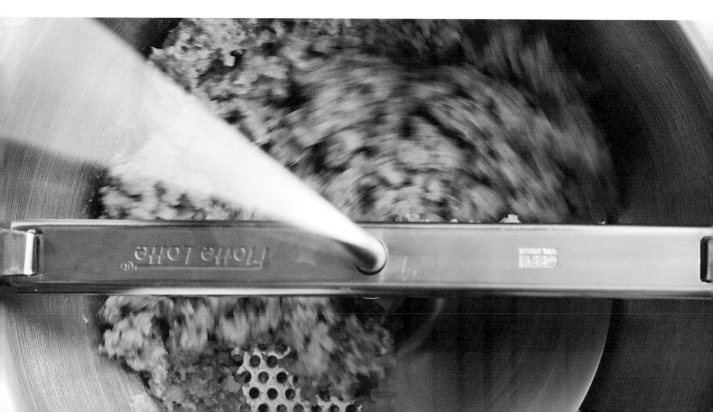

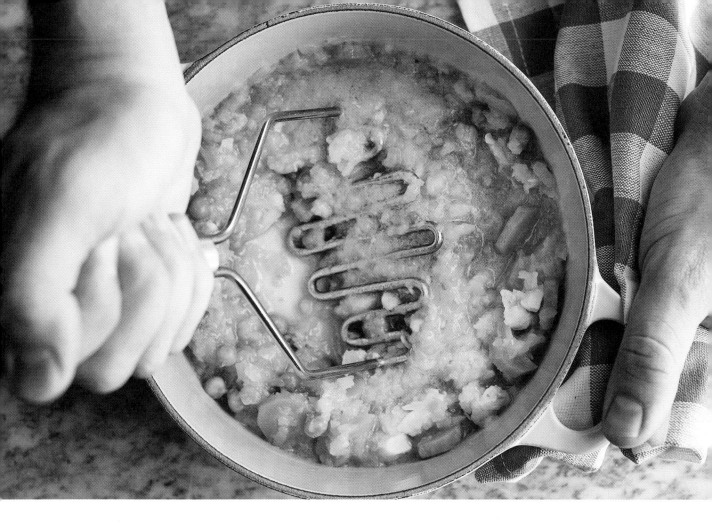

CHICKEN, CARROT, GINGER AND BUTTERNUT CASSEROLE .... Makes 8 portions

This is a great chicken recipe. The ginger adds a new level of flavour and is super way of introducing interesting flavours and spices to your baby's food. We've used chicken thighs because they're higher in good fats and iron, but you can use chicken breasts too. Remember that they cook faster, so adjust the cooking time accordingly.

2 tablespoons butter
1 small onion, finely chopped
½ teaspoon grated fresh ginger
200g peeled and grated butternut
100g peeled and thinly sliced carrot
150ml chicken stock
100g deboned chicken thighs,
  quartered
½ cup (75g) fresh peas

- Melt the butter in a saucepan and gently fry the onion and ginger until soft.
- Add the butternut, carrot and stock and simmer with the lid on for 10 minutes.
- Add the chicken and the peas, and simmer for a further 10 minutes or so.
- Pour everything into a food processor and blend to the desired consistency, or mash it with a potato masher or simply just chop things with a knife for a coarser texture.
- Keep a portion to use now and freeze the rest in ice cubes for later use.

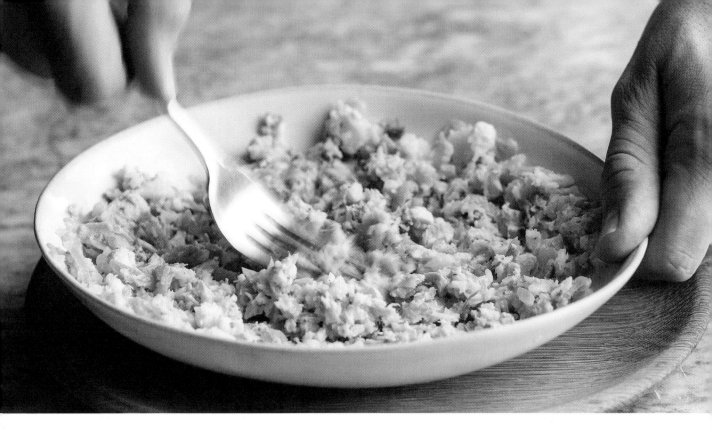

MINI-ME FISH-AND-BROCCOLI PIE WITH SWEET POTATO AND CHEESE TOPPING .... Makes 8 portions

This recipe is designed for a growing baby, but if it's prepared a little chunkier it's perfect for the whole family. Add a little spinach for extra veggies.

For the pie:
2 tablespoons butter
1 onion, finely chopped
1 carrot, peeled and grated
150g broccoli, chopped
1 leek, finely sliced
1 bay leaf
200g white fish (hake or sustainably
   fished cod) fillets, skinned and cubed
   – no bones
100g salmon trout fillets, skinned and
   cubed – no bones
150ml cream or vegetable stock
1 teaspoon chopped parsley

For the topping:
500g peeled and diced sweet potato
water, for boiling
2 tablespoons butter
50g grated mild Cheddar cheese

TO MAKE THE PIE:
- Melt the butter in a saucepan and gently fry the onion, carrot, broccoli and leek with the bay leaf until soft.
- Add the fish and the cream/stock and simmer for 8 minutes until the fish is cooked but still soft. Stir in the parsley.
- Remove the bay leaf and blend or mash together until the desired consistency is reached.

TO MAKE THE TOPPING:
- Boil the potatoes until tender. Drain and mash with the butter until smooth.
- Stir in the cheese.

TO ASSEMBLE:
- Place the fish mixture in freezer-proof ramekins, and add the sweet potato topping.
- Keep a portion to use now and freeze the rest for later use.

BEGINNER BEEF STEW WITH CARROTS AND SWEET ONIONS .... Makes 6 portions

This is a delicious recipe and can be made for the whole family. The key is to cook it slowly until the meat is very tender. Adjust the recipe times depending on the meat you're using.

1 tablespoon butter
1 onion, chopped
1 clove garlic, crushed
3 stalks fresh thyme, leaves only
150g cubed beef shin (or cut of your choice), bone removed
2 teaspoons tomato paste
200g peeled and diced sweet potato
175g peeled and sliced carrots
250ml chicken stock

- Melt the butter in a saucepan over a medium heat. Add the onion and gently fry until very soft.
- Add the garlic and thyme and cook for 1 minute.
- Add the beef and fry until it starts to brown slightly.
- Add the tomato paste and cook for 1 minute.
- Add the remaining ingredients and simmer over a gentle heat for 60-90 minutes, with the lid on. Once the meat is very soft, the stew is done. If the liquid cooks away, add a little more chicken stock.
- Pour everything into a food processor and blend to the desired consistency. As your baby gets used to more lumpy food, this stew is ideal mashed with a potato masher or just chopped with a knife.
- Keep a portion to use now and freeze the rest in ice cubes for later use.
- Increase the quantities appropriately if cooking for the whole family, and set aside the family's portion before blending.

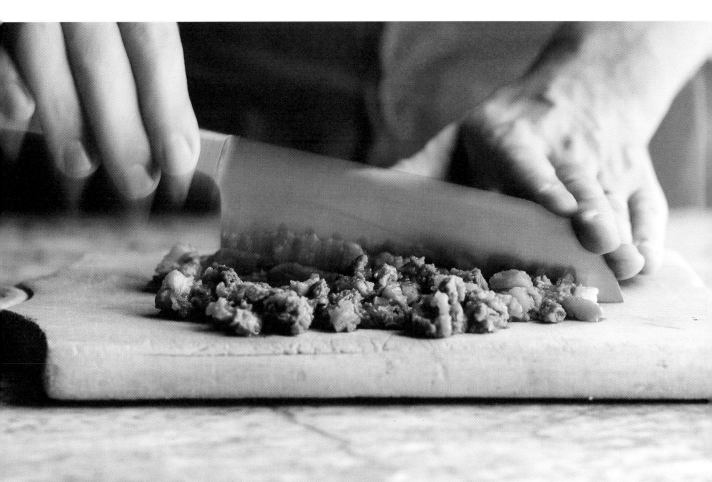

LAMB AND VEGETABLE STEW WITH GARLIC, ROSEMARY AND BROWN RICE

Makes 6 portions
Prep time: 20 mins
Cooking time: 90 mins

This is another delicious recipe that can be made for the whole family. Take particular care to cook the lamb slowly until it is beautifully soft so that there are no texture problems.

2 tablespoons butter

1 onion, finely chopped

1 leek, finely chopped

1 stalk celery, finely chopped

1 clove garlic, crushed

2 sprigs rosemary, leaves finely chopped

175g lamb shoulder, cubed

2 tablespoons tomato paste

200g peeled and diced potato

200g peeled and sliced carrot

350ml chicken stock

1 cup (200g) cooked brown rice (optional)

- Melt the butter in a saucepan over a medium heat. Add the onion, leek and celery and gently fry until very soft.
- Add the garlic and rosemary and cook for 1 minute.
- Add the lamb and fry with everything until it starts to brown slightly.
- Add the tomato paste and cook for 1 minute.
- Add the remaining ingredients, except the rice, and simmer over a gentle heat with the lid on, for about 60-90 minutes. Once the meat is very soft, the stew is done. If the liquid cooks away, add a little more chicken stock.
- Pour everything into a food processor and purée to the desired consistency. As your baby gets used to more lumpy food, this stew is ideal mashed with a potato masher or a fork.
- If you're adding the brown rice, stir it in now.
- Keep a portion to use now and freeze the rest in ice cubes for later use.
- Increase the quantities appropriately if cooking for the whole family, and set aside the family's portion before blending.

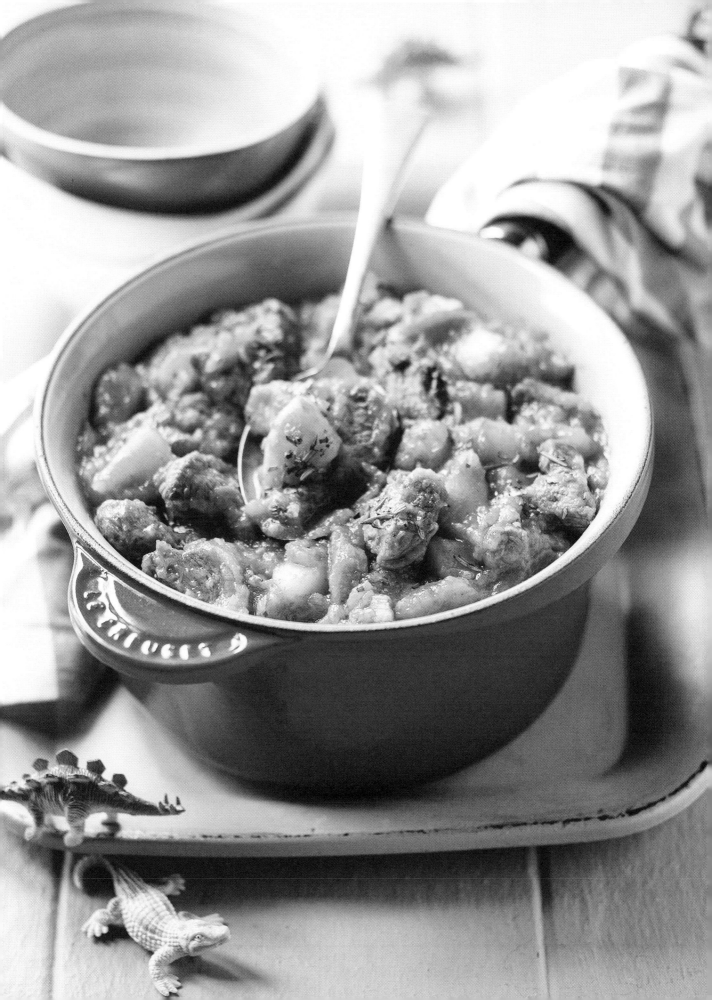

FRUITY CHICKEN BITES WITH FRESH PARSLEY AND CRÈME FRAÎCHE

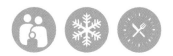

Makes 20 bites
Prep time: 10 mins
Cooking time: 20 mins

These soft and delicious chicken bites will be an absolute winner with your baby, and he can eat them himself. They are also great as a grown-up snack, so don't be shy with the quantities.

2 tablespoons butter
1 onion, finely chopped
1 carrot, peeled and grated
1 apple or pear, peeled and grated
300g chicken breast, cubed
2 teaspoons chopped parsley
about 4 tablespoons coconut oil
  for frying
crème fraîche, for dipping

- Heat the butter in a pan and gently fry the onion and carrot until soft.
- Using a sieve, squeeze as much water as you can out of the apple or pear.
- Place the chicken in the bowl of a food processor and add the cooked onion mix, apple and parsley. Pulse gently until the mixture is well combined but not too smooth.
- Heat a generous amount of coconut oil in a pan and, using a tablespoon, drop spoonfuls of mixture into the pan. Cook until golden brown, then turn them over with a spatula. Once golden on both sides, they are done.
- Drain them on kitchen paper, allow them to cool and serve them with a bowl of crème fraîche for dipping. The perfect finger food!

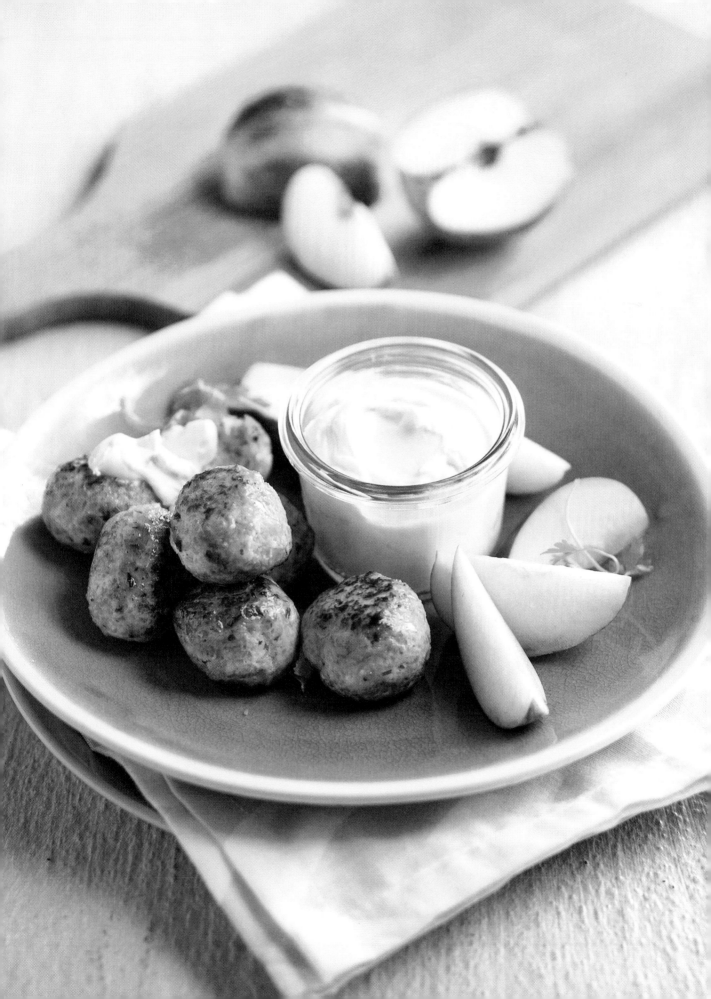

SALMON WITH BROCCOLI AND CHEESE SAUCE

Makes 5 portions
Prep time: 20 mins
Cooking time: 30 mins

Here's another dish for your growing baby that you'll find yourself tucking into. As a bonus, it includes a really straightforward broccoli-and-cheese-sauce recipe.

For the sauce:
1 tablespoon butter
1 onion, finely chopped
1 carrot, peeled and grated
3 tomatoes, skinned and chopped
1 cup (250ml) cream
½ cup (50g) grated Cheddar cheese
1 teaspoon fresh dill, finely chopped
200g cooked broccoli, chopped

For the fish:
350g salmon fillet, skin and bones removed
2 teaspoons butter, softened

- Preheat the oven to 180°C.

TO MAKE THE BROCCOLI AND CHEESE SAUCE:
- Melt the butter in a saucepan and gently fry the onion, carrot and tomatoes until soft and the acid has cooked from the tomatoes. This should take about 10 minutes.
- Pour in the cream and simmer for 5 minutes, stirring continually. Remove the sauce from the heat and stir in the cheese, dill and broccoli.

TO MAKE THE FISH:
- Place the fish on a greased baking tray and spread the butter over the top. Bake for 8 minutes while the sauce is cooking.
- Flake the fish into the sauce and mix well together. It's ready to eat.

ALTERNATIVELY:
- For older kids, you don't have to cook the fish separately and flake it into the sauce; rather, place the fish in a greased ovenproof dish, top with the sauce and bake it all together for the same amount of time as the recipe calls for. Also, serve the broccoli whole as we have done in the picture and bake it with the fish and sauce.

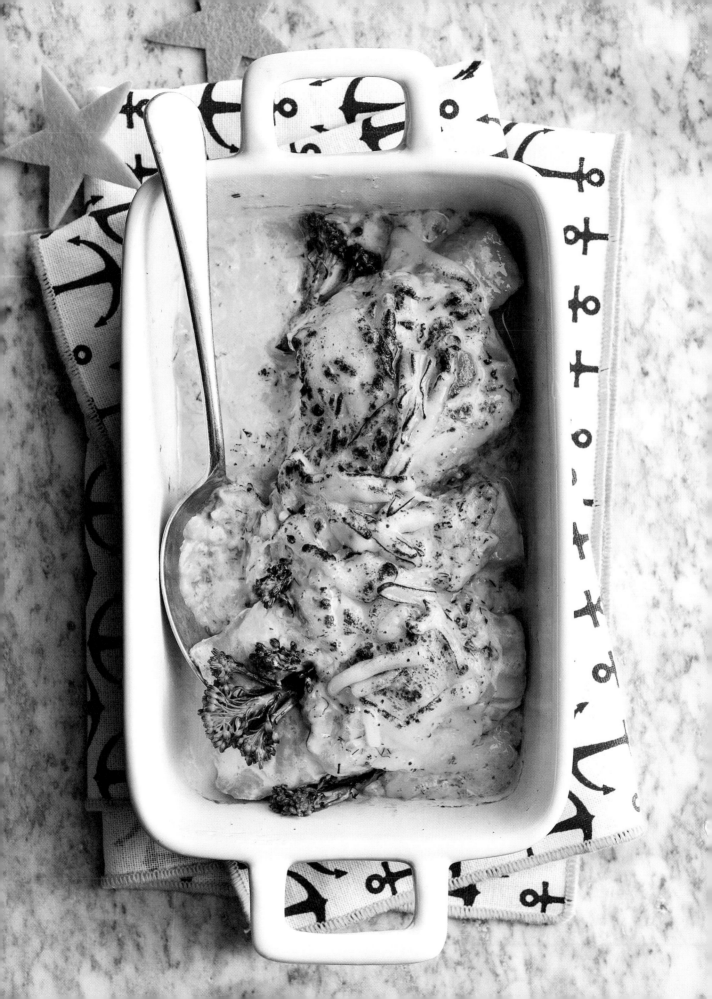

BAKED SWEET POTATO WITH CHEESE, VEGGIES AND BACON

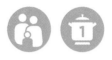

Makes 1 portion
Prep time: 20 minutes
Cooking time: 30 mins

This is a quick, easy and delicious meal, and perfect if you have a baked sweet potato left over from the night before. You could even get into the habit of cooking an extra sweet potato when you're having them for dinner.

1 baked sweet potato

1 teaspoon butter

½ cup chopped veggies such as onion, carrot, courgette, mushroom, peppers, aubergine, cauliflower, beans – basically what you have in the fridge

2 rashers bacon, finely chopped (for older kids)

2 tablespoons cream cheese

a sprinkle of chopped fresh parsley

2 tablespoons grated Cheddar

- Preheat the oven to 180°C.
- Slice the sweet potato lengthways, spoon out the flesh and set it aside in a bowl. Keep the potato skin, too.
- Heat the butter in a small frying pan and gently fry the chopped vegetables until soft.
- Pour the cooked vegetables into the bowl with the sweet potato filling. Add the cream cheese and parsley and mix well.
- Spoon the vegetable mix back into the potato skin and top with the grated cheese.
- Place the filled sweet potato on a baking tray and bake for 15 minutes to heat through.
- Let it cool to the correct temperature – then lunch is ready!

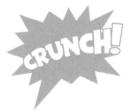

START BY JUST USING VEGETABLES OR MAYBE A LITTLE TINNED TUNA, AND ADD SOME FRIED BACON FROM ABOUT 1 YEAR OLD

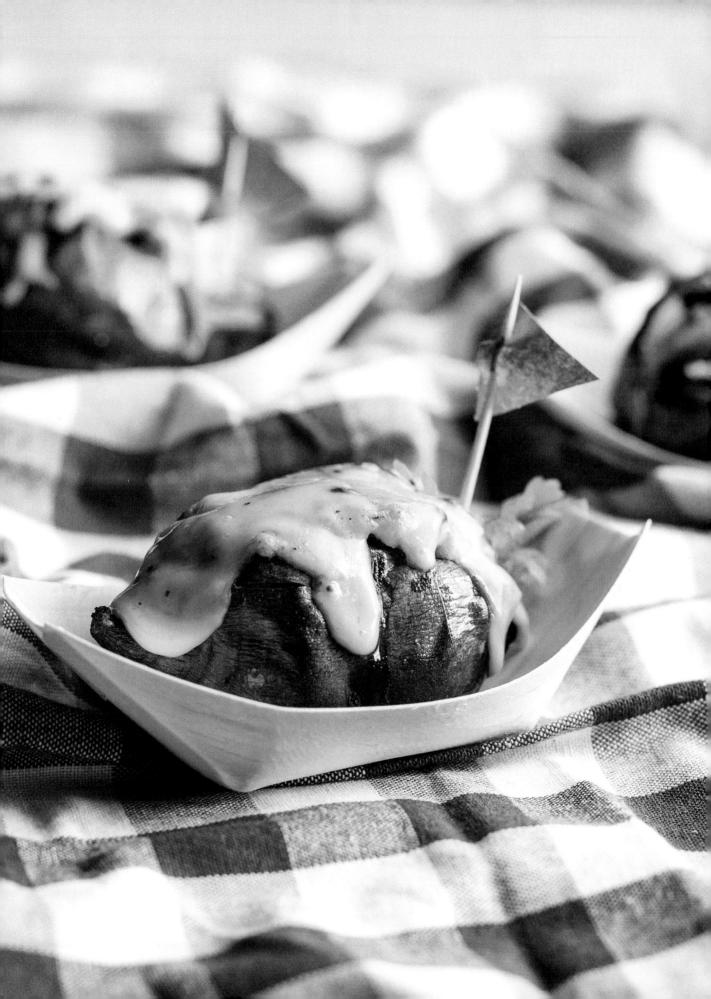

MASCARPONE CHICKEN WITH BASIL-AND-TOMATO SAUCE

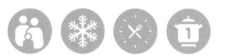

Makes 5 portions
Prep time: 10 minutes
Cooking time: 25 minutes

Mascarpone is good to use when you're introducing your baby to dairy. It's high in fat and very tasty. This is another dish that's delicious enough to be a meal for the family; just add a dash more seasoning and serve it on courgette noodles with some Parmesan.

For the chicken:
1 tablespoon butter
200g deboned chicken thighs, sliced into 3

For the sauce:
2 tablespoons butter
1 onion, finely chopped
1 carrot, grated
1 stalk celery, finely chopped
1 leek, finely chopped
1 clove garlic, crushed
½ cup (50g) grated pumpkin
2 courgettes, washed and grated
2 x 400g tins whole peeled tomatoes, blended
125g mascarpone
1 tablespoon chopped basil

FOR THE CHICKEN:
▪ Heat the butter in a frying pan and fry the chicken strips until cooked through. Remove from the pan and chop them up to the size your baby is eating.

FOR THE SAUCE:
▪ Heat the butter in a saucepan and gently fry the onion, carrot, celery, leek and garlic until soft.
▪ Add the pumpkin, courgettes and tomatoes and simmer for about 25 minutes until the sauce thickens and the acid is cooked out of the tomatoes.
▪ Remove the sauce from the heat and stir in the mascarpone, basil and chicken.

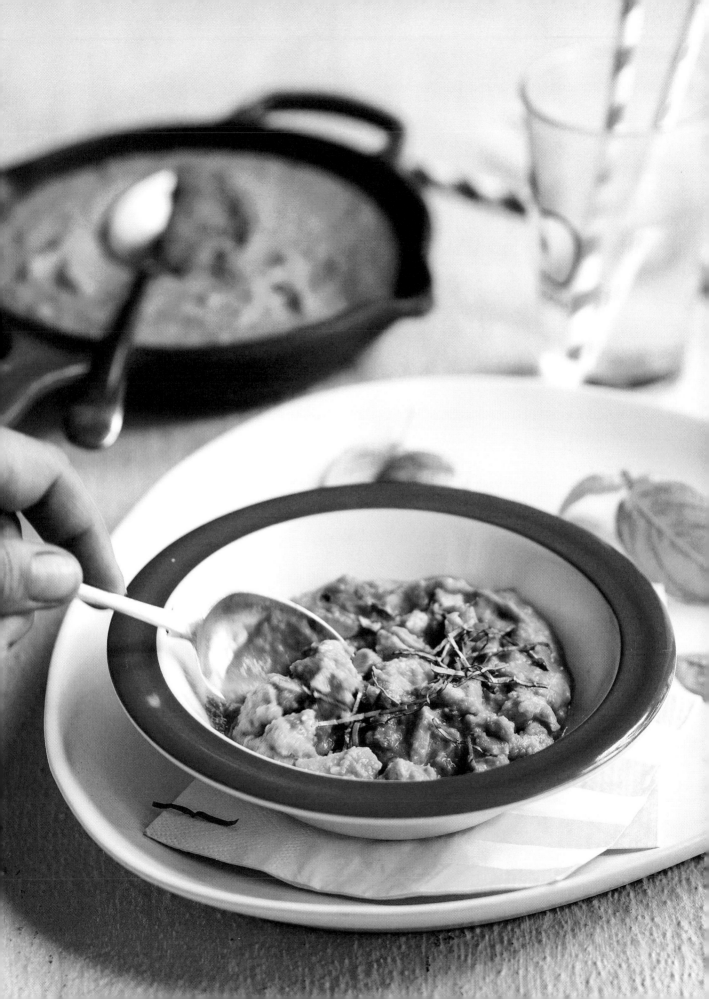

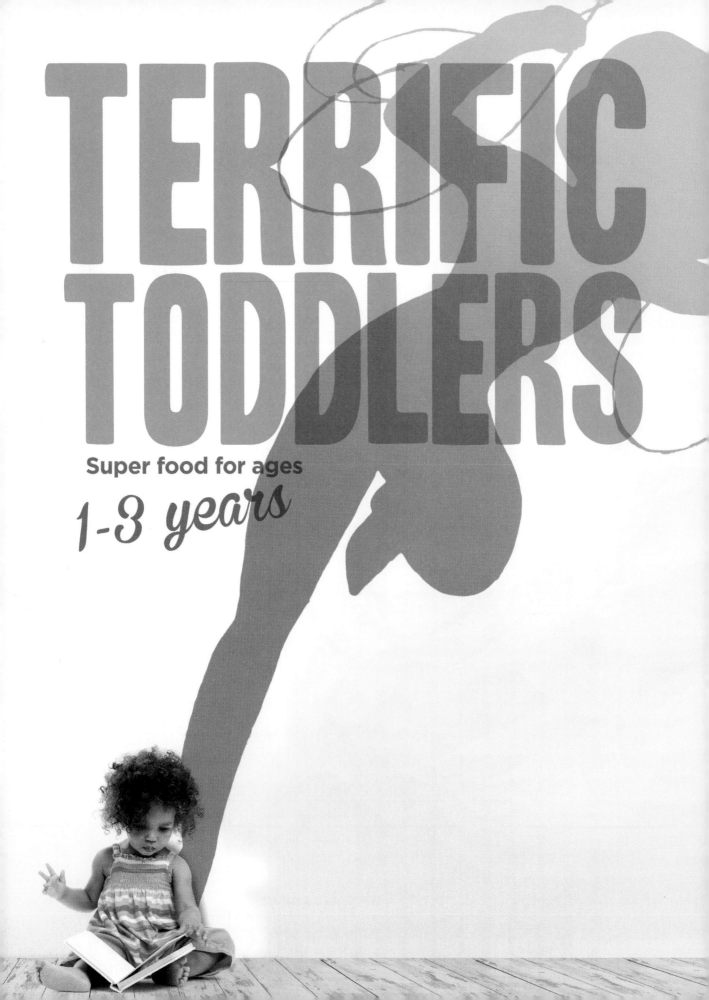

TERRIFIC TODDLERS

Super food for ages

1-3 years

By the age of one, your developing superchild will likely be weaned onto a variety of solids. From 9 to 12 months, her (or his) menu will hopefully have grown at a steady rate, and now as she enters toddlerhood it's time to continue this process and introduce her to as varied a range of REAL foods as possible. The more tastes she's introduced to at this stage of her life, the more likely she will grow up loving food, and the more likely she will avoid any fussy-eating phases. Then again, even the greatest toddlers can be stroppy and unpredictable – there's a reason they call it "the terrible twos" – so there are no guarantees at this age. Despite your best intentions, years 1 to 3 are often the most difficult stage to get eating regimes right. Good luck!

WHAT'S GROWING ON?

Your child's first growth spurt should be past by the age of 1, and another one will kick in after age 3, but her need for a nutritional, balanced diet remains constant. Even though growth slows during toddlerhood, there are plenty of important physical and mental developments during this time. You will become increasingly aware of her flourishing personality and her particular needs, and it's important to maximise her potential with the right dietary and lifestyle choices.

Key at this stage is once again brain development, an ongoing process that will typically continue until early adulthood but is unremitting right now. By age 2, your toddler's brain will already be about 80% the size of an adult brain. Her brain cells – literally increasing by the thousands every minute – communicate through messenger chemicals called neurotransmitters, which are formed from amino acids, the building blocks of protein. In other words, protein is an essential brain requirement (both now and later).

SUPER FOODS

We've said it before, but it bears repeating (over and over!): your aim as a parent should be to raise a healthy, well-nourished child who is at less risk of obesity and enjoys eating a wide variety of healthy, tasty, nutritious foods; in other words, not "beige foods". Bearing in mind that the dietary world of a toddler (usually) expands at a rate of knots, it's vital to set the best trends as soon as possible. With that in mind, consider the following critical guidelines.

Children need fat for healthy growth and development

The right fat is vital for healthy development of your toddler, so it's important not to think of fat as "bad". (This should go without saying by this point, a fundamental of the Real Meal Revolution that applies to children and adults alike.) Because they are energy-dense, fats are particularly useful for people with small stomachs (children); they are important for growth; they provide an array of important vitamins; and they play a role in wound healing.

If you need more convincing, consider this fact: around 60% or more of the brain is comprised of fat. In particular, omega-3 fatty acids are brilliant for brain development and "positively associated with changes in cognitive or behavioural performance".[1] Omega-3s aren't manufactured in the body, though, so make sure your child is getting enough in her diet, from the likes of salmon, sardines, mackerel and other oily fish, as well as beans, nuts, seeds and even grass-fed beef. Nuts and seeds are great for kids but are still choking hazards at this age, so feed them crushed, chopped or as nut/seed butters.

Avocados also provide healthy fat (and are handy as dips), as do meat (fattier cuts) and chicken (skin on), and dairy products like milk, yoghurt and cheese (all full cream). You can add olive oil or butter to increase the energy content of a meal. Along with other saturated animal fats besides butter – such as lard, tallow, duck fat and ghee – these are the healthy and delicious fats needed to power the brain.

Dangerous trans fats, typically found in processed food and oils made from seeds, beans and corn, are not included on this list, and should be avoided. (See *The Real Meal Revolution* for more on good fats versus bad fats.)

Protein is a huge plus

Protein is vital for the healthy development of your young child, particularly animal protein due to its high iron and zinc content and because it supplies all the essential amino acids. Consider just two factors for toddlers:

- Animal protein is rich in an amino acid called tryptophan, which is important in maintaining adequate serotonin levels. Studies have shown that increased serotonin levels brought about by tryptophan supplements "can decrease quarrelsomeness and increase agreeableness in everyday life". Admittedly these studies were conducted on adults, but the idea of a less quarrelsome and more agreeable toddler is certainly an appealing one! [2]
- When children are deprived of B12-containing foods before the age of 6 – a phenomenon that is prevalent in vegans, and more likely in vegetarians – related problems can manifest in children *years* after the deficiency has been rectified (through eating a carnivorous diet, for example). This can lead "to impaired cognitive performance" in adolescence. [3]

In short, make sure your child gets some animal protein at every meal. Around 10-20% of the total calories of a meal should be made up of protein (animal and non-animal), but don't get too hung up on measuring things; allow your child to guide you.

Kids and veggies

Many adult followers of low-carb high-fat eating don't eat enough vegetables. With children this phenomenon can be multiplied, as they tend to steer clear of leafy greens. Offer vegetables with every meal, and try to include a range of different colours, as each broad hue – red/purple, orange/yellow, white and green – seems to indicate different nutritional properties. They also make for a bright and exciting plate, which helps them to actually get eaten. See more tricks overleaf. (And for more details on the nutrition of vegetables see p332.)

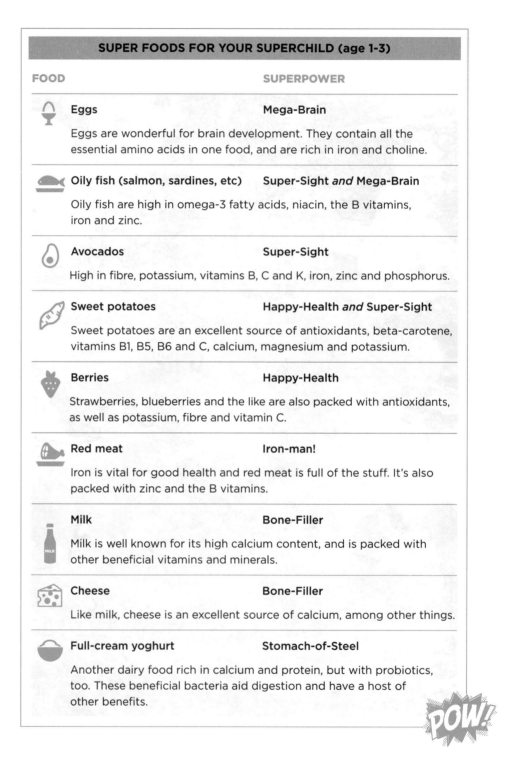

SUPER FOODS FOR YOUR SUPERCHILD (age 1-3)

FOOD	SUPERPOWER
Eggs	**Mega-Brain**
Eggs are wonderful for brain development. They contain all the essential amino acids in one food, and are rich in iron and choline.	
Oily fish (salmon, sardines, etc)	**Super-Sight** *and* **Mega-Brain**
Oily fish are high in omega-3 fatty acids, niacin, the B vitamins, iron and zinc.	
Avocados	**Super-Sight**
High in fibre, potassium, vitamins B, C and K, iron, zinc and phosphorus.	
Sweet potatoes	**Happy-Health** *and* **Super-Sight**
Sweet potatoes are an excellent source of antioxidants, beta-carotene, vitamins B1, B5, B6 and C, calcium, magnesium and potassium.	
Berries	**Happy-Health**
Strawberries, blueberries and the like are also packed with antioxidants, as well as potassium, fibre and vitamin C.	
Red meat	**Iron-man!**
Iron is vital for good health and red meat is full of the stuff. It's also packed with zinc and the B vitamins.	
Milk	**Bone-Filler**
Milk is well known for its high calcium content, and is packed with other beneficial vitamins and minerals.	
Cheese	**Bone-Filler**
Like milk, cheese is an excellent source of calcium, among other things.	
Full-cream yoghurt	**Stomach-of-Steel**
Another dairy food rich in calcium and protein, but with probiotics, too. These beneficial bacteria aid digestion and have a host of other benefits.	

POW!

FIGHTING OFF COLDS

There's nothing quite like a round of sniffles to bring down the family. With their immune systems still developing, young children are prone to sickness – and if you're tired and run down chances are you are, too. A well-balanced diet certainly helps to ward off lurgies; conversely, there's a reason the kid who eats only ice cream for dinner tends to get sick more often... We recommend keeping levels of the following up, especially during flu season:

- **Zinc:** It has been shown to reduce the duration of the common cold, and it may even help prevent it.[4] Good sources are meat, seafood, seeds and pulses.
- **Vitamin C:** Not quite the magic bullet our mothers would have had us believe, but it's still worth keeping up a regular supply of citrus fruit (and sweet potatoes), as vitamin C is believed to shorten and reduce the severity of colds.
- **Antioxidants:** Thought to boost the immune system, antioxidants are present – not coincidentally, perhaps – in zinc and vitamin C, as well as selenium. Foods high in selenium include Brazil and other nuts, mushrooms, seeds, eggs and cottage cheese.
- **Chicken soup:** Though it has not been definitively proven to help sick children, there is some evidence (beyond old wives' tales) that chicken soup can cure the symptoms of the common cold. More to the point, the World Health Organization recommends it for sick children as a soothing remedy.

KRYPTONITE FOR KIDS

It should go without saying by this point, that you should be doing your best to avoid junk food; that is, "bad" processed foods such as takeaway burgers, sweets and biscuits. Equally, so-called "good" processed foods – the ones we've been taught in the past to believe are healthy – are off limits. That's anything described as "low fat" or "low salt", and anything high in carbohydrates. Don't forget: it's all about eating REAL food.

The master villain – you and your child's nemesis – is, of course, sugar. To a toddler, sugar is the devil because it lines the sweet path to adult obesity and future diabetic problems. (See p23 and from p306.) At this age the addiction to sweet things can happen extremely quickly, perhaps within a few meals even, so try to pre-empt addiction by avoiding sweet things whenever possible and only offering real food. In the long run you'll have a healthier, happier child and you'll be a happier, saner parent. That said, don't despair if your child already has tasted (and loved) sugar. You *can* retrain her eating habits. See, for example, the "treat" recipes included in these pages (from p226) that you can make and store for those special occasions, none of which contain added sugar.

In general, follow these suggestions:

■ Be wary of fruit; it can be high in sugar. (See Healthy Eating Habits, opposite.)

■ Avoid all carbonated drinks *and* fruit juices. Normal sodas are packed with sugar, as we've seen, while "diet sodas" generally come with a raft of potential problems due to the sugar substitutes used. Fruit juices, meanwhile, tend to be particularly high in fructose, which is turned to fat in the liver and affects the brain directly to stimulate the overconsumption of calories. Rather teach your kid to drink (inexpensive, healthy) water or homemade flavoured drinks instead. (See p252-255 for recipes.)

■ Toddlers shouldn't be drinking tea or coffee. Besides being unnecessary, the idea of giving a toddler any measure of caffeine is... well, let's just say, unwise.

■ If dairy is in the diet, ensure it's full-cream. Children shouldn't be consuming "low-fat" milk. (No-one should!)

■ Steer clear of soy. It's a Real Meal no-no, best avoided by both kids and adults.

■ Be careful with grains. As we've noted already, we don't advocate Banting for children in general, and we're aware that, from a practical point of view, there's no denying that simple-to-prepare grains can make life easier for busy parents. But there is growing evidence to suggest that grains, both refined or whole, are best avoided, as discussed later (see p335). In the meantime, if you do go grain we suggest using small amounts of unrefined non-gluten varieties, such as quinoa, millet, buckwheat, oats (look out for steel-cut oats) and brown rice.

KRYPTONITE CRAVINGS AND THEIR ALTERNATIVES	
KRYPTONITE	**SUPERHERO ALTERNATIVE**
Potato chips	Vegetables crisps – see p218
Sweets	Homemade fruit leathers – see p228
Ice cream	Homemade ice cream – see p56
French fries	Sweet potato fries – see p134
Rusks	Homemade rusks – see p230
Fruit juice and soft drinks	Flavoured drinks – see p252-255
Ketchup	Homemade ketchup – see p294
Chicken nuggets	Coconut chicken strips – see p134

HEALTHY EATING HABITS

Various nutritional guidelines recommend feeding smaller energy-rich meals regularly, perhaps every three hours, to toddlers because of their relatively high energy requirements compared to their small stomachs. If you prefer to feed your toddler three times a day, then top up in between with snacks when she's hungry. But be careful that she doesn't get into the habit of grazing all day, in which case she may not be hungry at meal times. Consider a snack something to chew on, such as a fruit or berries, chopped nuts, cheese or a small stick of biltong. A meal should be wholesome and nutrient-rich, and include a protein, a supply of healthy fat and vegetables.

Fruit snacks are recommended twice a day at most, totalling one serving. A serving is one medium-sized apple, orange, pear or banana, or two apricots, plums or kiwi fruits. Do your best to offer the less sweet fruits, such as berries, pears and apples, to delay as much as possible the onset of a sweet tooth. Despite your best efforts, chances are your child will discover sweet foods at some point, but restraint at this age will bring great benefits later on.

Bearing in mind her critical need for fat and protein, if your child has taken a particular liking to, say, beef or lamb or another specific fat, don't try to persuade her otherwise; allow her to eat up. There's little risk of her eating too much meat, fat or veg, or drinking too much water, at this age. Rather watch out for junk food, sugar and refined carbs that kids will happily overindulge in.

As a rule you shouldn't try to overfeed or underfeed your toddler; be led by her. Always have enough for her to sample, to experiment with and to eat her fill, but don't force-feed.

TRICKS FOR TRICKY TODDLERS

Remember that you're the adult and your child – developing superchild though she may be – is still in nappies: even though she may seem to have your number, you really are the boss.

Use the tricks of the trade

As an example of kids being outsmarted, commercial food producers do it every day in the way they market their foods. Children are far more likely to eat anything – including revolting processed food – if presented in a colourful bowl or accompanied by a fairy fork or a bright sticker. It may seem obvious, but you can do the same – just make sure you're putting good, healthy food in the bowl and on the fork!

Always keep it fun

Kids need their food to be fun – which is why parents have been making train-chugging and jet-flying noises forever just to get their toddlers to open their mouths... The more fun you make food for your child, the more she will want to partake and experiment. It's amazing how innovative presentation can suddenly make a lowly green bean, for example, a thing of great excitement.

Use different colours, textures, shapes and sizes to make food interesting. Leafy greens are important, but don't forget to add some carrot or red and yellow peppers to brighten up the plate. Design faces with her food; present it on a tray so she can use her hands and make a mess. In general, let her discover and have fun.

Keep distractions to a minimum

Turn off the TV and other loud appliances. Create a relaxed, unhurried environment. Let her focus on the food and go at her own pace. This isn't just about consuming food; it's a learning process that involves a stimulating environment, choice making, the discovery of new tastes, textures and colours.

Allow her to make a mess (within reason). The more she associates mealtime with fun, the more she'll enjoy eating healthy, good foods.

Say no to bribery

Using non-nutritious snacks or desserts to bribe a child into eating a certain food will encourage her to reject more food the next time around. Don't be the crooked cop! Instead, encourage her to eat one mouthful of each food on the plate, and praise her when she tries something new. Yes, it's easier said than done, but a veggies-for-sweets trade-off is a vicious circle that's going to backfire in the end.

Use the art of disguise to introduce new foods

Disguise disliked or new foods in other foods you know your child likes. An old trick is to blend carrots and other disliked vegetables into a meat sauce rather than chopping them into noticeable pieces (works for the whole family), but there are far simpler options. Try sticking a little piece of celery into a piece of cheese, or wrapping a bit of tomato in some ham: simple!

When introducing a new food, start with smaller amounts and increase it meal by meal until she's used to the new taste. Toddlers will frequently reject new foods, so always be patient at meal time. (But you're a parent; we don't need to tell you about patience, do we?)

That said, don't worry if your child doesn't like every food you give her; it doesn't mean she's going to grow up to be a fussy eater. She may not like everything, but then *you* probably don't either. When dealing with something as important as nutrition, it can be easy to become prescriptive. Don't lose sight of the fact that your child is a little person with individual needs and tastes, as real and unique as your own.

Use butter and salt for flavour

A regular complaint from parents is the difficulty of getting their kids to eat their veggies. Besides hiding them in other foods, the easiest way to overcome this is to cook the vegetables in butter and salt. Butter and salt are delicious, and you shouldn't be afraid to use either.

That said, the correct dosage and use of salt remains somewhat controversial. Simply by steering clear of processed foods, your children will be avoiding a huge potential supply of sodium on a daily basis, but some nutritionists are still wary of salt. International recommended daily allowances of salt for ages 1-3 tend to vary from 2 grams (National Health Service, UK) to 2.5 grams (National Health and Medical Research Council, Australia).

Our recommendation: feel free to cook with salt, but don't overdo it on the plate; you want your children to taste the flavour of the food, not just salt.

Pre-empt party sugar-bingeing – if you can

Toddler birthday parties can be a nightmare to navigate, with platters of sandwiches, chips and sweets that just overflow with refined carbs and sugars... Don't despair, and don't think you're going to keep your little one from merrily tucking in. Let her have her fun and consider it a rite of growing up – but do what you can to limit the damage. Before you leave for a birthday party, let her eat her fill of (healthy) food she likes, so that she has less space for the party food later.

If you offer chocolate, go dark

If you want to introduce your child to chocolate, start off on very dark chocolate; the bitterer, the better. If she only knows 70% dark chocolate (or even 85%), she may well find regular chocolate too sweet when she tries it. Sneaky, hey?

EGGY BREKKIES

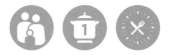

Makes 1-2 portions
Prep time: 5 mins
Cooking time: 5 mins

Eggs are a super food for your growing toddlers, and they make the perfect breakfast choice. Quick to cook and very versatile, they can also be a great vessel for hiding secret crunchy veggies.

CHEESY SCRAMBLED EGGS

1-2 eggs
2 tablespoons cream
1 tablespoon butter
1 spring onion, finely sliced
¼ cup (25g) grated Cheddar cheese

- In a bowl, whisk the eggs and cream together. You can add a little salt if you'd like.
- Heat the butter in a small frying pan and gently fry the spring onions until soft.
- Pour in the whisked eggs and cream. As the eggs begin to cook, give them a good scramble with a spoon or spatula.
- When the eggs are just about cooked, quickly stir through the grated cheese and spoon into a favourite bowl. The eggs may need to cool slightly before serving.
- Note: Two eggs may be too much food for a toddler so practise responsive feeding; stop when he seems full.

MY FIRST OMELETTE

2 eggs
2 tablespoons milk
2 tablespoons butter
¼ cup (25g) grated cheese

For the veggies:
a few slices of carrot, red pepper and courgette cut into moon and star shapes with a cutter

- Cook the vegetable shapes in some boiling water until soft. Drain and set aside.
- In a bowl, whisk together the eggs and milk.
- Melt the butter in a frying pan and pour in the egg mix.
- Cook on a low heat until the egg is cooked through, then sprinkle over the cheese. Scatter the veggie shapes over the top and keep on the heat until the cheese has melted.
- We served the omelette open so the shapes are visible, but fold it over if you prefer and pop it on a plate.
- Note: As above, two eggs may be too much for a toddler so practise responsive feeding.

BOILED EGGS WITH CHEESE COURGETTE DIPPERS

1 courgette, quartered lengthways
1 tablespoon melted coconut oil
2 tablespoons grated Parmesan or Cheddar cheese
¼ teaspoon dried thyme
1 egg

- Preheat the oven to 180°C.
- Place the courgettes on a rack over a baking tray and brush with coconut oil. Sprinkle with Parmesan and dried thyme.
- Bake for 15 minutes until lightly golden.
- While the courgettes are baking, cook the egg in boiling water for 8 minutes. As your child gets older, you can serve him softer eggs that need less boiling time.
- Serve the boiled egg in an egg cup with the dippers on the side and perhaps a cherry tomato or two.

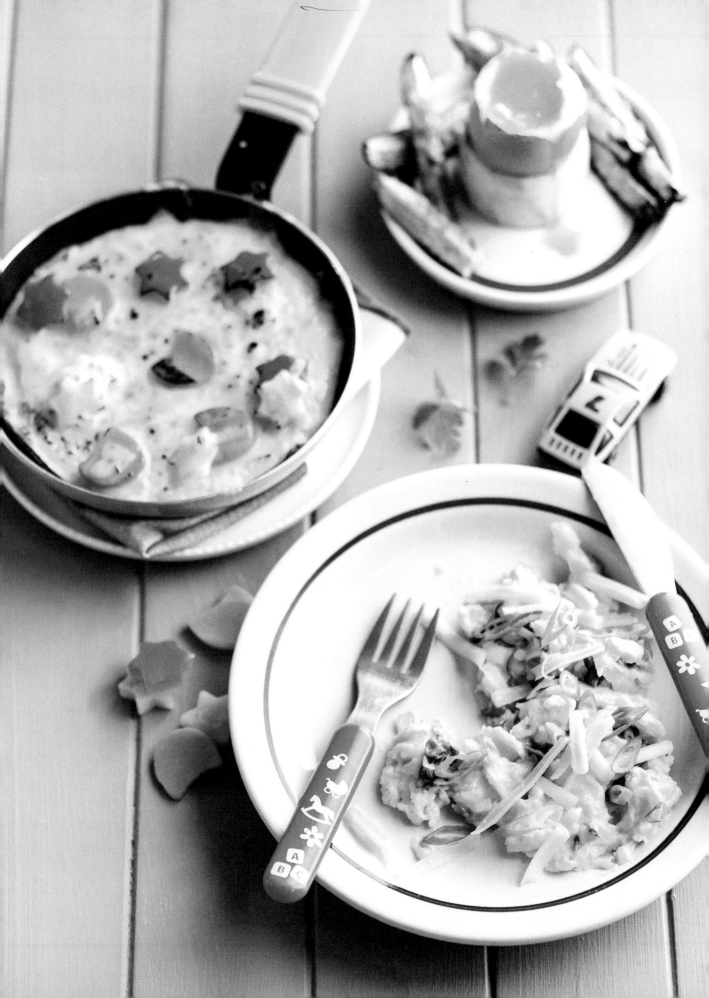

AWESOME OATS

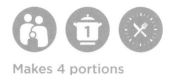

Makes 4 portions

What better breakfast than a bowl of oats? These recipes are a little more interesting than the plain version, and incorporate some new and exciting flavours. Keep an eye on the consistency and blend according to the texture your child prefers. Although oats make a filling breakfast, we recommend you serve them only once a week or so. Opt for high-quality organic oats if possible.

MANGO-AND-COCONUT OATS

Prep time: 5 mins
Cooking time: 15 mins

³/₄ cup (120g) steel-cut organic oats
1 cup (250ml) coconut milk
1 cup (250ml) water
½ teaspoon vanilla extract
pinch of ground cinnamon
130g peeled and diced mango
  (about 1 mango)

- In a small saucepan combine the oats, coconut milk and water. Cook gently over medium heat, stirring occasionally, until the mixture comes to the boil. Cook for about 5 minutes until the oats start to soften.
- Stir in the vanilla, cinnamon and mango and cook for a further 3 or 4 minutes, until the mango is warmed through.
- Take the oats off the heat.
- Using a hand-blender, blitz the oats until the mango is smooth and combined, and allow to cool before serving.
- We added some cut-out mango shapes to make breakfast a little more fun.
- As your child gets a little older, you needn't blend the oats as much, but it is still worth doing to incorporate the mango into the porridge. Play it by ear and be guided by your child.

BEGINNER BIRCHER

Prep time: 15 mins
Rest overnight

³/₄ cup (120g) steel-cut organic oats
½ cup (125ml) milk
1 cup (250ml) water
1 apple, peeled, cored and grated
⅓ cup (90g) plain Greek yoghurt
¼ cup (37g) fresh blueberries

- In a bowl, mix together the oats, milk and water. Cover and pop into the fridge to soak overnight. This will soften the oats.
- Stir in the remaining ingredients the following morning. Give the porridge a blitz using a hand-blender to incorporate the blueberries.
- As your child gets a little older, you needn't blend the oats as much, and you can top the porridge with a spoonful of extra yoghurt and some fresh blueberries.

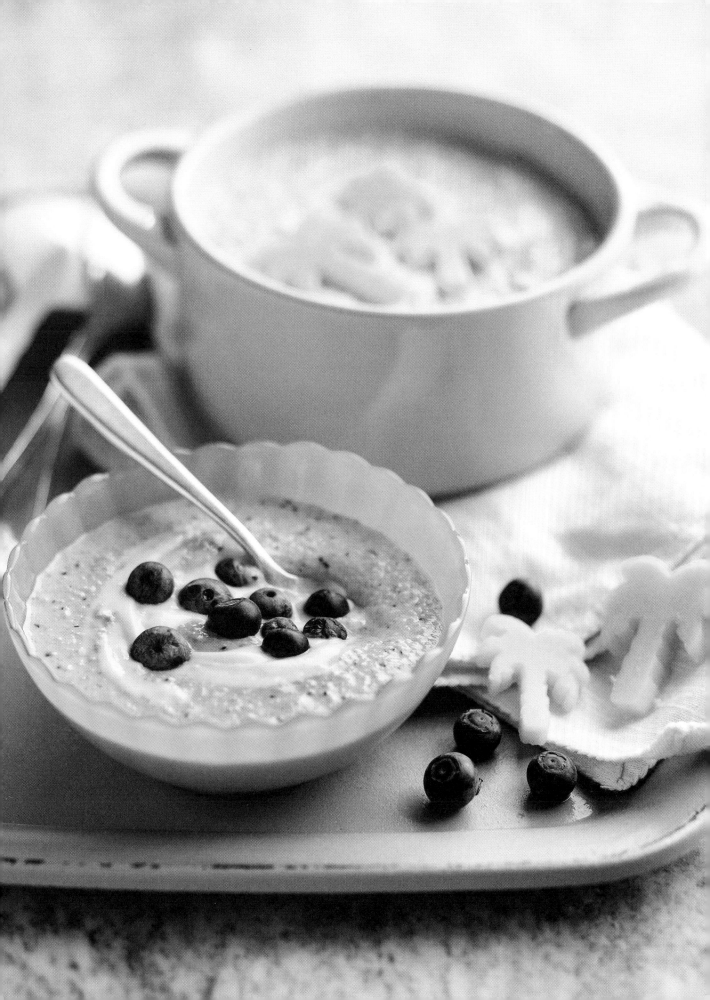

PERFECT PORRIDGE

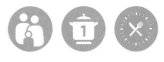

Makes 4-6 portions

Breakfast is the most important meal of the day and porridge is a comforting, filling staple. Here are some alternatives to using the simpler (and less nutritious) grains of the past.

CHOCOLATE PUDDING CHIA PORRIDGE

Prep time: 10 mins
Rest overnight

3 tablespoons chia seeds
1 cup (250ml) almond, coconut
 or cow's milk
2 tablespoons cocoa powder
¼ teaspoon vanilla extract
1 banana, peeled and sliced
plain yoghurt to serve

- Stir together the chia seeds and milk in a bowl. Cover and soak for at least an hour, preferably in the fridge overnight.
- Add the remaining ingredients to the bowl and blend until smooth. Serve with a dollop of yoghurt and some sliced banana.
- The chia seeds may be a bit tricky when your baby is little, so you may want to strain them out. The yummy chocolate pudding flavour will have him hooked though, so it may be a breakfast staple very soon!

BAKED SWEET POTATO PORRIDGE

Prep time: 10 mins
Cooking time: 30 mins

1 cup (200g) cooked and mashed
 sweet potato
1 banana
1 cup (250ml) milk
3 egg yolks

- Preheat the oven to 160°C.
- Place all the ingredients in a bowl and blend together using a hand-blender until smooth.
- Grease 6 ramekins and place them in a deep roasting tray. Divide the mixture between the 6 ramekins. Pour boiling water into the roasting tray so that it comes about a third of the way up the ramekins. This method is known as baking in a water bath or bain-marie.
- Bake for 25 minutes until the porridge has set. Remove from the oven and remove the ramekins from the water. Allow them to cool a little before serving.
- This porridge can be served hot or cold and can also be frozen. A delicious addition to your growing child's breakfast menu!

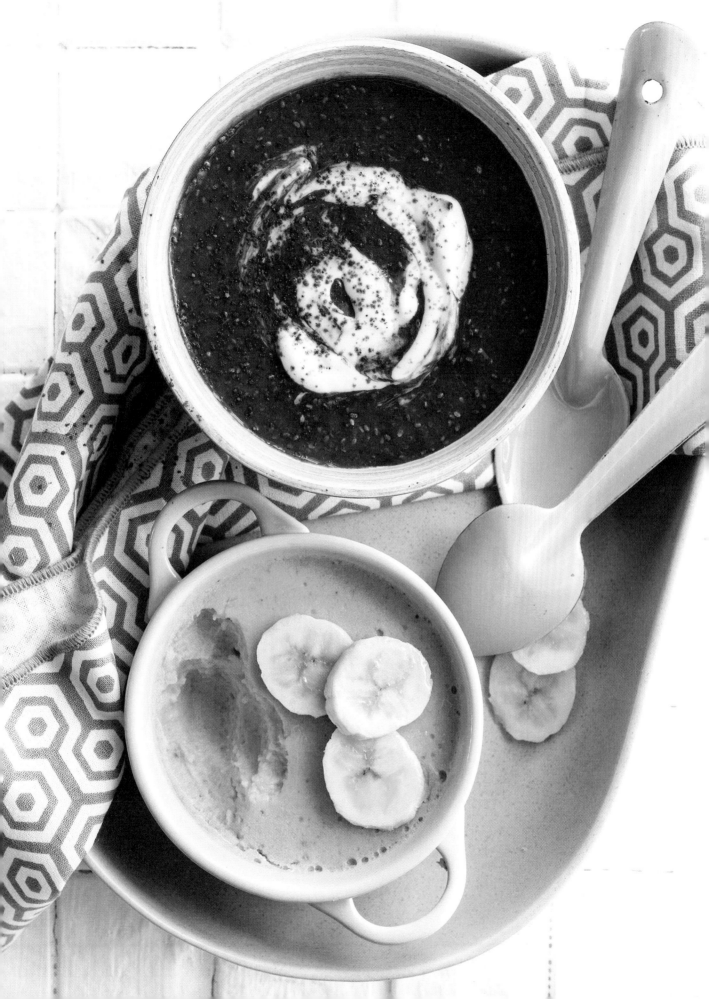

AVO-AND-BERRY BREAKFAST SUNDAE WITH A DUSTING OF COCOA

Makes 1 portion
Prep time: 5 mins

When you need to rustle up a healthy, fun breakfast in a rush, look no further than this quick-and-easy number. As your child gets a little older, add some nuts or even a few tablespoons of homemade granola (p156) to liven it up.

¼ avocado, diced
¼ cup (75g) plain yoghurt
a handful of fresh raspberries
1 teaspoon cocoa powder

- Layer the avocado, berries and yoghurt in a bowl or glass to create the sundae, and finish off with a dusting of cocoa.
- If raspberries are unavailable, use another seasonal fruit.

MAKE IT EXCITING BY USING OLD-FASHIONED, FUN-COLOURED SUNDAE GLASSES – BREAKFAST WILL FEEL LIKE A REAL TREAT!

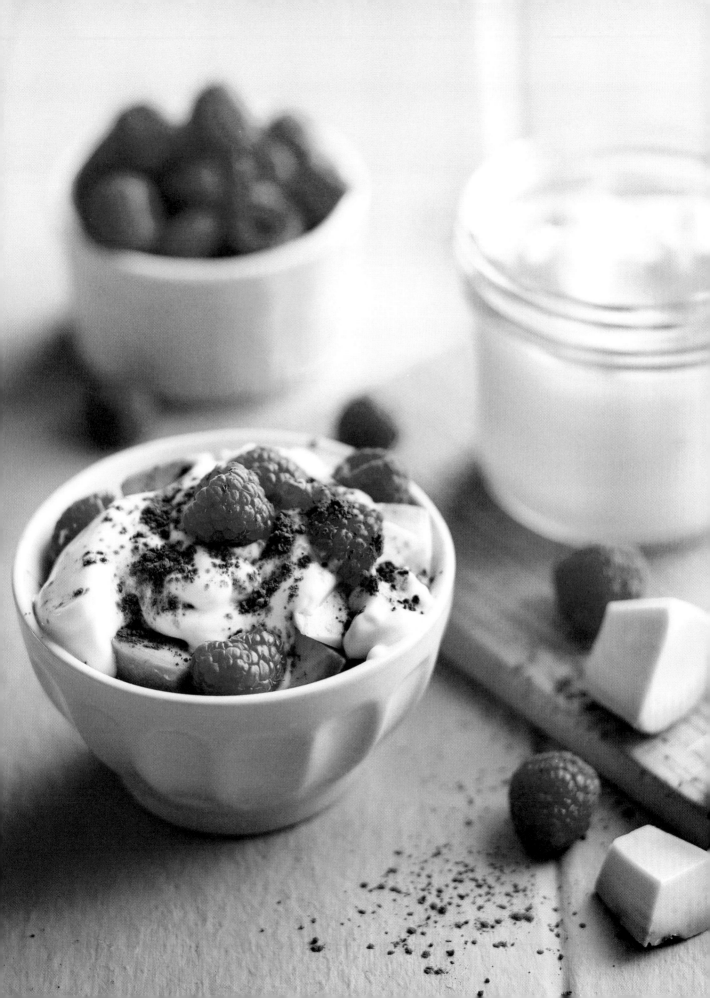

CAULIFLOWER-AND-CHEESE TOTS

Makes about 50
Prep time: 20 mins
Cooking time: 30 mins

Bite-sized cauliflower cheese! Could this be the greatest invention ever? They may look like a pain to make, but they're actually very easy, and they're so delicious they're unlikely to even make it onto a plate. Remember to eat them while they're hot!

2 tablespoons cream
2 tablespoons butter
450g cooked cauliflower
2 egg yolks
1 cup (100g) grated Cheddar cheese
1 teaspoon baking powder
4 egg whites
homemade ketchup to serve (p294)

- Preheat the oven to 180°C.
- Line two baking trays with silicone baking paper.
- Melt together the cream and butter.
- Place the cooked and drained cauliflower into the bowl of a food processor with the melted cream and butter, and blend until fine. Remove from the food processor and place in a mixing bowl. Allow to cool completely.
- Once the cauliflower mixture is cold, stir in the egg yolks, grated cheese and baking powder.
- Whisk the egg whites until stiff.
- Fold ¼ of the egg whites into the cauliflower mixture, followed by the rest.
- Using a round nozzle, fill a piping bag with the cauliflower mixture and pipe little tots onto the lined baking tray. Make them about 3cm long, and leave a little space between each one.
- Bake for 15-20 minutes until they are golden.
- Serve immediately with homemade tomato ketchup.

IF YOU DON'T HAVE A PIPING BAG AND NOZZLE, MAKE THE TOTS USING TWO TEASPOONS; SCOOP WITH ONE, AND USE THE BACK OF THE OTHER TO SCRAPE OUT THE TOT

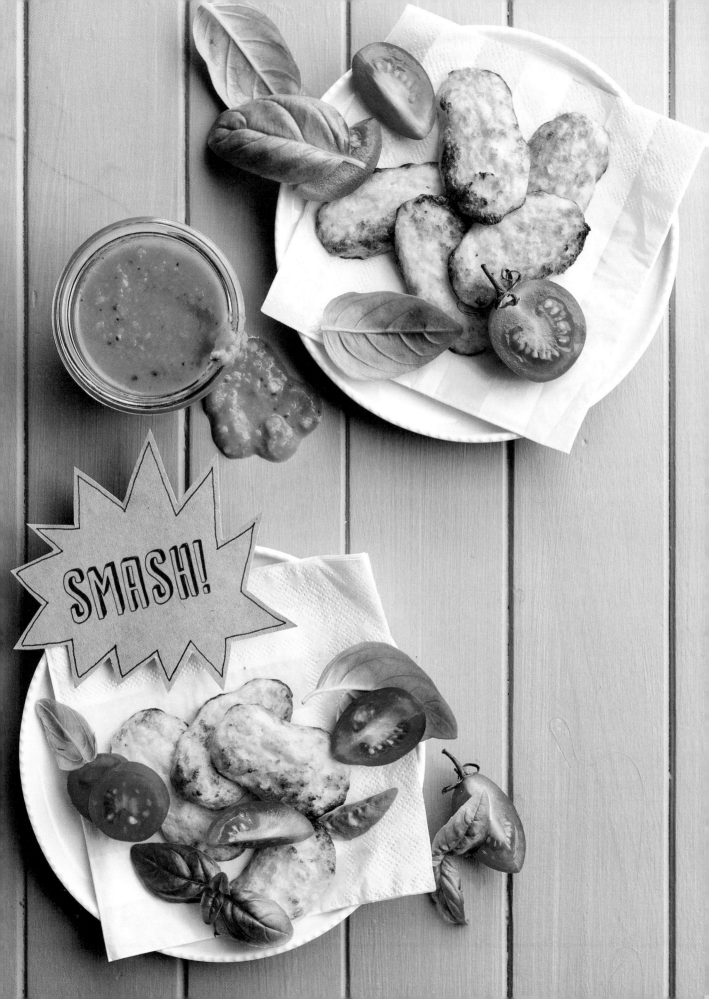

KIDDIES' KEDGEREE

Makes 8-12 portions
Prep time: 20 mins
Cooking time: 30 mins

Kedgeree is a dish that was originally served for breakfast in the Indian colonies in a bygone time, but we suggest trying this recipe for lunch or dinner. It's a light, fresh meal and a great introduction to the world of spices for your little one.

1 bay leaf

2 peppercorns

175g haddock, skin and bones removed

175g hake, skin and bones removed

3 tablespoons butter

2 onions, finely chopped

1 clove garlic, crushed

1 teaspoon mild curry powder

300g cauliflower, blitzed in a food processor to resemble rice

½ cup (50g) fresh peas, cooked

2 tablespoons lemon juice

2 tablespoons chopped flat-leaf parsley

3 eggs, boiled and quartered

- Place a pot of water on the stove and add the bay leaf and peppercorns. Bring it to the boil, add the fish and simmer for 5 minutes until just cooked. Remove the fish from the water, drain and flake into quite big chunks, then set aside.
- Heat the butter in a large frying pan and add the onions. Fry on a gentle heat until they start to turn golden.
- Add the garlic and curry powder and fry for another minute.
- Add the cauliflower and peas and gently fry for a further 10 minutes.
- Stir in the lemon juice, parsley, fish and eggs.
- Season with a little salt if needed, and serve.

INSTEAD OF THE CAULI-RICE, USE COOKED BROWN RICE FOR SOMETHING DIFFERENT

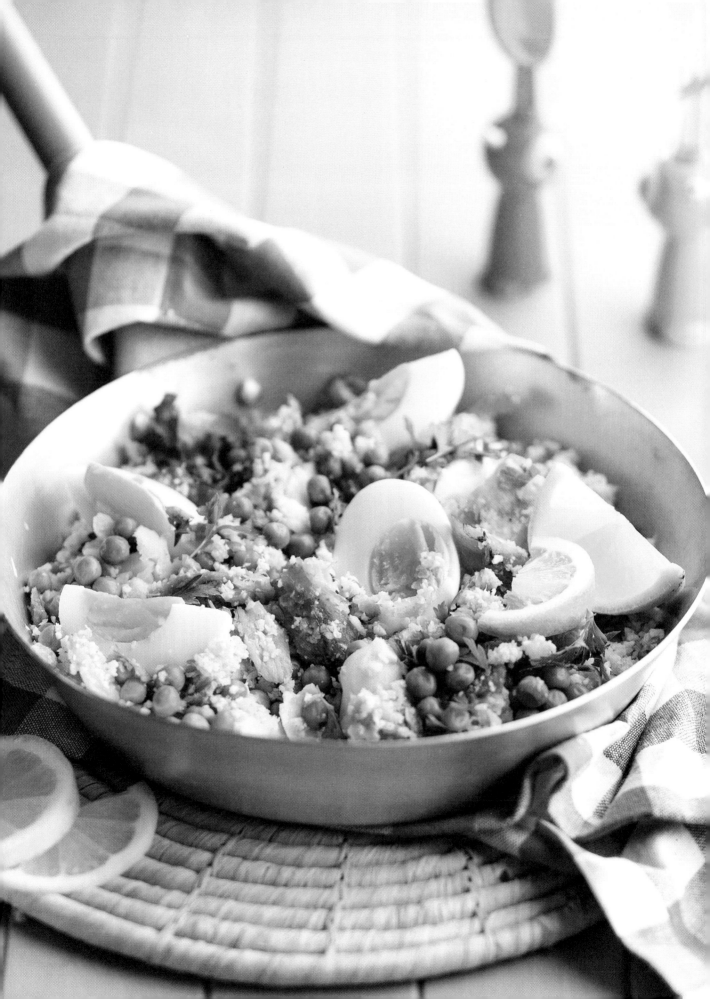

SOUP IT UP!

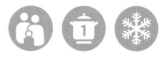

Makes 8 portions

These soups freeze like a dream, so make a big pot of each and freeze them into family-sized portions for those chilly winter days. There's nothing more comforting than a steaming cup of soup – from toddler to grown-up, the whole family will love these recipes.

'LEARNING TO COUNT' CHICKEN SOUP

Prep time: 15 mins
Cooking time: 90 mins

2 tablespoons butter
1 onion, finely chopped
1 large carrot, peeled and chopped
1 large leek, halved lengthways,
   washed and sliced
1 stick celery, finely chopped
1.5 litres water or chicken stock
   (chicken stock if you want a strong
   chicken flavour)
1 bouquet garni (5 sprigs of fresh
   thyme, 4 sprigs of parsley and 2 bay
   leaves tied in a bundle with string)
1 whole chicken
a little salt for seasoning

For the garnish:
slice 3 carrots and cut out numbers
   using number cutters

- In a soup pot, melt the butter and gently fry the onion, carrot, leek and celery until soft.
- Add the water or chicken stock, bouquet garni and the whole chicken.
- Gently simmer for 1 hour. Using a slotted spoon, skim off any scum that rises to the top.
- Using tongs, remove the chicken from the soup then let the pot simmer for another hour or so.
- Shred the chicken off the chicken carcass and set aside.
- When you're ready to serve the soup, remove the bouquet garni, add the shredded chicken and the number carrots, and simmer for a final 5 minutes.
- Season with a little salt and serve. (Extra salt isn't necessary when using a commercial chicken stock.)

BROCCOLI-AND-SPINACH SOUP WITH CHEDDAR CHEESE

Prep time: 10 mins
Cooking time: 20 mins

2 tablespoons butter
1 medium onion, roughly chopped
1 stalk celery, finely chopped
1 leek, halved lengthways, washed
   and finely chopped
2 medium garlic cloves, crushed
1 litre chicken stock
500g broccoli florets, roughly chopped
2 cups (60g) baby spinach
150g grated Cheddar cheese
a little salt for seasoning

- Heat a soup pot over a medium heat and add the butter. Gently fry the onion, celery and leek until soft. Add the garlic and cook for 1 minute.
- Add the chicken stock and bring the soup to the boil.
- Add the broccoli and simmer for 8 minutes until soft.
- Throw in the spinach and cook for a further minute.
- Take the soup off the heat, add the cheese and blend until smooth.
- Season with a little salt and serve.

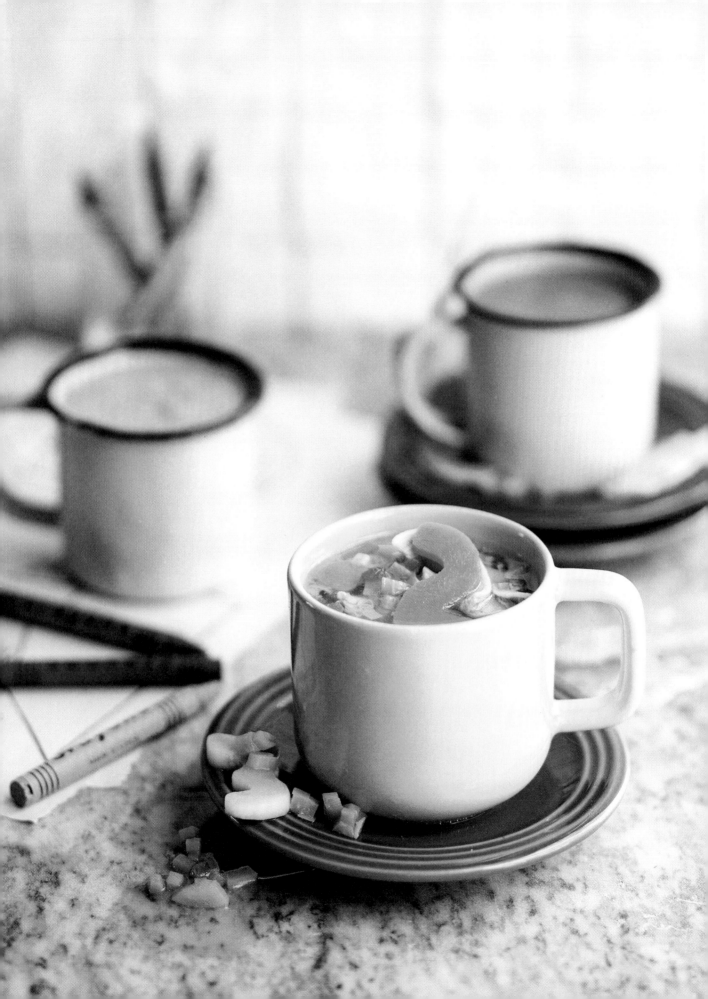

TOMATO-AND-SWEET-POTATO SOUP (pictured on previous page)......

Prep time: 15 mins
Cooking time: 35 mins

2 tablespoons butter

1 large onion, finely chopped

1 stalk celery, finely chopped

1 carrot, peeled and grated

1 clove garlic, crushed

1 tablespoon tomato paste

1 x 400g tin whole peeled tomatoes, blended

2 sweet potatoes (about 400g), peeled and diced

1 apple, peeled, cored and grated

500ml vegetable or chicken stock

¼ teaspoon ground nutmeg

a little salt for seasoning

chopped parsley (optional)

- Melt the butter in a large pot.
- Gently fry the onion, celery, carrot and garlic until soft.
- Add the tomato paste and fry for 1 minute.
- Make sure that you have blended the tinned tomatoes and add the remaining ingredients to the pot.
- Simmer for about 30 minutes, until the sweet potato has softened completely.
- Season with a little salt and blend the soup until smooth using a hand-blender.
- Serve with a little chopped parsley if you like.
- This soup will freeze like a dream, so any leftovers can go straight into the freezer.

MOZZARELLA DIPPERS ....

Prep time: 5 mins
Cooking time: 15 mins

1 cup (120g) grated mozzarella

- Preheat the oven to 180°C.
- Line a baking tray with non-stick silicone paper.
- Make little lines of grated cheese on the baking tray about 10cm long and 2cm wide. Make sure to leave some space between each because they spread.
- Bake for about 15 minutes, until they are bubbly and golden. Remove from the oven and allow to cool and crisp. Serve with the tomato-and-sweet-potato soup.
- These can be kept in an airtight container for a few days and are a delicious snack.

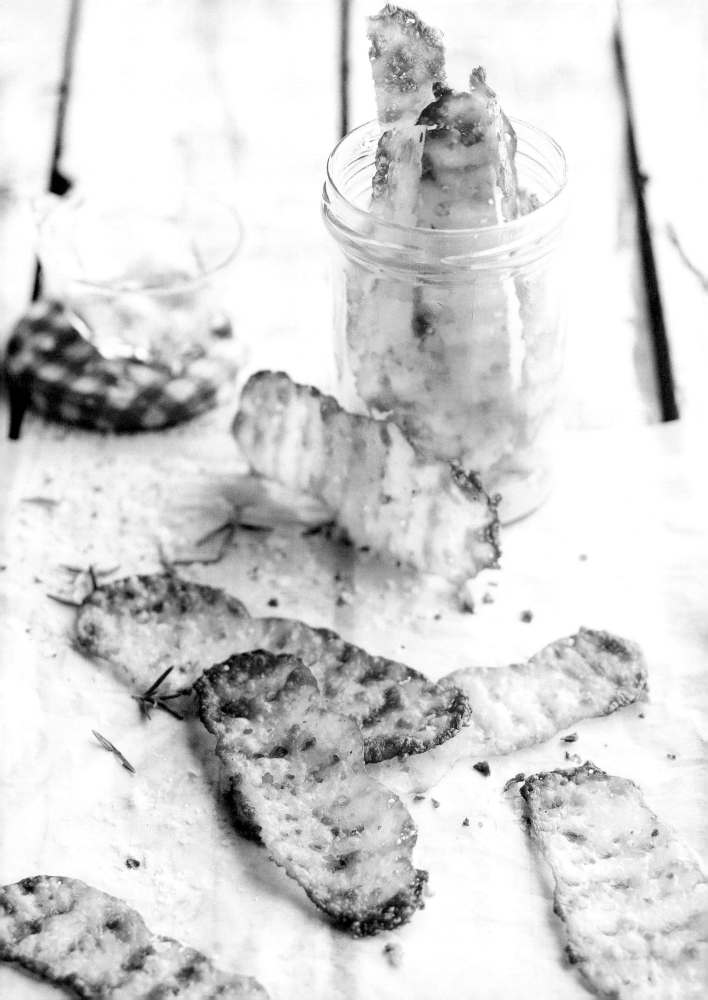

TUNA CUPS

Makes 12 portions
Prep time: 10 mins
Cooking time: 25 mins

These little babies are a doddle to make, especially if you have leftover sweet potato. We've mixed in spring onion and lemon zest, but you can get creative with chopped veggies and other herbs. They make a perfect lunch served with chunky vegetables or a salad.

4 tablespoons melted butter

2 x 170g tins tuna in spring water, drained

3 spring onions, thinly sliced

2 tablespoons finely chopped fresh coriander

300g cooked, mashed sweet potato

½ teaspoon lemon zest

2 large eggs

a little salt for seasoning

- Preheat the oven to 180°C.
- Grease the cups of a 12-cup muffin pan with half the melted butter.
- Mix the remaining ingredients together in a bowl and season with a little salt. Pour the remaining melted butter into the mixture.
- Divide the mixture between the muffin cups and flatten each a little using the back of a spoon.
- Bake for 25 minutes until golden brown and starting to crisp.
- Serve with a simple salad of cucumber, tomato and avo, and some crème fraîche.

TINNED TUNA IS A BRILLIANT STAPLE TO KEEP IN THE CUPBOARD FOR CONJURING UP THOSE MIRACLE MEALS

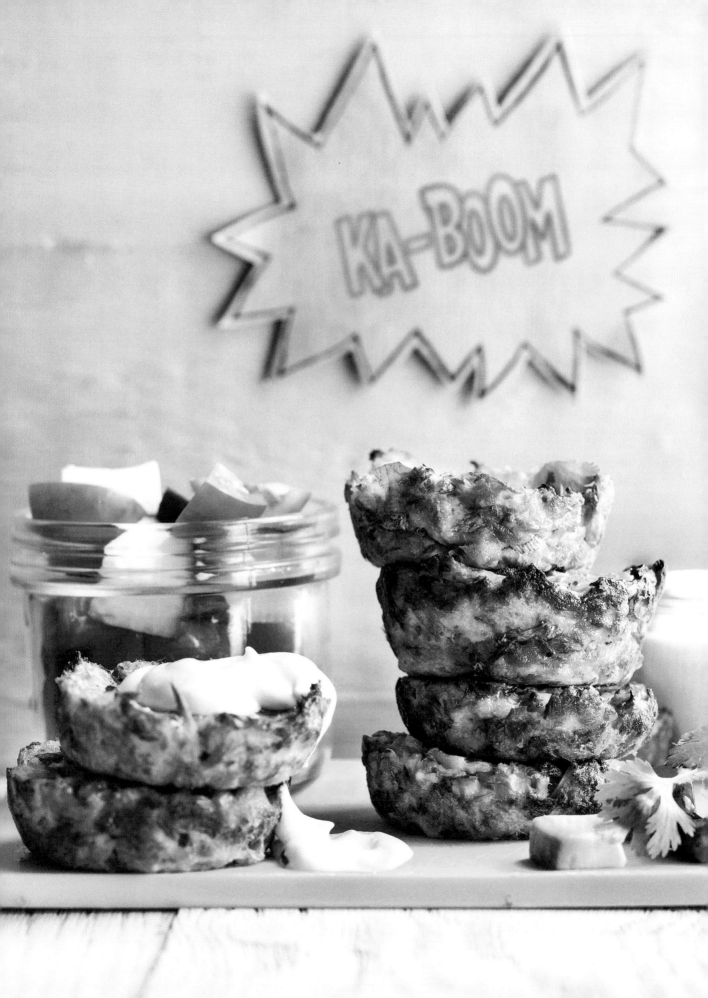

CHICKEN, SPINACH AND CHEDDAR CANNONBALLS

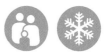

Makes 4 portions
Prep time: 25 mins
Cooking time: 45 mins

These cannonballs are great for the whole family and come with a basic tomato sauce that's worth keeping in your recipe arsenal. You can swap the Cheddar for feta (when junior is ready), and the courgette noodles can be made from carrots if you prefer.

For the cannonballs:
2 tablespoons butter
1 carrot, finely grated
1 onion finely chopped
1 cup (30g) tightly packed baby spinach leaves
300g chicken breast fillets, cubed
½ cup (50g) grated mild Cheddar cheese
3 tablespoons coconut oil or butter

For the tomato sauce:
2 tablespoons butter
1 onion, finely chopped
1 stalk celery, finely chopped
1 clove garlic, crushed
1 x 400g tin whole peeled tomatoes, blended
1 cup (250ml) water
2 tablespoons cream cheese
1 tablespoon chopped basil

For the noodles:
4 courgettes, thinly shredded or cut into noodles

TO MAKE THE CANNONBALLS:
- Heat the butter in a pan and gently fry the carrot and onion until soft. Add the spinach and cook for 2 minutes until soft. Take off the heat and allow to cool.
- Blitz the onion mix and chicken in a food processor until smooth. Add the cheese and give it one last blitz. Add a little salt if needed.
- Roll the chicken mixture into walnut-sized balls.
- Heat the coconut oil or butter in a pan and fry the chicken on a medium heat until golden brown on all sides. Set aside and keep warm.

TO MAKE THE TOMATO SAUCE:
- In a saucepan melt the butter and gently fry the onion, celery and garlic until soft.
- Add the blended tomatoes and water and gently simmer for 25 minutes until the acid has cooked from the tomato and the sauce has thickened slightly.
- Remove from the heat and stir in the cream cheese and basil.

TO MAKE THE COURGETTE NOODLES:
- Boil the courgettes for 1 minute in boiling water, and drain.

- To serve, place the courgette noodles in a bowl and top with the sauce and cannonballs.

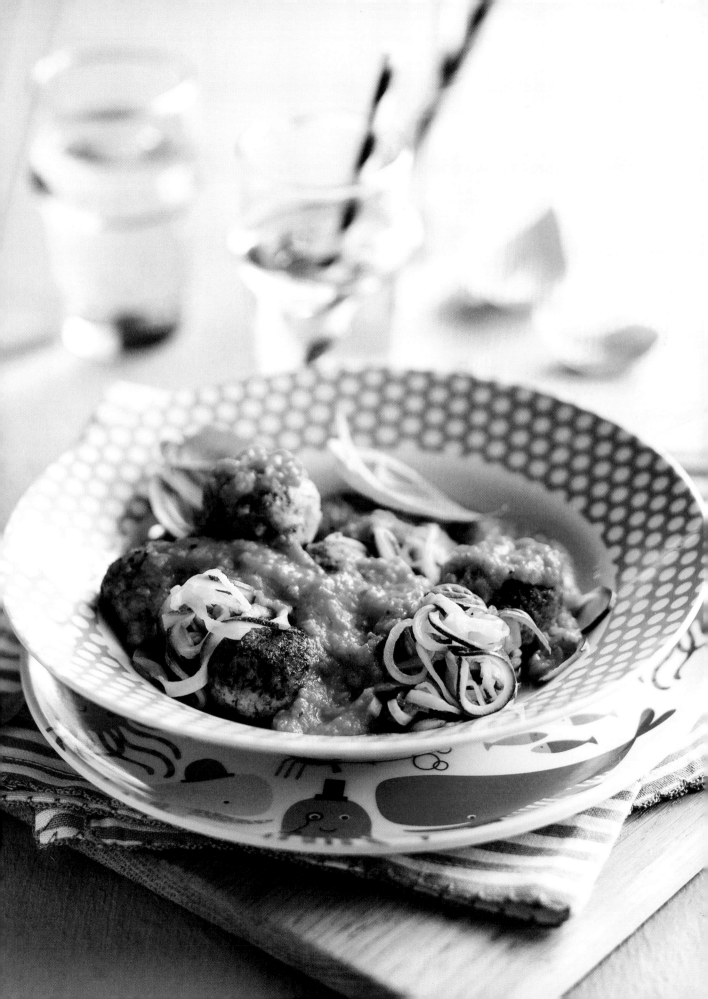

MINI MOUSSAKA – AUBERGINE STUFFED WITH MINTED BEEF AND CHEESE

Makes 6 portions
Prep time: 15 mins
Cooking time: 45 mins

These moreish moussakas may be too spicy for a beginner eater, so perhaps halve the spice to start – the whole family will love them either way. The mince recipe also makes a great quick bolognaise, because it doesn't need to cook for ages; just leave out the aubergine and cheese.

3 large aubergines, halved
3 tablespoons coconut oil, melted

For the mince:
4 tablespoons butter
2 medium onions, finely chopped
2 cloves garlic, crushed
300g beef mince
½ teaspoon ground cumin
½ teaspoon ground coriander
½ teaspoon ground cinnamon
4 tablespoons cream cheese
1 tablespoon chopped mint
1 tablespoon chopped parsley
salt for seasoning
1 cup (100g) grated cheese
mint, to garnish

TO MAKE THE AUBERGINES:
- Preheat the oven to 180°C.
- Place the halved aubergines on a roasting tray and drizzle with the coconut oil.
- Roast for 30 minutes, until the aubergines are soft in the centre. Remove and spoon out the centre of the aubergines, keeping the skins on the tray. Set aside.

TO MAKE THE MINCE:
- Cook the mince while the aubergines are roasting.
- In a large frying pan, melt the butter and fry the onions on quite a high heat. Cook until the onions are golden, then add the garlic and cook for 1 more minute.
- Add the mince and fry until it is browned and cooked through.
- Add the spices and fry until they are toasted.
- Stir in the cooked aubergine flesh, the cream cheese and chopped herbs. Season with a little salt.
- Using a spoon, fill the hollow aubergines with the mince mixture and top with grated cheese.
- Roast the filled aubergines for a further 15 minutes until the cheese is bubbly and golden.
- Garnish with mint leaves and serve with a chunky salad.

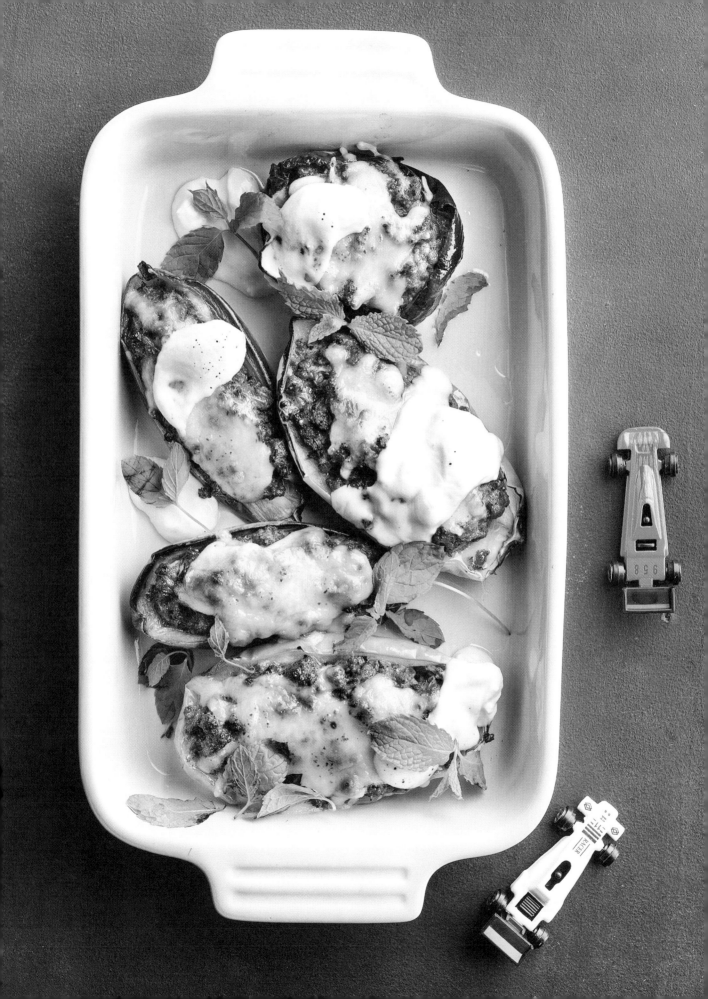

COCONUT CHICKEN STRIPS WITH SWEET POTATO FRIES

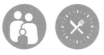

Makes 4 portions
Prep time: 20 mins
Cooking time: 30 mins

These sweet potato fries are likely to disappear in a flash, so make more than you think you'll need. The crunchy coconut chicken strips are also a delicious basic that can be easily incorporated into a salad or served with veggies.

For the fries:
2 large sweet potatoes, cut into fries
2 tablespoons coconut oil, melted
a little salt for seasoning
homemade mayo to serve (p301)

For the chicken strips:
½ cup (60g) coconut flour
2 eggs, whisked
1 cup (80g) desiccated coconut
coconut oil for frying
2 chicken breast fillets, sliced
  lengthways into 1cm strips

TO MAKE THE FRIES:
- Preheat the oven to 180°C.
- Line a baking tray with silicone paper. Place the sweet potatoes on the baking tray and brush well with coconut oil.
- Bake for about 20 minutes, until they start to brown, then turn them over to cook for another 10 minutes.
- Sprinkle with a little salt and serve immediately.

TO MAKE THE CHICKEN STRIPS:
- Place the coconut flour, whisked eggs and desiccated coconut into three separate bowls. Dip the chicken strips into the coconut flour, followed by the egg and finally the desiccated coconut.
- Heat the coconut oil in a frying pan and fry the chicken strips on a medium heat until golden.
- Serve with homemade mayo and the sweet potato fries.

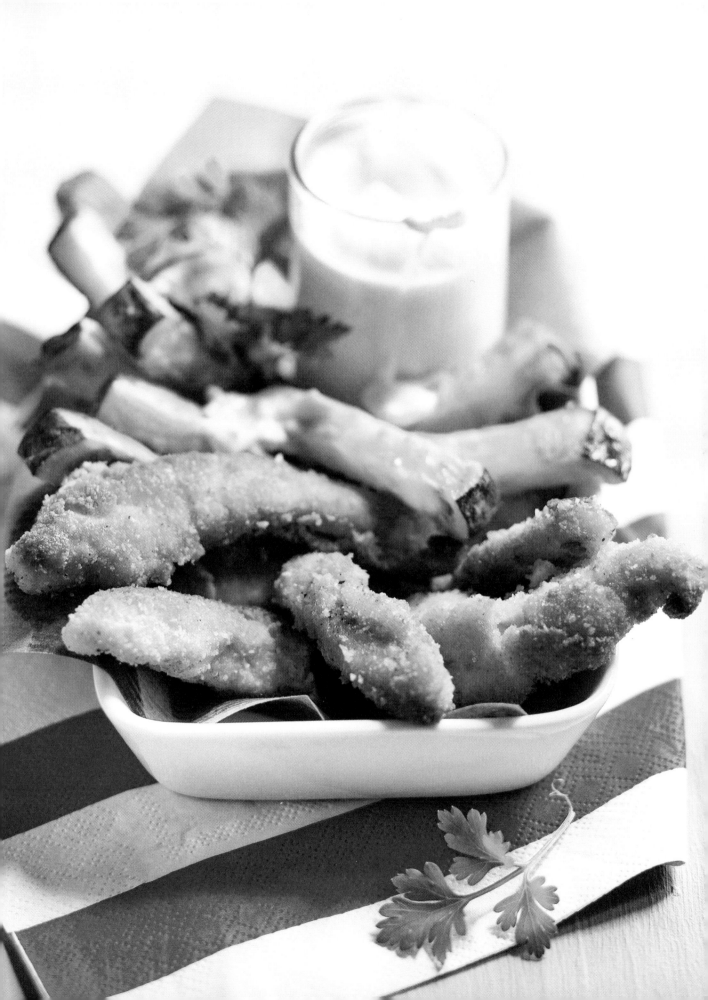

LAMB TAGINE

Makes 6 portions
Prep time: 25 mins
Cooking time: 2 hrs

Take your toddler on his first culinary journey to Morocco with this simple tagine, and the whole family can come along for the ride. Although there are quite a few spices in it, the taste isn't too strong and the sweetness of the apricots makes it perfect for the beginner gourmand.

6 tablespoons butter

500g cubed leg of lamb or shoulder, seasoned with a little salt

1 large onion, chopped

1 large carrot, peeled and grated

1 clove garlic, crushed

½ teaspoon ground ginger

½ teaspoon ground cumin

½ teaspoon ground coriander

½ teaspoon ground cinnamon

½ teaspoon ground paprika

1 x 400g tin whole peeled tomatoes, blended

1 cup (250ml) chicken stock

50g dried apricots

Flat-leaf parsley or chopped chives to garnish

- Melt half the butter in a casserole dish and fry the cubed lamb, a little at a time, until golden brown. Set aside.
- Add the remaining butter if necessary, and fry the onion and carrot until soft. Add the garlic and fry for a minute with the spices.
- Pop the lamb back in and pour in the blended tomatoes, chicken stock and dried apricots. Reduce the heat and simmer very slowly for 1½ - 2 hours, until the lamb is soft.
- Garnish with flat-leaf parsley or chopped chives and serve with some cauli-couscous.

ADD SOME ROASTED CUBED AUBERGINE OR PUMPKIN TO BULK UP THE VEGGIES

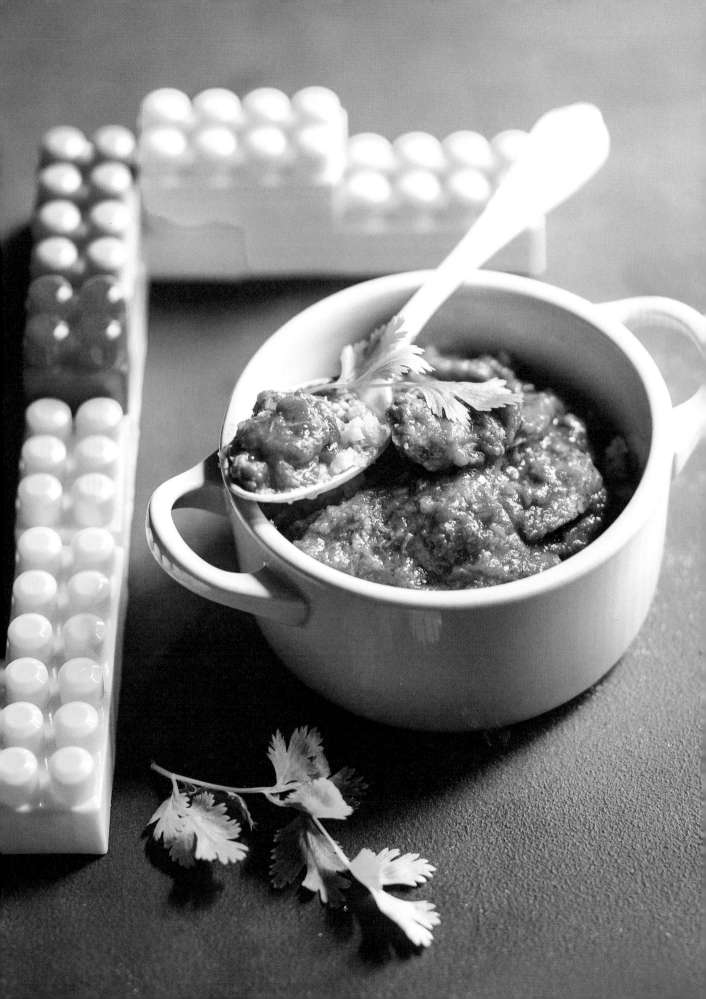

INCREDIBLE
KIDS

Super food for ages

3-13 years

If you thought surviving the terrible twos was something, have we got news for you: welcome to the thunderous threes, the freak-out fours and the flippen horrible fives. (Insert your own more-adult words, as you see fit.) Although parenting may seem like an uphill battle at times, you're an old hand by now, and of course the joys of seeing your bundle of joy transform into a complex, personality-filled little human far outweighs the annoyance of seeing him or her turn his nose up at your latest kitchen creation. As your toddler transforms into a little kid and then a bigger kid, your job as parental nutritionist gets easier in certain ways and harder in others. Cooking separate meals is no longer necessary because he can eat with the grown-ups (mostly), but as he spends more time at school and with friends you may find it harder to keep him eating the right things. Make the effort because it's worth it in the long run. Next thing puberty will arrive and you won't know where the time went…

WHAT'S GROWING ON?

From pre-school to high school, children still grow at a rate of knots, causing parents throughout the world to cry out, "Where's my baby gone?!". Until puberty, he or she should shoot up at around 5 or 6 centimetres a year, though it's less a steady extension than fitful spurts that come from month to month and even week to week. (Kids grow more in spring, apparently, FYI.) No matter their rate of growth, their energy needs remain high at all times. You need to ensure that, as much as possible, you're giving your child the nutritious choice as opposed to the convenient choice.

As he gets older, you'll find yourself relinquishing some of the nutritional control you once maintained. All sorts of external factors will start to influence his diet, from a favourite TV programme to more frequent kids' parties to a vegetarian best friend (gasp!). Which is a reminder to you to a) instil in him good habits as early as possible so that he chooses good foods when the choice is his alone, and b) never stop making the effort to prioritise his nutrition.

So what should you be giving your not-so-little-one to eat on the odd occasion that he listens to you? It's pretty much the same as what you gave him as a toddler, just bigger quantities:

- Plenty of protein, including meat, fish and eggs;
- Lots of legumes and vegetables, with fruits in moderation;
- Sufficient dairy (but see Dairy Query on p144);
- Healthy fats at every meal.

Growing pains

One of the downsides of growing is growing pains. Children can start complaining about them from as young as three, and though we don't know what causes them, we do know that the pain involved is not actually related to the growing process – but that's not to say that the pain your child is experiencing isn't very real; it is. One of the possible causes is reduced bone strength, and there are several remedies that may help relieve the pain.

Try:

- **Vitamin D:** low vitamin-D levels have been linked to growing pains[1] – so get your kid outside to soak it up the natural way from the sun (just don't forget the suncream), or consider a supplement.
- **Milk and dairy:** consuming more calcium helps support healthy bones.
- **Magnesium-rich foods:** magnesium – found in leafy greens, fish and bananas – helps to increase bone density.

- **Potassium-rich foods:** a shortage of potassium in the diet may lead to an imbalance between sodium and potassium, which is not ideal for optimum bone health. Potassium is common in fruit and vegetables.

Avoid:
- **Soft drinks:** yet another excuse to avoid (sugar-laden) commerical soft drinks is their contribution to poor bone strength, due to the combination of caffeine and phosphoric acid.

COMMON CHALLENGES

Fast healthy breakfasts

Healthy breakfasts are a must, and low-carb high-fat eating is filled with delicious eggy delights that are a wonderful way to power up at the start of the day – if you've got a bit of time to spare. But what about *fast* healthy breakfasts? As in, something your 7-year-old can get together while you're trying to snap out of your pre-coffee morning zombiefication? Once upon a time, that's where breakfast cereals came in, but as we now know, the majority of them make for the worst kind of refined-carb high-sugar meal-in-a-bowl; they are, in fact, exactly *not* what your kids should be eating. (See p26-27 and p337.)

For those times when cooking a full-blown breakfast of champions for the whole family just isn't feasible – probably most weekdays, for the average parents out there – make your life easier by planning ahead.

Some good breakfasts on the go include:
- Our amazing low-carb granola. Perhaps best to limit it to once a week, but at least that's Monday morning out the way. See p156.
- A smoothie pre-made the night before with yoghurt, fruit, vegetables, berries and nuts – because it's good to get a protein boost in there. See p154.
- Full-cream Greek yoghurt with nuts and berries – already made up and ready for takeaway if necessary.
- Plain old fresh fruit. Load up on berries.
- Boiled eggs. Okay, your 7-year-old (probably) isn't making this one, but it's boiling water with an egg in it; it literally takes ten minutes from start to finish. And you know how much we love eggs...
- Lastly, if you must fall back on cereal – because sometimes you've just got to get by – then try to opt for whole grains such as quinoa, millet and oats. Add a protein and some fat to keep those blood-sugar levels under control.

Vegetable avoidance

So your child has declared war on vegetables. Don't worry; you're not alone. Whether it's stubbornness or stupidity, many children will do anything to avoid eating what's good for them. Take comfort that he'll probably grow out of it, but in the meantime you'll need to delve into the bag of tricks you first used on your toddler.

- Make vegetables palatable. Seriously, who wants to eat boiled broccoli when you can cook it in butter and cover it with cheese?
- Offer them as snacks with dips. Even the staunchest carnivore will give crudités a chance if they're offered with tasty dips like tzatziki, hummus, pâté or even peanut butter.
- Use them to bulk up your soups.
- Go sweeter if necessary. Sweeter veg is usually better tolerated – and you're not likely to kick off a sweet tooth with sweet potato, sweet corn or peas. Sneak them into salads and he won't even know.
- Disguise vegetables in stews and mince dishes. An oldie but a goodie.
- Keep trying. The no-eating-veggies stage really is a parental rite of passage.

The sugar trap: other people's children (at other people's houses)

The frustration levels can be infinite when you do everything humanly possible to ensure your child avoids those sugary drinks and refined carbs only to have your best efforts shot to pieces by Johnny's mommy who "gave me *three* vanilla chocolate fudge cupcakes!"

The reality is, you can't control what your child eats when he's not in your immediate vicinity. Accept it for what it is. And make the most of the fact that you *can* control what he eats at home. If he doesn't eat sugar, refined carbs and processed foods when he's in your care, then he's less likely to want to eat them when he's at that after-school play date with Johnny – or, at the very least, will want to eat less of them.

To stack the cards more heavily in your favour, fall back on the trick we learnt last chapter: before you send your kid off to a play date or party, fill him up with a nutritious meal. Make it something he really likes, and with any luck he won't have much room left over when the sweets come out.

If you're hosting the party, don't be afraid to stick to your house rules of healthy eating; it doesn't mean you can't have a whole lot of eating fun and deliciousness, as you'll see in the Snacks & Treats and Party Food sections coming up. (See from p226.)

Sweet alternatives

As you know if you've read this far, the guiding principle of this book is to blend the best up-to-date scientifically endorsed nutritional information with the practicalities of feeding your child. Maybe you didn't start him off on a no-sugar diet and you've just come around to the idea (better late than never, we say). Perhaps, as he's got older and more accustomed to eating with the grown-ups, you need to integrate his taste buds with those of the family just a little (though the healthier option would be to integrate the family's with his). Or perhaps, despite your best efforts, your child just likes sweet things. Whatever the case, you may want to know how to bring a bit of sweetness into his diet without compromising all that we've suggested so far.

Fruit: The obvious first choice, and we have, for instance, used fruit to flavour our homemade drinks (see p252-255) and suggest it as a snack option. Berries always come highly recommended. Don't forget, however, that we don't recommend too much fruit in general due to its high natural sugar content.

Honey: Both as an addition to foods and in cooking, honey often makes a good substitute for sugar, and we've used it in a number of our recipes. It also has proven health benefits attributed to its phenolic compounds, and is considered a super food by many nutritionists due to its antibacterial, antioxidant, anti-tumour, anti-inflammatory and antiviral properties.[2] It is, however, particularly high in fructose and glucose, so don't overdo it.

Natural sweeteners: Then there are the sweeteners. In general we prefer to steer clear of sweeteners but, if you must, two of the more preferable options are erythritol and stevia. The former is probably the better tasting of the two, while the latter may have active health benefits.

Erythritol is a naturally occurring sugar alcohol with a minty aftertaste. About as sweet as table sugar, it contains significantly fewer calories and has a less volatile effect on blood-sugar levels. It has the added advantage of being less damaging on the teeth than sugar, and it doesn't cause the bloating and diarrhoea in children that is sometimes associated with other sugar alcohols.

Stevia, a low-calorie sweetener derived from a basil-like South American plant, has gone through the legal wringer to get fit-for-consumption approval; the European Commission, for instance, only approved it in 2011. But not only is it apparently safe, it contains a variety of nutrients, including folic acid and vitamin C, and may in fact have antioxidant, antimicrobial and antifungal properties. It is stable at high temperatures, which makes it good for baking. [3]

Using these and other options, and steering clear of sugar, you can still go to town with an amazing array of treats and snacks. But as with all sweet foods, we must caution against using sweeteners regularly to avoid the risk of your child becoming accustomed to the taste. Try to consider them as ingredients in treat foods only.

DAIRY QUERY

Dairy is an occasionally problematic branch of the Real Meal Revolution food philosophy. We are certainly pro-dairy – as long as it's full cream – and we agree with the commonly held nutritional advice to include it as a healthy part of a child's diet. But it seems undeniable that in certain children (and later adults) dairy products can lead to health issues such as asthma, eczema, increased mucus, and ear, nose and throat problems. This is most likely due to dairy-specific proteins, while the lactose in dairy can have an ill effect on the gut of those who are lactose intolerant. There also appears to be some evidence that dairy's reputation as the essential ingredient for healthy bone formation is not all it's cracked up to be; other calcium-containing foods are probably just as good. [4]

As a result, we suggest monitoring your child's reaction to dairy products. If you suspect there's a problem, opt for the better tolerated dairy foods: yoghurt instead of milk, and sheep and goat products instead of cow products. The clinical evidence seems to support this route, so see what works. If there is a true anaphylactic response, it is unlikely any dairy will be tolerated. Consider cutting out dairy entirely, and bear in mind that a calcium supplement may then be needed.

A WORD ON...

Soft drinks

One soft drink every now and then can't be that bad, right? Uh-oh. Don't be tempted down that path, for there lies the surest way to destruction. Or future health problems, at least.

If our thought experiment in the introduction isn't fresh in the memory (see from p24), let us remind you: soft drinks, simply put, are the quickest way to get your child hooked on sugar. They will destroy their teeth, their bones and their overall health. We cannot emphasise just how bad they are. And unfortunately most fruit juice isn't great either, so be wary if you go that route; dilute with water and limit serving sizes. Rather offer your child water or homemade flavoured drinks (see p252-255). If you do it from the start, he will never miss sugary drinks. And heed this tip: as the parent, it's much easier to enforce this if you lead by example.

Caffeine

You pick up your child from school and before you can ask him about his day he's suggesting you stop off for a "grande chai tea latte with extra foam". Say what? Yes, there's your child "growing up" again, and being influenced by people who aren't you...

Perhaps you could do with a post-lunch green tea or coffee yourself, but should your child be having caffeine? There are no clear guidelines on caffeine consumption for children, but we believe children should not consume it. Because of their body size, children are far more susceptible to the adverse affects of caffeine, such as interrupted sleep, nervousness, anxiety, restlessness and the need to urinate more often. Never mind the peeing, that potential lost sleep alone is just not worth it. Caffeine can also cause stomachaches and headaches. Remember that there are other sources of caffeine, such as chocolate and soft drinks.

So that's a no to the grande chai tea latte with extra foam. Still, there's nothing stopping you from getting him a grande *decaf* chai tea latte with extra foam. Apart from, possibly, your tolerance for ordering obnoxious sounding beverages.

Supplements

Generally speaking, if your child is getting enough iron, protein, vegetables, fruit and dairy, he'll be getting all the vitamins and minerals he needs and won't require a supplement. This is one of the benefits of eating a properly balanced diet.

As mentioned previously, however, vitamin D may help if your child is experiencing growing pains. And if he's on a restricted diet then he may also require a supplement. (Calcium for no dairy, for example.) Again, however, we recommend you consult your paediatrician or doctor before taking the supplement route.

SIMPLE OMELETTES

Makes 1-2 portions
Prep time: 5 mins
Cooking time: 5 mins

Once you've mastered the art of making omelettes, they're a fantastically quick and easy way to make breakfast for the kids. They also provide a great way to sneak veggies into their diet. Younger children may not manage a full omelette, so let them stop when they're full.

1 tablespoon butter
2 large eggs
3 tablespoons grated cheddar cheese

- Heat the butter in a small frying pan and grease it well.
- Whisk the eggs in a bowl and pour them into the hot, greased pan. Move the pan around to spread the mixture out evenly. Cook on a medium to low heat.
- When the omelette begins to cook and firm up, top one half with grated cheese.
- Allow the cheese to melt a little then use a spatula to ease around the edge of the omelette and fold it in half.
- Slide the omelette onto a plate and leave for a few seconds for the cheese to melt and for the omelette to cool slightly before serving.

SOME FLAVOUR SUGGESTIONS:
HAM AND CHEESE
CHEESE AND TOMATO
CHICKEN AND PINEAPPLE
LEFTOVER ANYTHING PLUS CHEESE (MINCE IS DELICIOUS!)

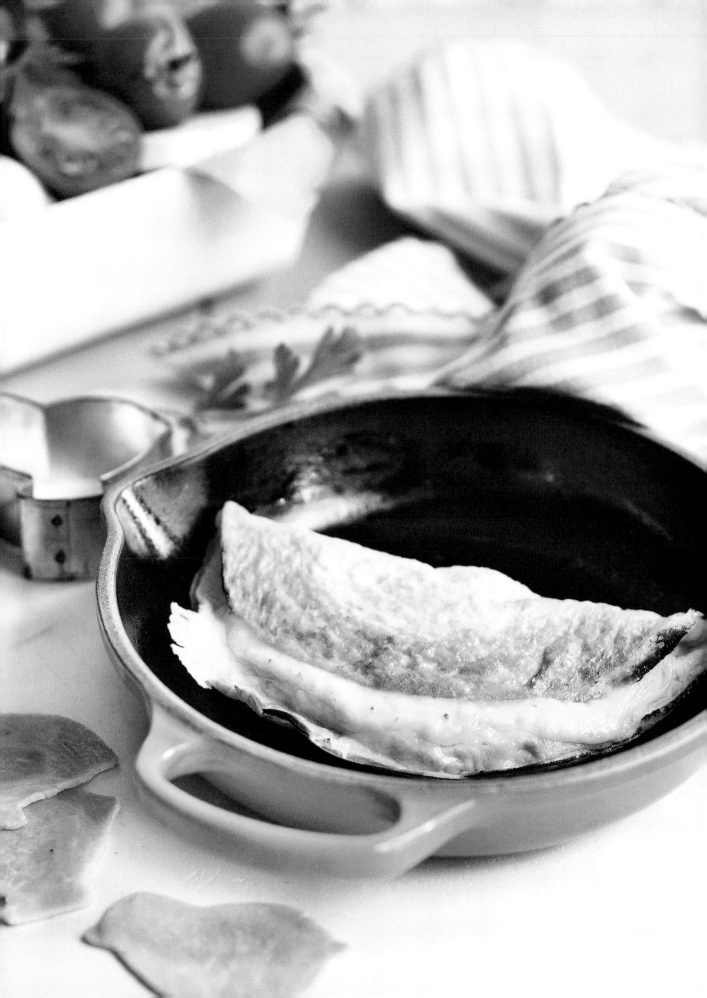

BLUEBERRY-AND-COCONUT BREAKFAST MUFFINS

Makes 10
Prep time: 15 mins
Cooking time: 30 mins

Think of muffins as a little work going a long way. They're a bit of a mission to make, but you can make a load in one go and they freeze like a dream – heat a couple quickly and you've got a great instant breakfast.

3 apples, peeled, cored and grated
4 eggs, at room temperature
¼ cup (60ml) melted butter
3 tablespoons honey
1 cup (80g) desiccated coconut
½ cup (60g) coconut flour, sieved
¼ cup (45g) flax seeds, ground in
  a coffee grinder
½ teaspoon sea salt
1 teaspoon baking powder
1 ½ cups (225g) fresh blueberries

- Preheat the oven to 180°C.
- Line a 12-cup muffin pan with muffin cups.
- Whisk together the wet ingredients in a bowl.
- Combine the dry ingredients in a separate bowl.
- Add the dry ingredients to the wet and mix until just combined.
- Immediately fold through the blueberries. The batter will thicken as it sits, so do this right away.
- Use an ice-cream-sized scoop with a lever (a ¼ cup or 60ml scoop) to fill 12 muffin cups. (If you don't use a scoop the tops won't be quite as round.)
- Bake for 25-30 minutes or until cooked through.

TO HEAT FROM THE FREEZER, JUST POP THE MUFFINS IN A MODERATE OVEN TO DEFROST AND WARM UP. BREAKFAST IS SERVED!

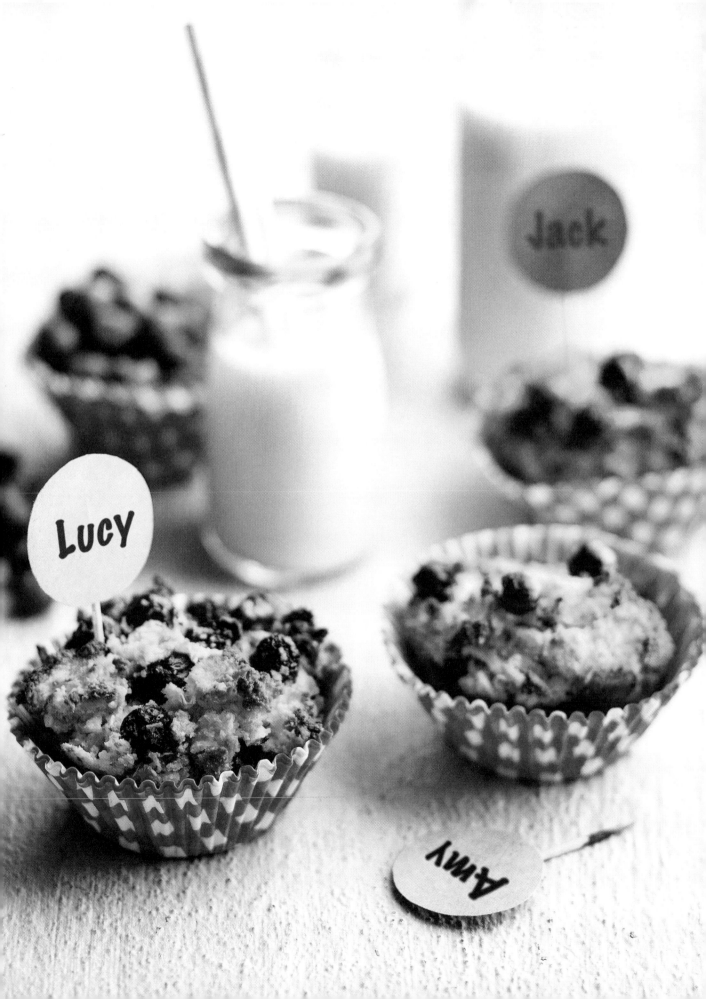

EGGY BREAD WITH FRIED BANANAS AND CREAM CHEESE OR YOGHURT

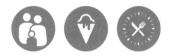

Makes 1 portion
Prep time: 5 mins
Cooking time: 10 mins

This is the low-carb answer to French toast – it's delicious, easy to make, and your kids can help you do it. Add a little crispy bacon for a more grown-up breakfast. Bake your own low-carb bread (see p296) or simply use a good store-bought loaf.

1 egg
1 tablespoon milk
1 slice low-carb bread
2 tablespoons coconut oil
2 tablespoons butter
1 banana, peeled and sliced
3 tablespoons cream cheese
  or yoghurt
a sprinkle of cinnamon

- Whisk the egg and milk together in a shallow plate with a rim.
- Submerge the bread in the egg mixture and coat it well on both sides.
- Heat the coconut oil in a frying pan with 1 tablespoon of butter. Lightly fry the sliced banana and set aside.
- Add the remaining butter to the pan and fry the eggy bread until it's cooked through and golden on both sides.
- Transfer the bread to a plate and top with the bananas, some cream cheese or yoghurt and a sprinkle of cinnamon.

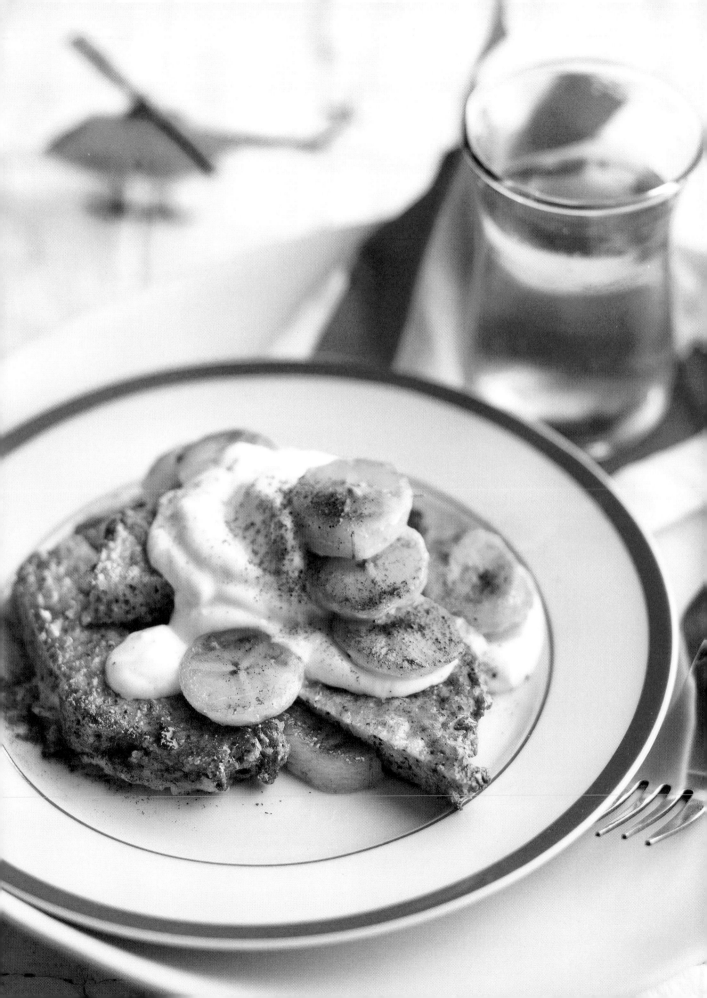

HAM-AND-VEGETABLE EGG CUPS

Makes 4 portions
Prep time: 10 mins
Cooking time: 25 mins

This recipe is a great way to use up leftover vegetables, especially roasted ones – you'll need a little more than a cup of cooked chopped veggies. Serving the egg cups in a ramekin with different dishes on the side makes for an interesting mix-and-match breakfast.

2 tablespoons butter
¼ pepper, diced
1 courgette, washed and sliced
¼ cup (60g) diced aubergine
½ onion, chopped or grated
8 slices ham or gammon
4 eggs
¼ cup (25g) grated cheese
homemade ketchup (p294) or diced tomato to serve

- Preheat the oven to 180°C.
- Heat the butter in a frying pan and gently fry the vegetables until soft. Remove from the heat and set aside.
- Line 4 greased 180ml ramekins with 2 slices of ham each.
- Divide the vegetable mixture between each ramekin.
- Break an egg into each ramekin and bake on a baking tray for 20 minutes.
- Top each egg with some grated cheese and return to the oven for a further 5 minutes.
- Serve with homemade ketchup or fresh diced tomato.

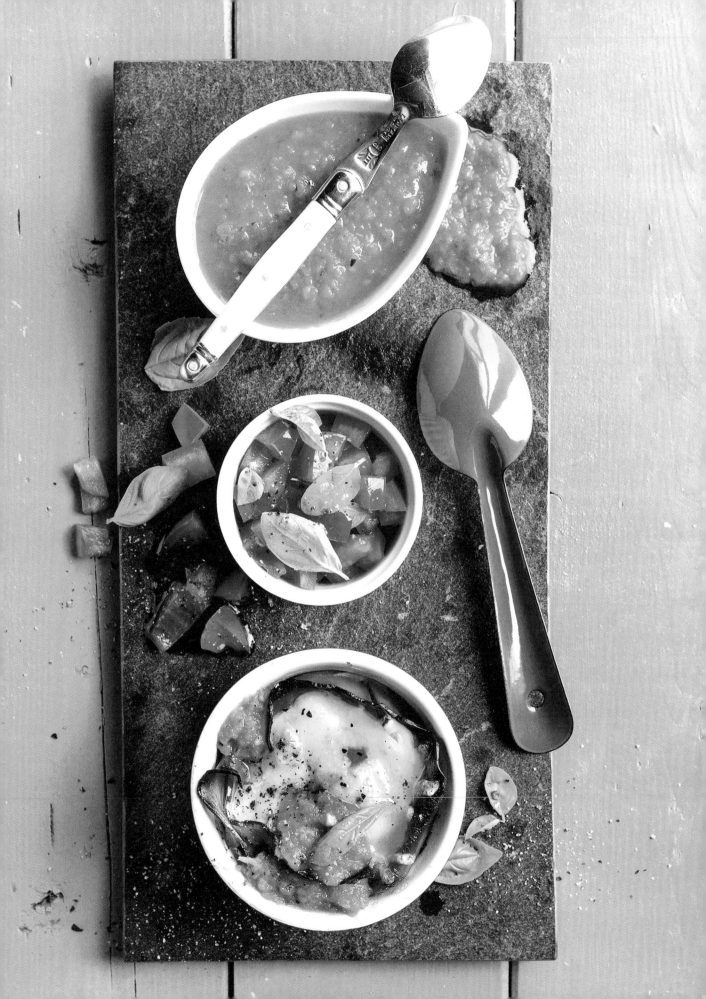

SUPERB SMOOTHIES

Makes 2 portions
Time: 5 minutes

Smoothies are a great way to get lots of nutrients into a glass and make it feel a bit like a milkshake. If you're late on the school run, you could give your kids their smoothies to drink in the car. Just make sure they don't spill...

PAPAYA, GINGER, COCONUT AND OAT SMOOTHIE

1 banana, peeled and chopped
½ cup (70g) papaya, peeled and cubed
1 teaspoon grated ginger
⅓ cup (80g) yoghurt
3 tablespoons oats, soaked in little
  coconut milk overnight
a handful of ice cubes

- Place all the ingredients in a blender or smoothie machine and blend until smooth.

ALMOND, BANANA AND COCOA SMOOTHIE

2 bananas, peeled and chopped
2 tablespoons cocoa powder
⅔ cup (170ml) unsweetened almond milk
a handful of ice cubes

- Place all the ingredients in a blender or smoothie machine and blend until smooth.

PEAR, AVOCADO, SPINACH AND MINT SMOOTHIE

1 pear, peeled, cored and chopped
½ avocado, skin removed and chopped
¼ cup (7g) baby spinach, tightly
  packed
small bunch mint leaves
⅓ cup (80g) yoghurt
a handful of ice cubes

- Place all the ingredients in a blender or smoothie machine and blend until smooth.

FOR A SCHOOL-LUNCH DRINK, FREEZE SMOOTHIES THE NIGHT BEFORE, THEN POP THEM INTO A LUNCH BOX IN THE MORNING. BY BREAK TIME THEY'LL BE STARTING TO MELT

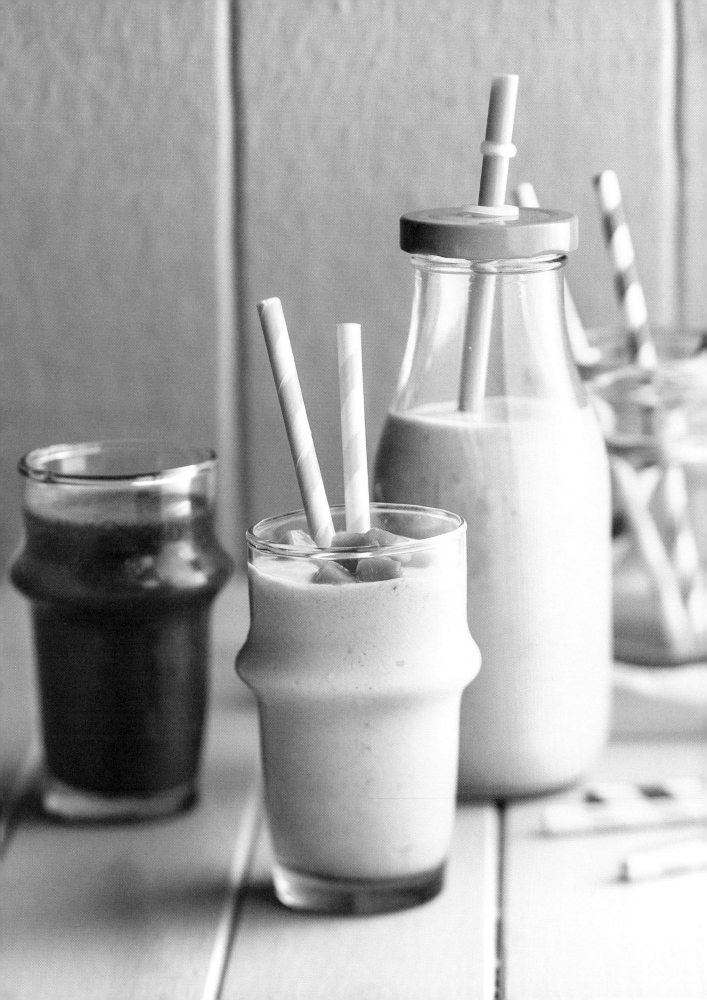

COLONEL CRUNCHY GRANOLA

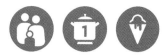

Makes 500g granola
Prep time: 15 mins
Cooking time: 3 hours

This granola is so tasty you'll be tucking into it before your kids have the chance. It does contain oats, though, so make sure you buy the right type and try to limit it to one breakfast a week. The good news is it keeps for weeks if you store it properly in an airtight container.

100g pecan nuts
100g raw, unsalted macadamia nuts
100g blanched whole almonds
½ cup (45g) oats
4 tablespoons butter
2 tablespoons honey
½ teaspoon ground cinnamon
½ teaspoon vanilla extract
½ cup (40g) desiccated coconut
100g dried pears, chopped

Optional:
3 tablespoons unsweetened cocoa powder
60g dark chocolate, chopped

- Preheat the oven to 110°C.
- Using a food processor, coarsely chop the nuts and then add the oats. Blitz together quickly.
- In a saucepan, gently melt the butter, honey, cinnamon and vanilla. If you're going to make chocolate granola, add the cocoa to the butter at this point.
- Pour the butter mixture into the food processor and pulse it once or twice to just combine the butter into the mixture. Add the coconut and pulse one more time.
- Spread the mixture onto a baking sheet and bake for 2-3 hours, until toasted and slightly golden.
- Remove from the oven and mix through the chopped dried pears.
- If you are making chocolate granola, allow it to cool and mix through the chopped chocolate.

THIS DELICIOUS GRANOLA GOES WITH SO MANY THINGS. FIRST UP, TRY GREEK YOGHURT AND SOME FRESH BERRIES. YOU CAN ALSO USE DIFFERENT DRIED FRUITS

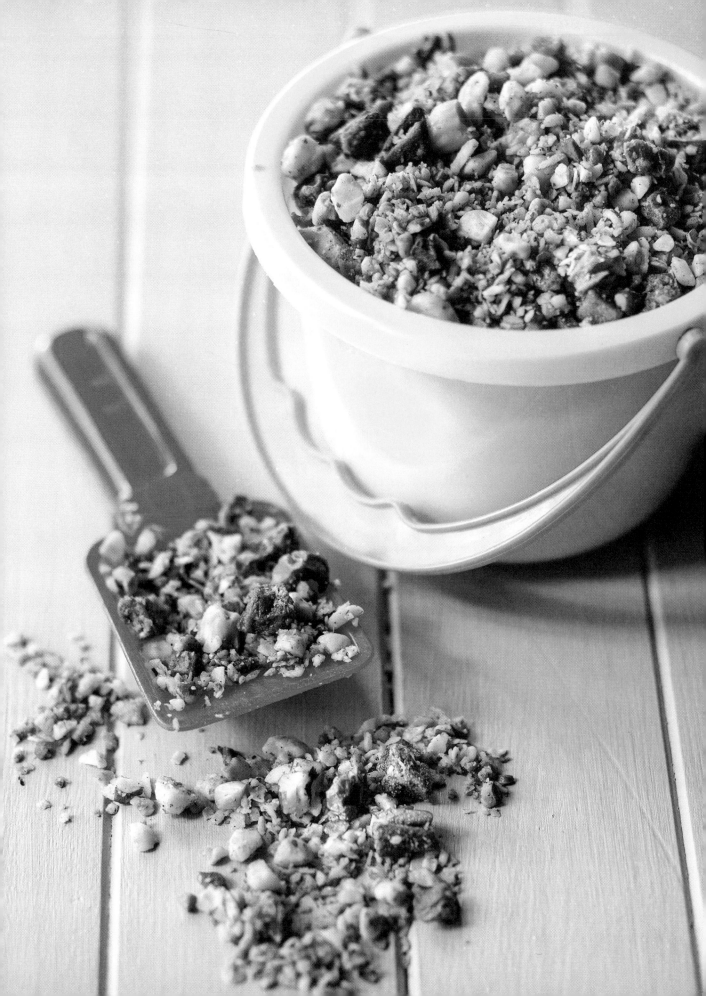

PUMPKIN NUT HOTCAKES WITH CINNAMON BUTTER

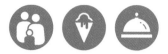

Makes 4 portions
Prep time: 10 mins
Cooking time: 15 mins

These American-style pancakes make for a yummy family breakfast treat. They're also good for using up leftover cooked pumpkin from the night before. The recipe works wonderfully well in a waffle maker too, so if you have one give it a go.

For the hotcakes:
2 eggs, separated
1 banana, peeled and chopped
1 cup (225g) cooked and mashed
   pumpkin
⅓ cup (85g) almond butter
½ teaspoon ground cinnamon
½ teaspoon mixed spice
⅓ cup (35g) almond flour
1 teaspoon baking powder
2 tablespoons melted butter
coconut oil or butter for frying
cream cheese to serve

For the cinnamon butter:
3 tablespoons melted butter
½ teaspoon ground cinnamon
50g chopped pecan nuts

- In a clean bowl, whisk the egg whites to soft peaks and set aside.
- Except for the coconut oil or butter and cream cheese, place the remaining ingredients and egg yolks into a food processer and mix until they are the consistency of a batter.
- Pour the batter into a bowl.
- Gently fold the egg whites through the batter using a metal spoon.
- Heat a little coconut oil and/or butter in a large pan to medium heat.
- Once the butter starts to sizzle, add spoonfuls of batter into the pan and cook until bubbles start to appear on the surface of the hotcakes.
- Flip the hotcakes over and cook until golden on both sides. Repeat with the remaining batter. (Note: because these hotcakes aren't made with gluten, they are quite delicate, so take care when flipping.)
- To make the cinnamon butter, simply melt the ingredients together.
- Serve the hotcakes with a few spoonfuls of cream cheese and a drizzle of cinnamon butter.

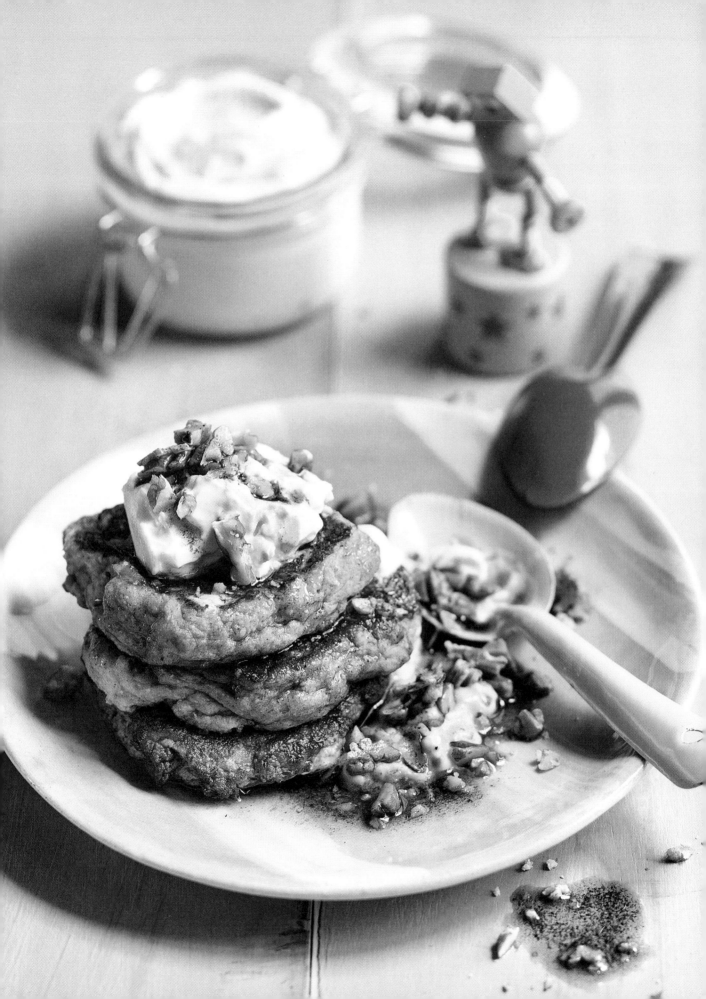

RATATOUILLE 'SHAKSHUKA' EGGS

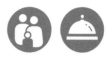

Makes 3-4 portions
Prep time: 20 mins
Cooking time: 35 mins

The recipe name may sound rather fancy, but it's a piece of cake to make and a great way to encourage family breakfasts. If you make the ratatouille in bulk and keep it frozen, you can put it all together in a matter of minutes.

For the ratatouille:
2 tablespoons butter
1 onion, chopped
1 aubergine, diced
1 yellow or red pepper, seeds removed and diced
4 courgettes, sliced or diced
125g button mushrooms, chopped
1 clove garlic, crushed
1 tablespoon tomato paste
1 x 400g tin chopped tomatoes, blended
½ cup (125ml) water
a handful fresh basil, chopped (optional)
a pinch of salt

In the pan:
3-4 eggs

- In a wide pan, melt the butter on a medium heat. Add the vegetables and gently fry until soft. Add the garlic and fry for a minute.
- Stir the tomato paste into the pan and fry for another minute or so. Add the tomatoes and the water and simmer slowly for about 20 minutes until the sauce thickens.
- Add the chopped basil and a little salt. At this stage, you could serve the ratatouille as a vegetable option with a dish or as a delicious Mediterranean sauce. (It freezes well, so hang on to the leftovers.)
- To complete the shakshuka, make hollows in the ratatouille mixture and crack in the eggs. Cover the pan with a lid and simmer for about 5-10 minutes, or until the eggs are cooked to your preference.
- Serve straight from the pan.

WHEN USING COLD OR FROZEN RATATOUILLE IN THIS DISH, MAKE SURE YOU HEAT IT WELL IN THE PAN BEFORE CRACKING IN THE EGGS

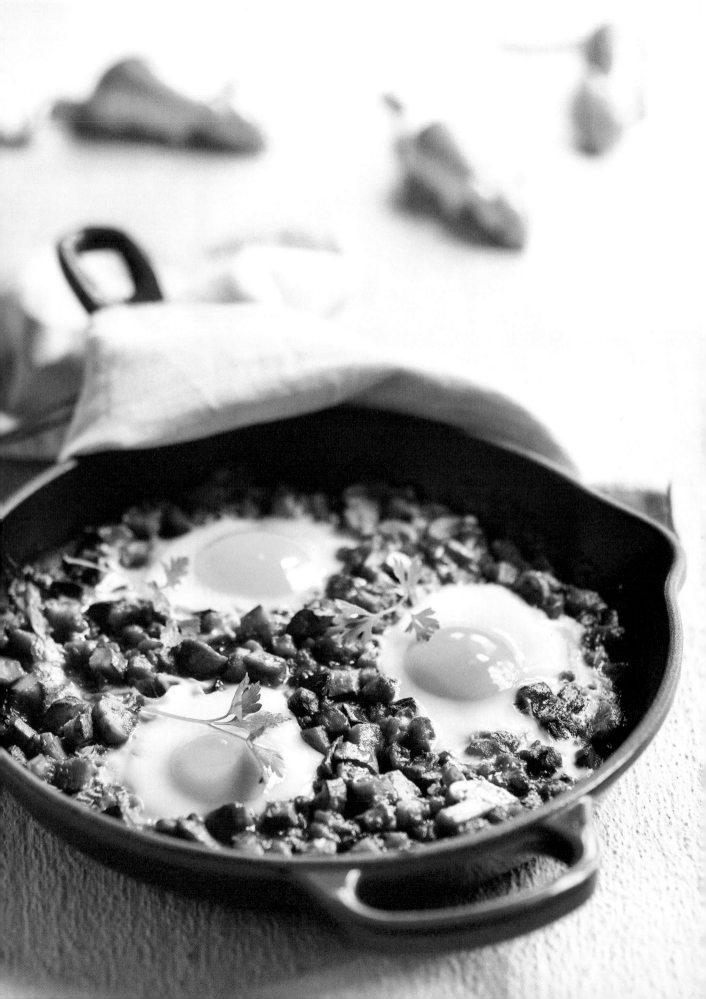

MEATY BREAKFAST BURRITO

Makes 6 portions
Prep time: 20 mins
Cooking time: 45 mins

A great beef mince is invaluable for family meals and is another dish worth making in bulk and popping in the freezer for a rainy day. If you've got ready-made mince, this recipe is quick to make and a real crowd-pleaser.

For the beef mince:
2 tablespoons butter
1 onion, finely chopped
2 celery stalks, finely chopped
1 carrot, peeled and grated
3 rashers bacon, finely chopped
2 teaspoons rosemary, finely chopped
1 clove garlic, crushed
400g beef mince
2 tablespoons tomato paste
1 x 400g tin chopped tomatoes, blended
½ cup (125ml) beef stock or water
1 bay leaf
salt to season

For the egg wraps:
6 eggs
butter for greasing the pan

To serve:
grated cheese
fresh avocado slices
coriander leaves
sour cream or cream cheese

TO MAKE THE MINCE:
- Heat the butter in a saucepan and gently cook the onion, celery, carrot, bacon and rosemary until soft. Add the garlic and cook for a minute.
- Sprinkle the beef mince into the saucepan, using a wooden spoon to separate it, and brown it on a higher heat.
- Stir in the tomato paste and fry for a few minutes.
- Add in the chopped tomatoes, stock or water and the bay leaf and simmer for 45 minutes, until the sauce has thickened and is a rich dark colour. Add a little salt to season.

TO MAKE THE EGG WRAPS:
- Whisk the eggs together.
- Place a frying pan on a low heat and grease it well.
- Pour in enough of the whisked egg to just cover the bottom of the pan. Swirl it around to fill any holes. If you use too much egg, the wrap will break when it's rolled.
- Cook the egg until it sets, then gently flip it over using a spatula and cook it on the other side for a minute or two.

TO MAKE YOUR BURRITO:
- Fill the egg wrap with some mince, grated cheese, avo, fresh coriander, sour cream and/or cream cheese, and roll it up to eat.
- For some extra deliciousness, top it with cheese and place it under the grill until it's a gooey, cheesy breakfast feast.

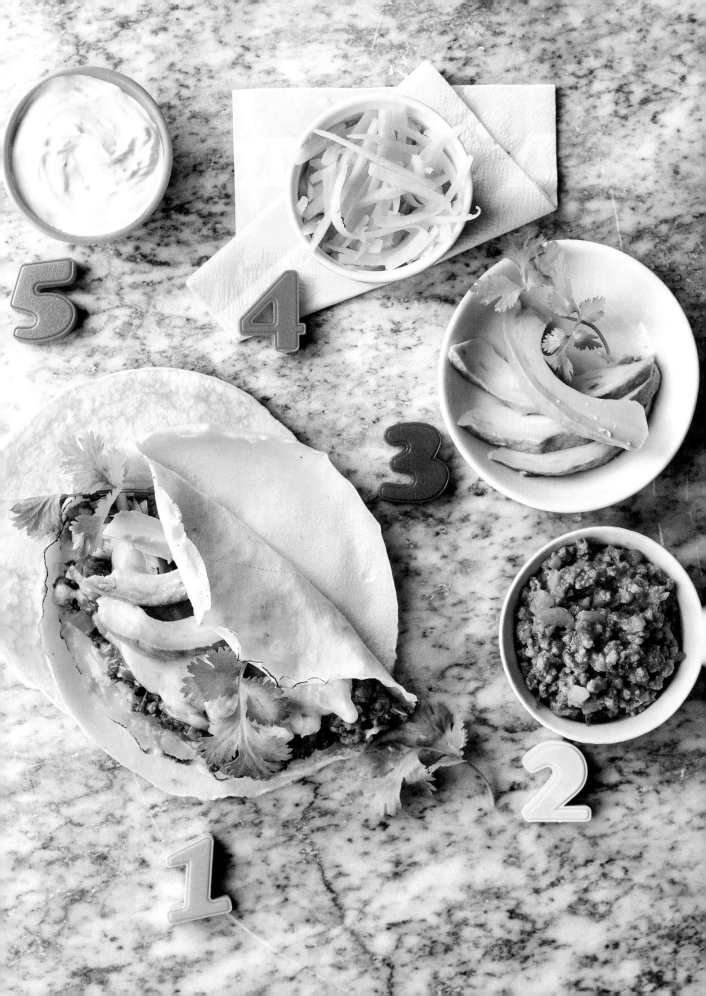

CHOCOLATE QUINOA WITH YOGHURT AND BUTTERY PEARS

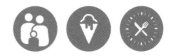

Makes 6 portions
Prep time: 5 mins
Cooking time: 25 mins

Quinoa is a grain-like plant that contains some carbohydrates, but it's also high in protein and jam-packed with the good stuff. It's a much healthier option than regular grains such as wheat, barley and rye. Still, consider this a treat rather than an everyday recipe.

1 cup (250g) quinoa
1 cup (250ml) water
200ml coconut milk
2 pears, peeled and grated
1 teaspoon orange zest
2 tablespoons cocoa
1 pear, cored and thinly sliced
2 tablespoons butter
yoghurt to serve

- Rinse the quinoa well in running water. (If you don't, it will taste bitter.) Drain in a sieve.
- Place the quinoa and water in a saucepan and simmer on low heat for 15 minutes. Watch that the water doesn't cook away entirely, in which case the quinoa can burn and stick.
- When the quinoa starts to open, add the coconut milk, grated pear, orange zest and cocoa and simmer for a further 5-10 minutes.
- You will know it's ready when the quinoa grains are puffy and have opened up.
- While the quinoa is cooking, melt the butter in a pan and lightly fry the sliced pear until cooked through and slightly golden.
- Serve the chocolate quinoa with a spoonful of yoghurt, scattered with the buttery pears and a sprinkle of cocoa.

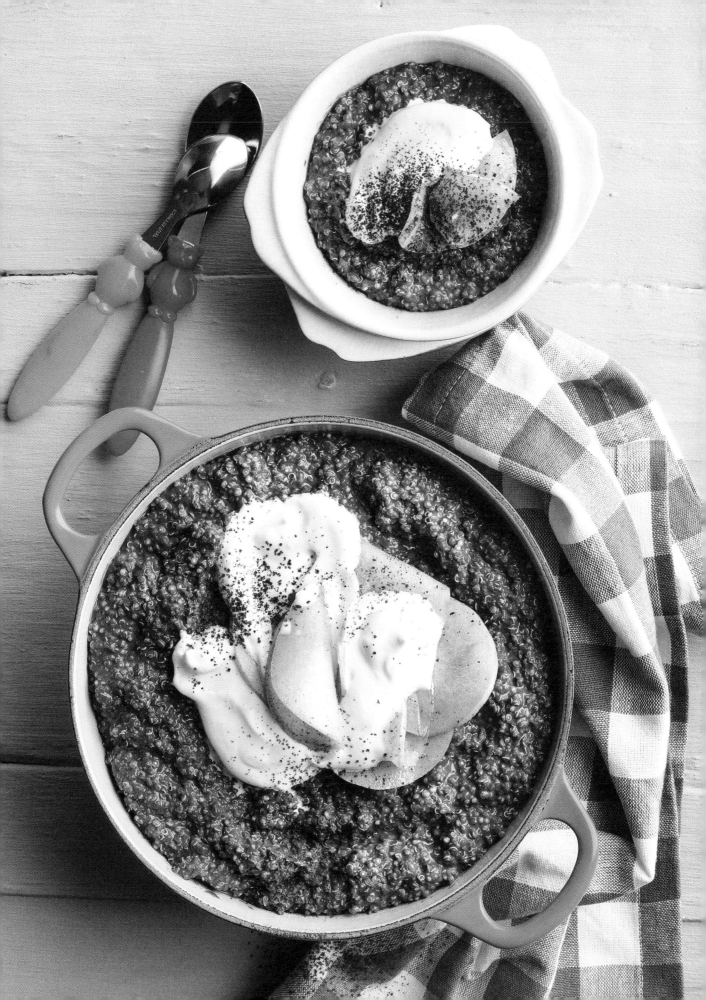

KIDDIES' 'CRUSTLESS' QUICHES

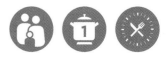

Makes 12
Prep time: 15 mins
Cooking time: 25 mins

Serve these quiches with some chunky veg or a quick salad and you have lunch in a flash. Any extras will be great in a lunchbox the next day. This is a clever way to use up cooked leftovers from the night before; we've used ham and cheese here, but feel free to try your own flavours.

2 tablespoons butter
1 onion, roughly chopped
250g ham, roughly chopped
4 eggs
2 egg yolks
500ml cream
salt and pepper
1 cup (100g) grated Cheddar

- Preheat the oven to 180°C.
- Melt the butter in a frying pan and gently fry the onion until soft. Add the ham and remove the pan from the stove.
- Whisk together the eggs, egg yolks and cream with a little salt and pepper.
- Grease a large 12-cup muffin pan.
- Spoon the onion-and-ham mixture into the bases of the muffin pan and sprinkle over the grated cheese.
- Pour the egg-and-cream mixture into each muffin cup until it is about 1mm from the top.
- Bake for about 25 minutes, until the egg mixture is set and the top is golden. Cool for 10 minutes and remove from the tin.
- Serve hot or cold.

THE KEY TO THIS RECIPE IS GETTING THE RATIO OF EGGS, YOLKS AND CREAM JUST RIGHT

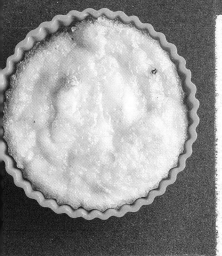
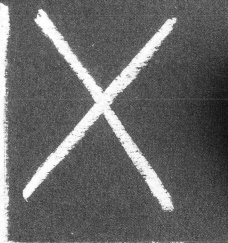
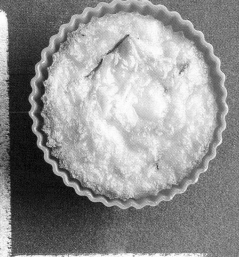
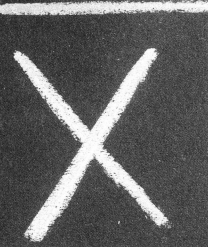
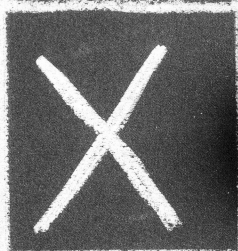
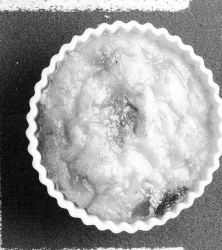
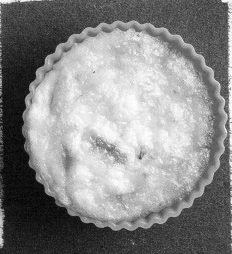
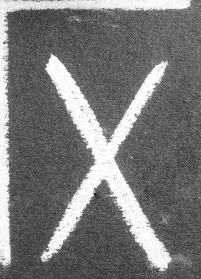
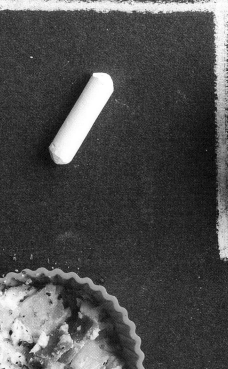

'CARRATE' CHICKEN NOODLE SALAD

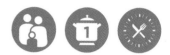

Makes 2 portions
Prep time: 15 mins

This is the perfect salad to throw together if you have some leftover roast chicken from the night before. We've used a Chinese slicer to cut the carrots and cucumber into noodles. If you don't have one, simply shred or julienne the ingredients.

For the dressing:
3 tablespoons tamari soya sauce
1 tablespoon sesame oil
1 tablespoon honey
1 tablespoon lemon juice

For the salad:
1 cup (125g) shredded roast chicken
1 large carrot, peeled and thinly sliced
  into noodles (or shredded
  or julienned)
¼ cucumber, peeled and thinly
  sliced into noodles (or shredded
  or julienned)
50g mangetout, thinly sliced
  (or shredded or julienned)
1 stalk celery, thinly sliced using
  a peeler
½ cup (50g) Chinese bean sprouts
1 teaspoon toasted sesame seeds

- In a bowl mix together the ingredients for the dressing, and set aside.
- To make the salad, place the chicken and vegetables in a bowl and mix together well.
- Toss through the dressing, sprinkle with the toasted sesame seeds, then serve immediately.

TIE THE CHOPSTICKS TOGETHER WITH STRING TO HELP TEACH YOUR KIDS HOW TO USE THEM

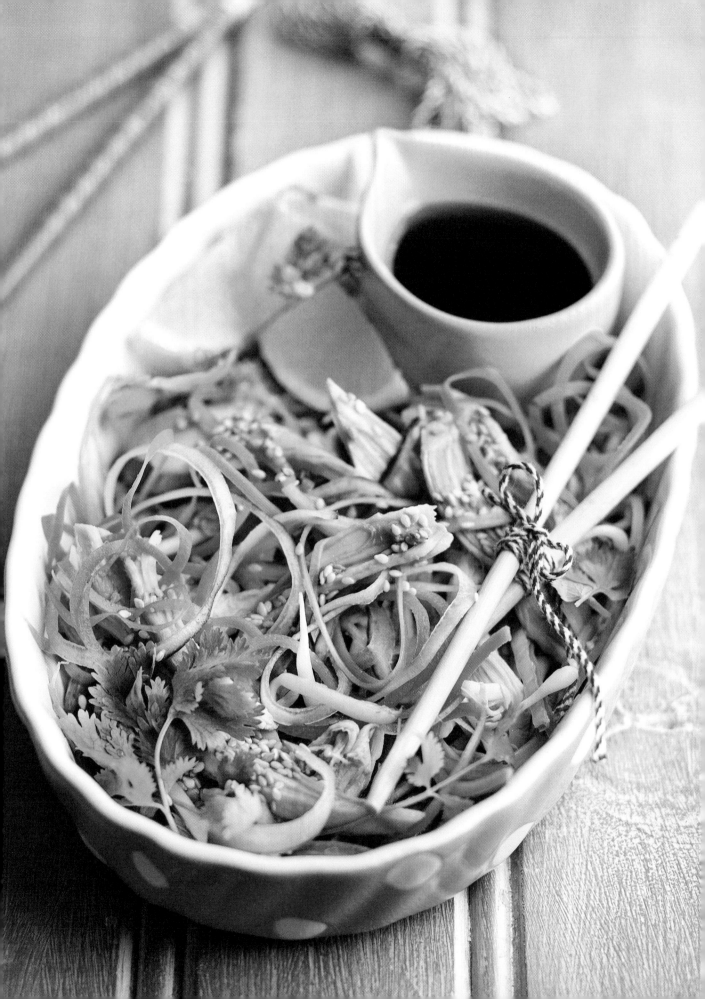

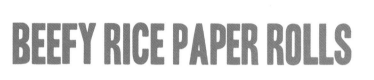

BEEFY RICE PAPER ROLLS

Makes 4 portions
Prep time: 30 mins
Cooking time: 10 mins

The rice paper for these rolls is what sets this apart from other dishes. It's a wafer-thin way of keeping the ingredients together, and you'll get the hang of using it easily enough. We've used seared steak in this recipe but it's also delicious with cooked chicken or grilled fish.

For the sauce:
1 tablespoon honey
1 tablespoon Thai fish sauce
1 tablespoon water
1 tablespoon lemon juice
1 teaspoon chopped coriander
a little chopped chilli (if your kids are older and like it)

For the rice paper rolls:
350g beef sirloin steak
salt and pepper
2 tablespoons butter
12 small rice paper rounds
½ cucumber, cut into batons or julienned
2 carrots, cut into batons or julienned
1 avocado, sliced
50g sugar snaps, thinly sliced
1 mango, peeled and cut into strips (optional)
½ cup (50g) Chinese bean sprouts
fresh mint leaves

TO MAKE THE SAUCE:
- Mix all the ingredients together in a bowl.

TO MAKE THE RICE PAPER ROLLS:
- Season the sirloin well with salt and pepper.
- Heat the butter in a frying pan and fry the sirloin for about 4 minutes on each side, until medium rare. Leave to rest for 5 minutes, then slice thinly.
- Lay out all the filling ingredients in front of you, with a bowl of warm water and a clean damp cloth nearby.
- Soak a rice paper round in the warm water for 30 seconds until it just begins to soften. Lay it on the damp cloth.
- Top the rice paper round with a selection of the meat, vegetables and herbs. Place them in the centre of the rice paper.
- Fold the far end of the rice paper over the filling to form a half circle, fold in both sides and roll everything into a cigar shape.
- Repeat with the remaining ingredients and serve with the sauce.

DON'T FORGET THAT RICE IS HIGH-CARB AND GENERALLY NOT ENCOURAGED, SO TRY NOT TO SERVE DISHES LIKE THIS TOO REGULARLY

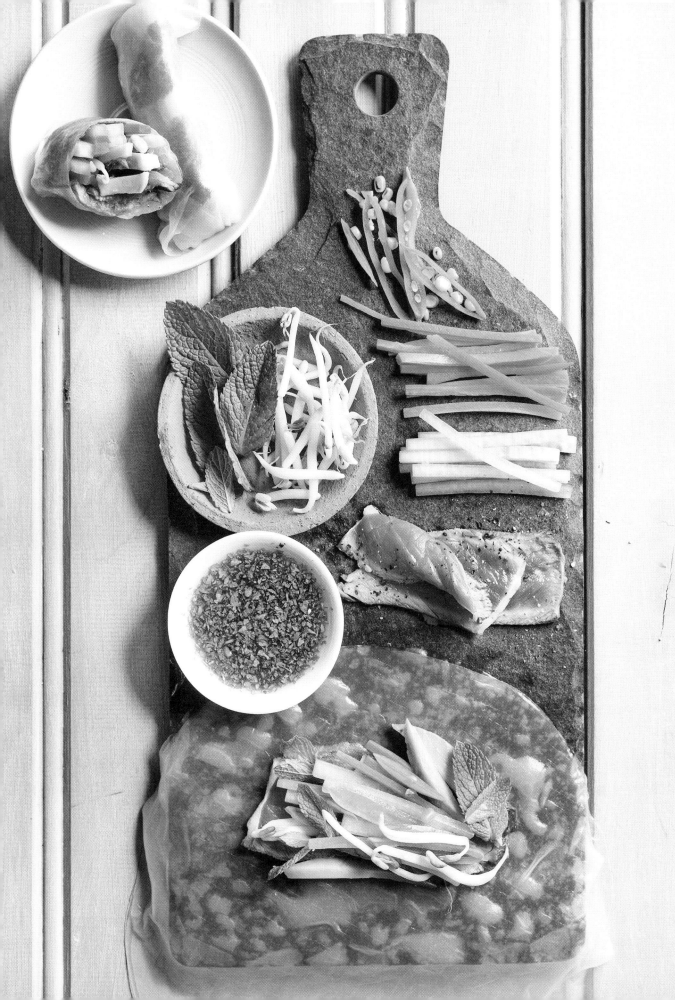

CHICKEN MAYO AND AVOCADO WRAPS

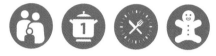

Makes 4 wraps
Prep time: 25 mins
Cooking time: 10 mins

The thing to master with these wraps is the pancake-like wrap itself. It takes a bit of time to work out the consistency, but this is such a versatile staple that it's worth the effort. We've gone for a simple chicken and avo filling using leftover roast chicken, but you could try almost anything.

For the wraps:
¼ cup (30g) coconut flour
⅓ cup (85ml) water
¾ cup (185ml) egg white
½ teaspoon salt
½ teaspoon mixed dried herbs

For the filling:
1 cup (125g) shredded roast chicken
¼ cup (60ml) homemade mayo (p301)
1 stalk celery, finely chopped
1 spring onion, sliced
2 gherkins, finely chopped
1 avocado, thickly sliced
½ cucumber, cut into batons
4 baby gem lettuce leaves

OTHER MUST-TRY FILLINGS ARE BEEF, MOZZARELLA AND TOMATO, AND BACON, CHEESE AND PINEAPPLE

TO MAKE THE WRAPS:
- Place the coconut flour into a bowl and mix in the water. Add in the remaining ingredients and blend using a hand-blender. Leave to rest for about 5 minutes.
- Grease a medium-sized frying pan and warm over a low to medium heat.
- Pour ¼ cup (62ml) of the batter into the pan and swirl it around to form a thin layer. If the mixture is a little too thick, use the back of a spoon to spread it in the pan. Cook until brown on the bottom, then carefully flip it to cook on the other side.
- Repeat with the remaining batter.

TO MAKE THE FILLING:
- Place the chicken, mayonnaise, celery, spring onion and gherkin in a small bowl and mix well.
- Spoon the chicken mixture down the centre of the wrap and top with the avocado, cucumber and lettuce.
- Roll up the wrap to enclose the filling. Cut in half and serve with a simple salad.

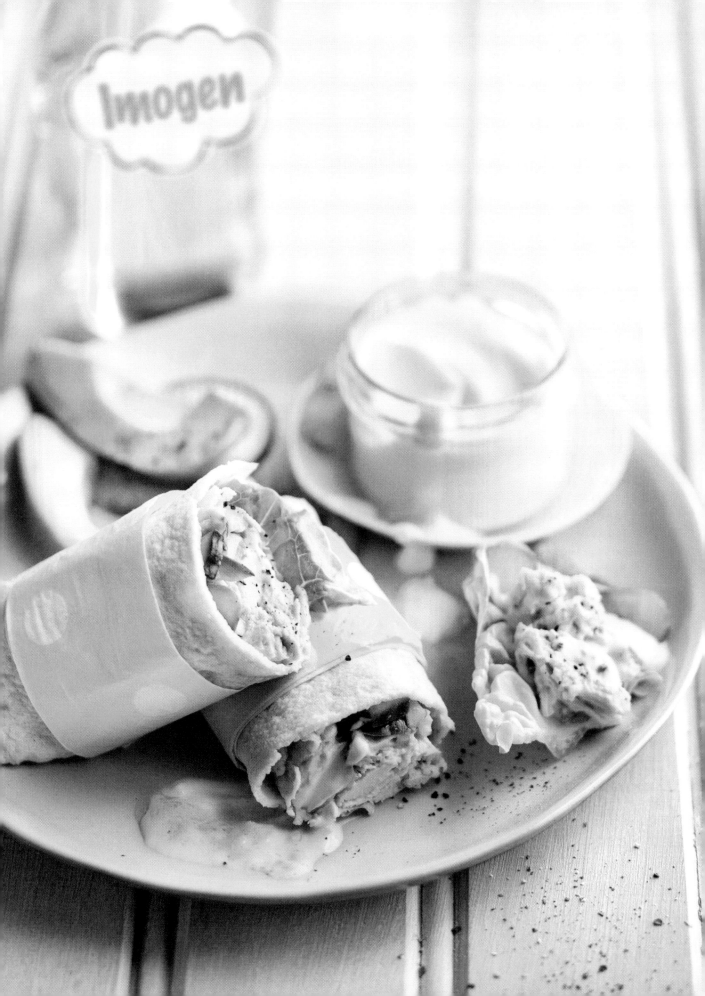

HAWAIIAN BEACHBALL MEATBALL BAKE

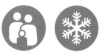

Makes 24 balls
Prep time: 25 mins
Cooking time: 35 mins

This is a yummy and versatile bake that serves a horde, and the pineapple gives it a bit of a twist – just make sure you squeeze out all the pineapple liquid. For a more complete meal, serve the bake with a quick salad.

750g beef mince

1 tablespoon grated fresh ginger

3 spring onions, thinly sliced

3 tablespoons chopped fresh coriander

3 tablespoons coconut flour

½ red pepper, trimmed, seeded and finely chopped

150g fresh pineapple, grated and the liquid squeezed out

2 eggs, lightly beaten

salt and pepper

coconut oil for frying

2 cups (500ml) homemade secret vegetable tomato sauce (p292)

1 cup (120g) grated mozzarella

- Preheat the oven to 180°C.
- Place the beef mince, grated ginger, spring onion and coriander in a bowl and mix together well.
- Stir through the coconut flour, red pepper, pineapple and eggs. Season with a little salt and pepper.
- Using damp hands, roll the mince into meatballs the size of golf balls.
- Heat the coconut oil in a frying pan over a high heat and toss the meatballs in the pan to give them good colour.
- These meatballs can be eaten straight from the pan with some homemade ketchup and a few veggies for a quick lunch. If that's the case, cook them for at least 5 minutes in the pan, so that the meat cooks through.
- To make the bake, lay the quickly fried meatballs in an ovenproof dish. Top with the secret vegetable tomato sauce and the grated cheese.
- Bake for about 25 minutes, until bubbling and gooey.

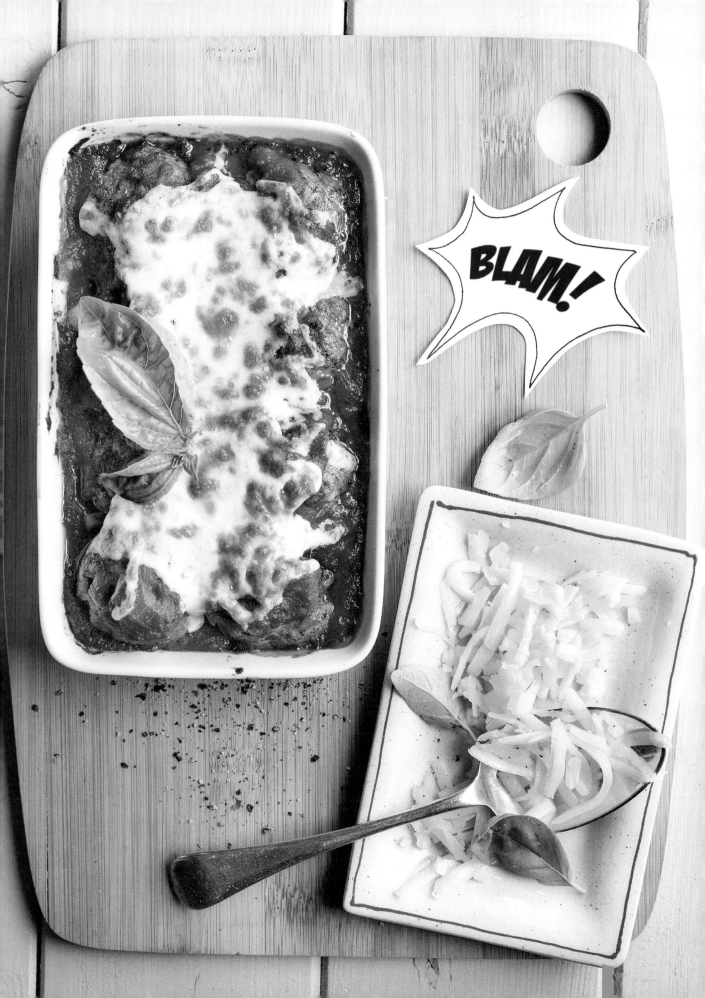

TUNA AND AVOCADO SHIPS

Makes 4 ships
Prep time: 10 mins

For lunch in a flash, this meal is a surefire winner. You can use this tuna mayonnaise recipe for so many things: salads, sandwiches, wraps, rolls and various other fillings.

2 x 170g tins tuna in spring water, drained
2 spring onions, finely chopped
$\frac{1}{4}$ cup (40g) chopped cucumber
$\frac{1}{4}$ cup (60ml) homemade mayo (p301)
$\frac{1}{4}$ cup (70g) double-cream Greek yoghurt
$\frac{1}{2}$ mango, peeled and roughly chopped (optional)
juice of half a lemon
1 tablespoon fresh chopped parsley
salt and pepper
2 avocados, halved and seeded

- Mix together all the ingredients except the avocado and season with a little salt and pepper.
- Spoon the tuna mixture into the cavity of the avocados, and serve.

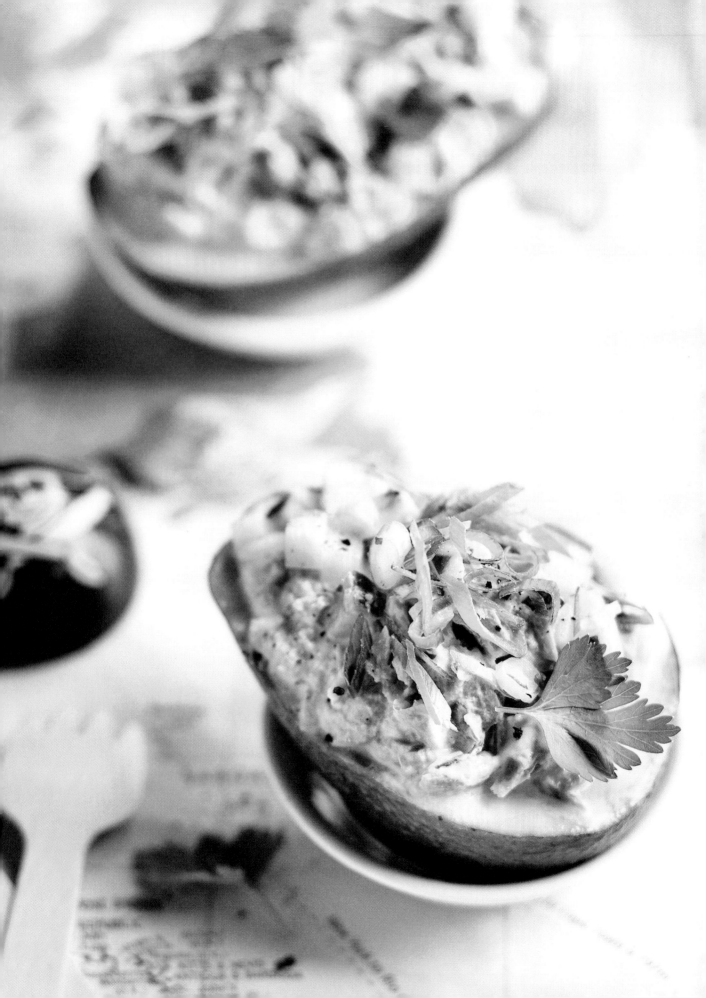

PESTO COURGETTI WITH PANNED TOMATOES AND GRATED CHEESE

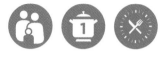

Makes 2 portions
Prep time: 10 mins
Cooking time: 10 mins

This recipe makes for a quick courgetti 'pasta'. We used a Chinese slicer for the noodles, which makes them feel authentic and really speeds up the process. If your kids aren't into basil pesto, try a gentler tomato pesto instead.

2 tablespoons butter

250g cherry tomatoes, halved

4 large courgettes, sliced thinly into noodles (or as you prefer)

6 tablespoons basil pesto (p301)

a drizzle of olive oil

3 tablespoons crème fraîche or cream cheese (optional)

2 handfuls of grated Cheddar or mozzarella

- Melt the butter in a pan and fry the tomatoes for a few minutes until soft and gooey.
- Add the courgette noodles to the pan and fry until soft.
- Take the pan off the heat and stir in the pesto. Add a little olive oil if you need it to coat the courgette noodles better.
- Stir through the crème fraîche for a creamy dish – not necessary, but delicious.
- Finally stir through a handful of grated cheese and spoon the courgetti into bowls.
- Top with the remaining grated cheese, and serve.

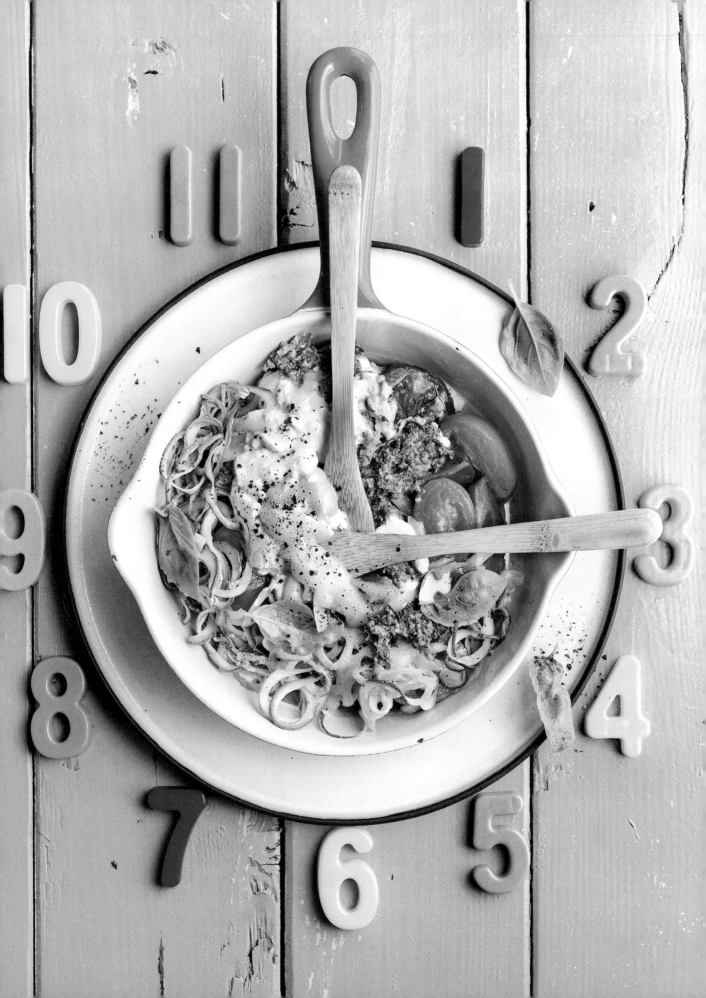

ROAST SWEET POTATO, PUMPKIN AND FETA CAULI-RICE TUMBLE SALAD

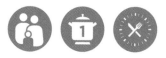

Makes 2-4 portions
Prep time: 20 mins
Cooking time: 45 mins

This is a delicious recipe that works equally well as a salad or as a meal. Add some grilled chicken to bulk it up into something more filling, and try it with other roasted veggies and perhaps some toasted almonds. A little Morrocan spice will turn it into a more sophisticated dish.

1 cup (150g) peeled and diced sweet potato (about 2cm diameter)

1 cup (125g) peeled and diced pumpkin (about 2cm diameter)

3 tablespoons coconut oil, melted

2 tablespoons butter, melted

salt and pepper

2 tablespoons pumpkin seeds

1 head cauliflower, blitzed to rice size in a food processor

2 tablespoons dried cranberries (optional)

a drizzle of olive oil

100g feta or grated mozzarella

- Preheat the oven to 200°C.
- Place the sweet potato and pumpkin on a roasting tray and drizzle with the coconut oil and melted butter. Season with salt and pepper.
- Roast for 35 minutes until soft and gooey.
- Pour the pumpkin seeds into the oven tray and pop it back in the oven for 2 minutes.
- Take the tray out of the oven again and add the cauliflower and dried cranberries. Give it all a good stir and put it back in the oven for a further 5 minutes.
- Take the tray out of the oven and drizzle with the olive oil and stir in the cheese. Check the seasoning before serving.

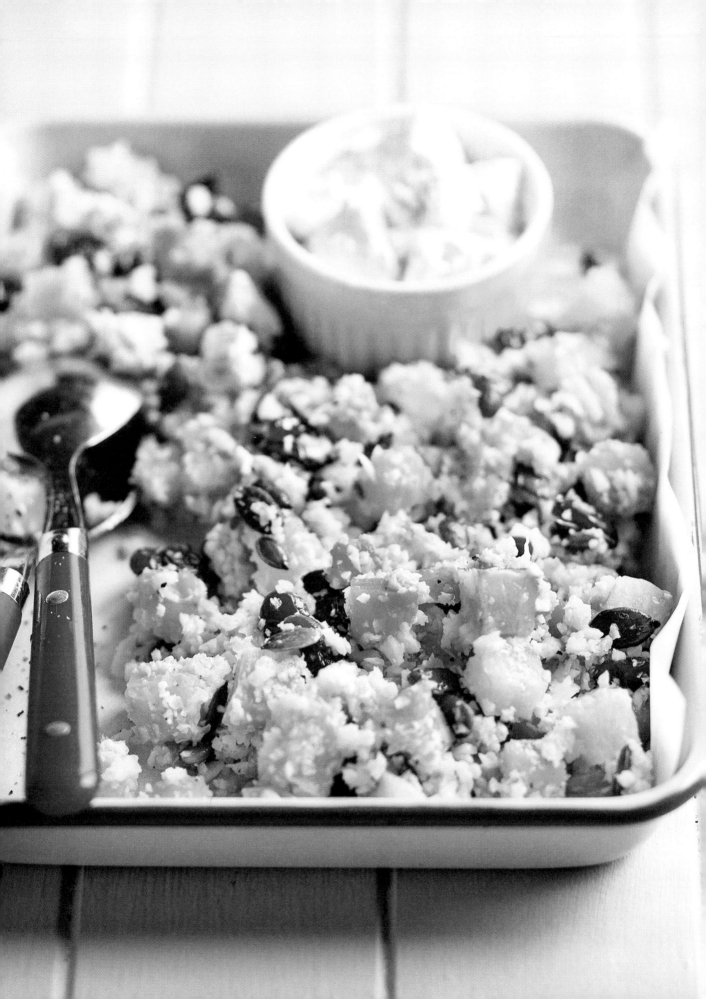

ROASTED CAULIFLOWER AND CHEDDAR SOUP

Makes 4-6 portions
Prep time: 10 mins
Cooking time: 45 mins

This soup is perfect for a chilly winter lunch. Serve it with a buttery Banting roll or some carb-free toast. We took it up a notch and made a grilled cheese-on-toast – extra cheesy and wonderful for winter!

1 onion, peeled and quartered
2 leeks, washed and roughly chopped
1 head cauliflower (about 400g),
  broken into florets
6 cloves garlic
3 tablespoons coconut oil, melted
salt and pepper
1 litre hot chicken stock
200g grated Cheddar

- Preheat the oven to 180°C.
- In a roasting tray, toss the onion, leeks, cauliflower and garlic in the melted coconut oil.
- Season with salt and pepper and roast until soft. Give it a toss every now and then while it's roasting. This should take about 45 minutes.
- Scrape the ingredients into a bowl and add the chicken stock and cheese. Blend until smooth. Add a little extra seasoning if you need to.
- If the soup cools too much during blending, reheat gently.

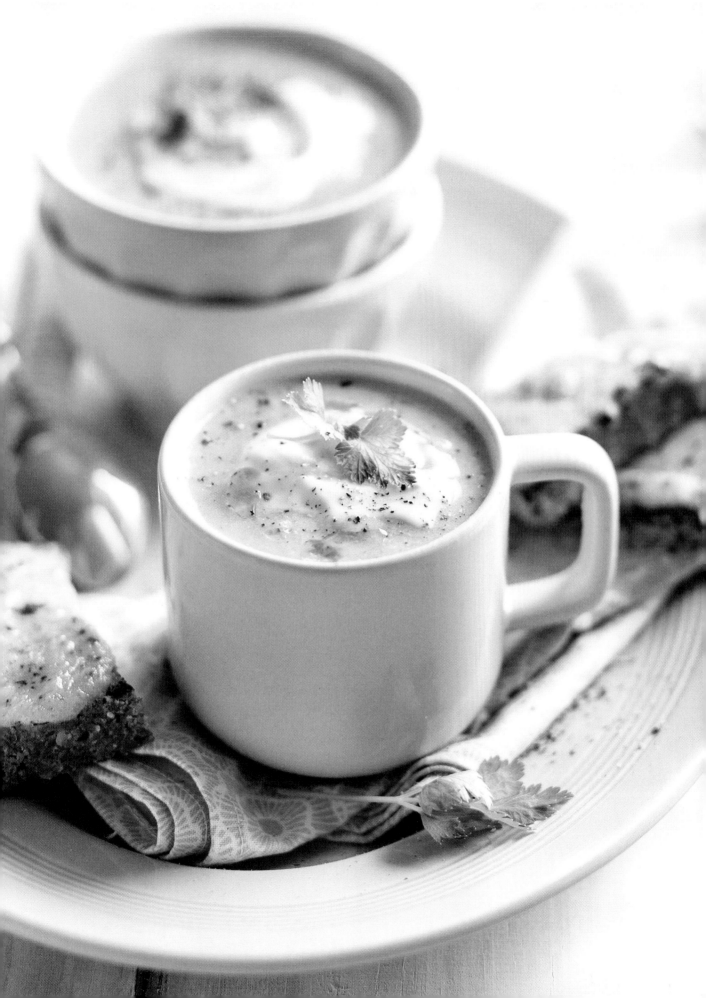

GRILLED AND ROASTED AUBERGINE AND MOZZARELLA OPEN SANDWICH

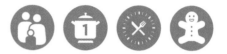

Makes 2 portions
Prep time: 10 mins
Cooking time: 40 mins

These open sandwiches are our answer to a quick 'pizza'. They're simple to make and absolutely delicious. We've gone with cheese and salami as the topping but you could also try ham and cheese, bacon, or even roasted tomato.

2 large aubergines, sliced 1cm thick lengthways
4 tablespoons coconut oil, melted
salt and pepper
½ cup (125ml) secret vegetable tomato sauce (p292)
a few slices of ham or salami (optional)
½ cup (60g) grated mozzarella
a few leaves fresh basil, torn (optional)

- Preheat the oven to 180°C.
- Place the sliced aubergine on a roasting tray and brush with the melted coconut oil. Season with a little salt and pepper.
- Roast the aubergine until soft and slightly browned. This should take about 30 minutes. Remove from the oven. (To speed up the cooking process, you could pan-fry the aubergines for 5 minutes until golden before moving to the next step.)
- Top each slice of aubergine with a little secret vegetable tomato sauce, sliced ham or salami (if you're using it) and grated cheese.
- Bake the topped aubergine slices in the oven for 10 minutes until the cheese is melted and bubbling. Garnish with a little torn basil if you're trying to be fancy.

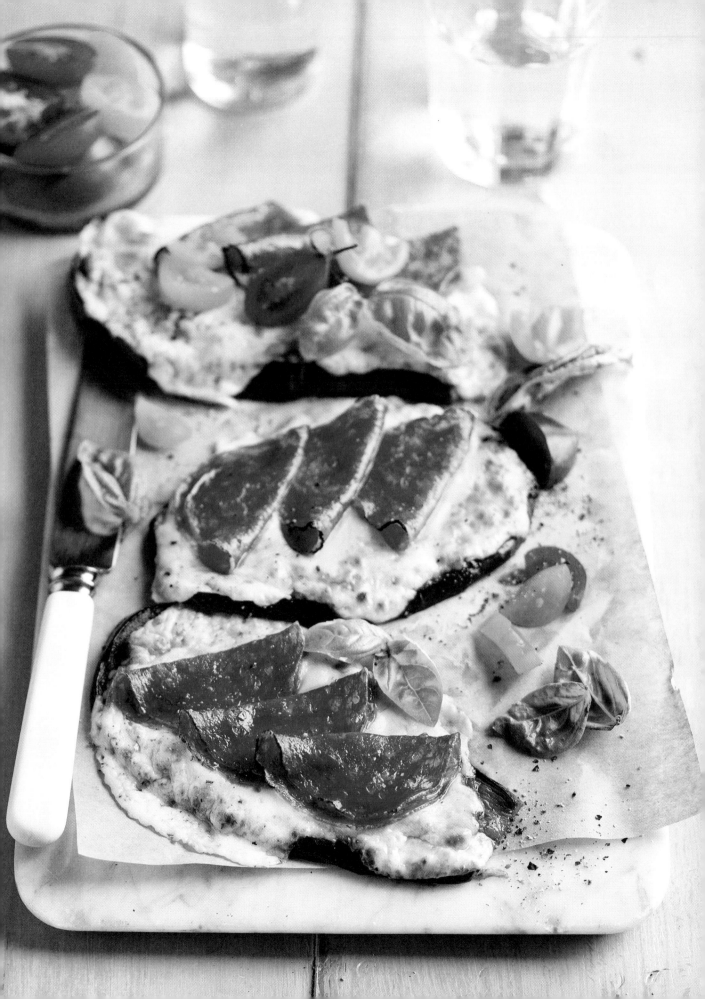

POWER PACKED LUNCHES

Remember the excitement of being a kid and opening your lunchbox to see what was inside? If you had a mum who knew her stuff it might've been the highlight of your school day. Even without the white-bread sarnies and sugar-dipped Twinkies of our past, you can make power-packed lunches that are brimming with flavour. We've put together 10 delicious and nutritious lunchboxes here; make as is or mix and match. And add biltong, salami sticks, chunks of cheese, pieces of fruit and veg, boiled eggs, nuts and other healthy (and fun) extras.

BBQ CHICKEN WINGS .... Makes 8 mini wings (about 2 portions)

4 chicken wings, halved
½ cup (125ml) homemade BBQ
  marinade (p295)

- Preheat the oven to 200°C.
- Toss the chicken wings in the BBQ marinade and place on a baking tray. Roast for 40 minutes until golden and crispy. Allow to cool before putting into the packed lunch.
- These are perfect cooked the night before.

QUICK COLESLAW .... Makes 4 portions

1 carrot, peeled and grated
1 cup (225g) shredded white cabbage
1 cup (225g) shredded red cabbage
4 tablespoons dried cranberries
⅓ cup (85ml) homemade mayo (p301)
salt and pepper

- Mix together all the ingredients and spoon into an airtight container. (If you don't have red cabbage, use white cabbage only.)
- This coleslaw can be made the night before.

SALAMI, CHEESE AND CUCUMBER ROLLS .... Makes 4 rolls

4 slices salami (non-processed)
1 tablespoon cream cheese
8 thin slices Cheddar
½ cucumber cut into matchsticks

- Lay the salami on a board and spread each slice with the cream cheese. Lay the Cheddar cheese over this and pile some cucumber in the centre. Roll the salami up and place in the packed lunch.
- Goes well with vegetable crisps (p218).

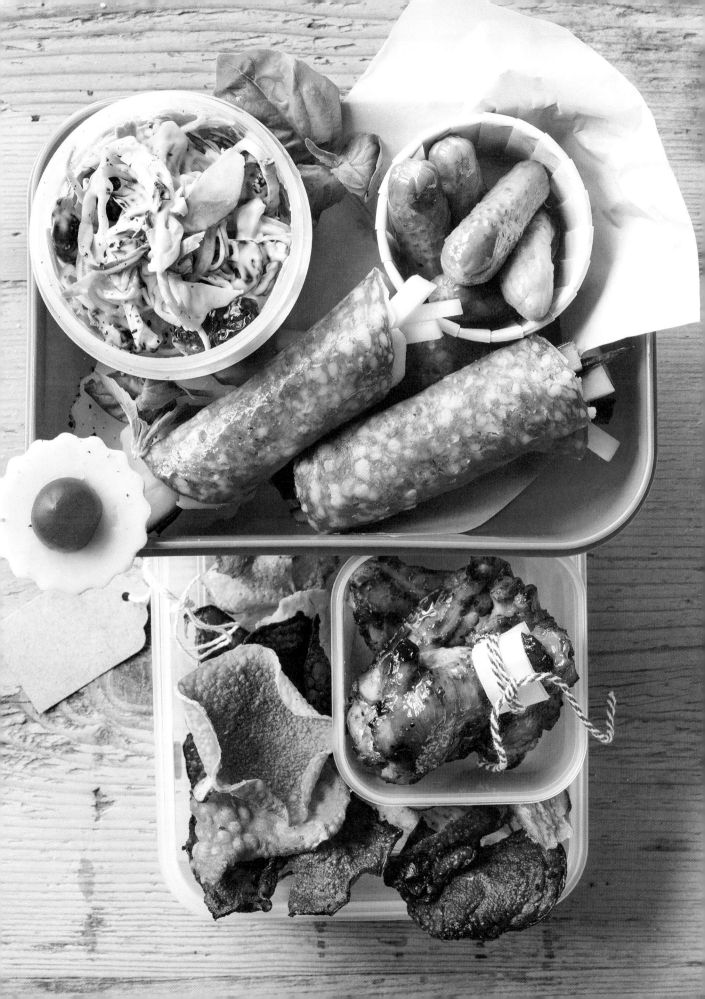

EGG MAYO SALAD

Makes 1 portion

2 hard-boiled eggs, mashed with a fork
2 tablespoons homemade mayo (p301)
1 teaspoon chopped chives
1 teaspoon chopped dill
salt and pepper

- Mix together all the ingredients and season with a little salt and pepper. Include some seed crackers in the lunchbox for dipping.

TUNA AND CUCUMBER SUBS

Makes 2

2 x ¼ cucumbers
1 x 170g tin tuna in spring water, drained well
3 tablespoons homemade mayo (p301)
2 spring onions, finely chopped
a few baby tomatoes, quartered
2 gherkins, chopped
salt, pepper and a squeeze of lemon

- Peel, halve and hollow out the cucumber pieces, and place them on some paper towel to draw out any excess liquid. Discard the cucumber innards.
- In a bowl mix together the remaining ingredients and season with a little salt and pepper. Spoon the tuna mix into the bottom of the hollowed-out cucumber subs.
- Use the top halves of the subs as lids and secure with toothpicks. Pack into a snug airtight container to avoid in-transit destruction.

HAM, APPLE AND CHEESE WRAPS

Makes 4 small wraps

4 slices ham (non-processed)
1 red apple, sliced – sprinkle a little lemon juice on it to stop it going brown
4 slices Cheddar

- Make little wraps using the ham as the wrapping and the cheese and apple as the filling. Secure with toothpicks.

FLAVOURED WATER

Water + fruit, veggies or herbs

- Water is the best choice for your kids to drink, but it can get a little boring. Zhoosh it up with some sliced fruit, veggies or herbs. We've added sliced orange and some mint leaves to the juice bottle in this packed lunch.

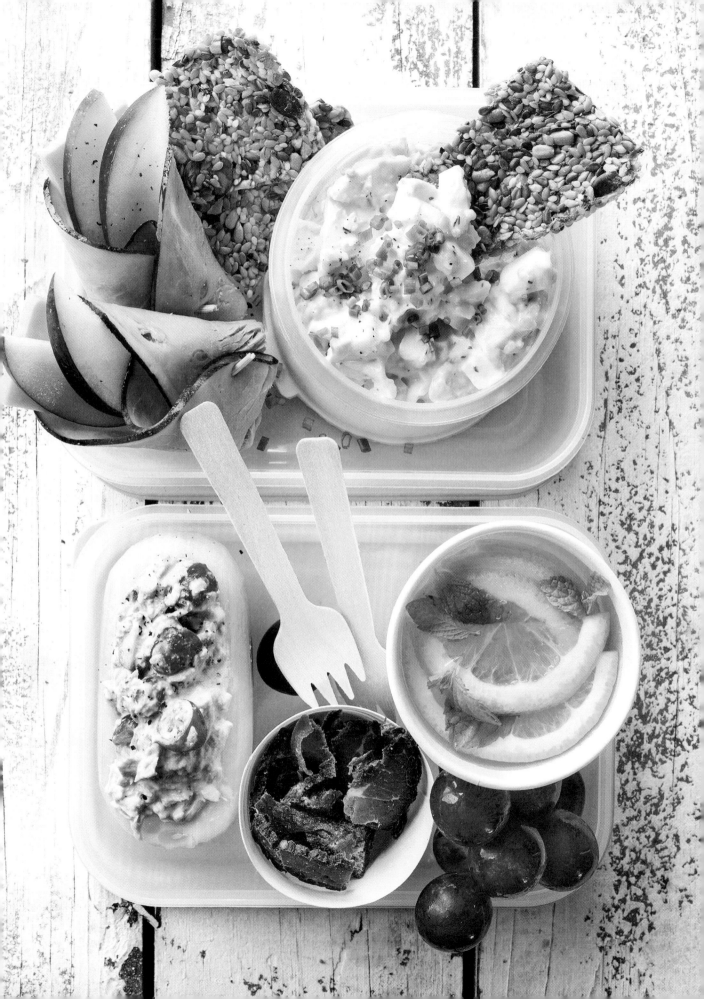

LITTLE EGG, SALMON, CREAM CHEESE AND CUCUMBER ROLLS .... Makes 2 egg rolls

a little coconut oil for greasing
2 eggs, beaten well with a pinch
  of salt
2 tablespoons cream cheese
¼ cucumber, sliced thinly using
  a peeler
50g smoked salmon
dill for garnish (optional)

- Heat a frying pan and grease it with a little coconut oil. Pour half the beaten egg into the pan and make a thin omelette, almost like a pancake. Wait for the egg to lightly brown on one side and flip it over to cook on the other. Repeat with the remaining egg mixture. Lay the omelettes out on a board.
- Spread the omelettes with the cream cheese and top with the cucumber and smoked salmon. Roll them up tightly into a cigar shape and slice into thick rounds. We put ours on skewers with a few cucumber stars.

PORK BANGERS WITH HOMEMADE KETCHUP .... Makes 2 portions

8 mini pork sausages (grain free)
4 tablespoons homemade ketchup
  (p294)

- Preheat the grill of your oven and place the bangers on an oven tray. Grill until golden, then turn over and repeat on the other side.
- These are perfect cooked the night before.
- Serve with homemade ketchup.

MUSTARD DIP WITH CRUDITÉS .... Makes 1 cup

225g cream cheese
2 tablespoons chopped chives
3 tablespoons wholegrain mustard
assorted dipping vegetables like
  carrots, celery, mangetout,
  cucumber, baby tomatoes

- Mix together the ingredients for the dip and season if necessary. Pop it in a small Tupperware in the lunchbox, along with the crunchy veggies.

BANANA, STRAWBERRY AND VANILLA SMOOTHIE .... Makes 1 smoothie

⅓ cup (85g) sugar-free vanilla yoghurt
2 tablespoons homemade granola
  (optional) (p156)
1 banana, peeled and roughly sliced
¼ cup (50g) sliced fresh strawberries

- Blend all the ingredients together until smooth. Pop into a bottle and place either in the fridge or the freezer until the kids are ready for school. (You can add a dash of milk if you think it's a bit thick.)

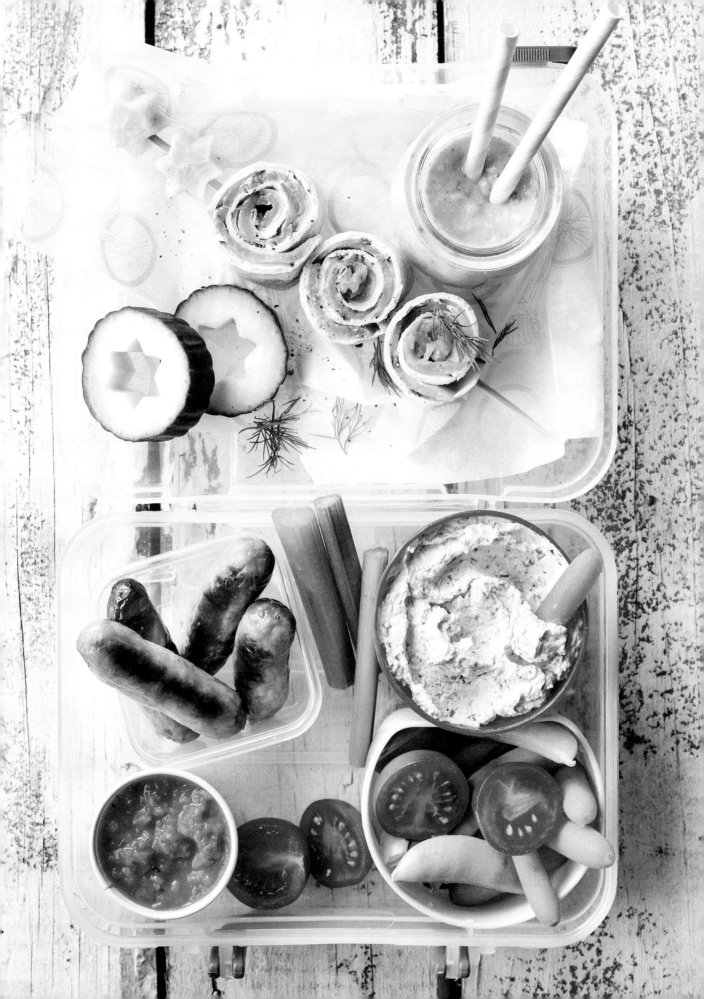

CHICKEN, APPLE AND YOGHURT SALAD IN LETTUCE CUPS .... Makes 2 portions

1 cup (140g) cubed roast chicken
1 red apple, cubed
¼ stalk celery, sliced
2 tablespoons homemade mayo
  (p301)
2 tablespoons Greek yoghurt
1 teaspoon chopped parsley
salt and pepper
a few baby gem lettuce leaves

- Mix together all the ingredients except the lettuce leaves, and season with a little salt and pepper. Spoon into an airtight container for your lunchbox and serve with the lettuce leaves. Don't forget to pack a spoon so your kids can fill the lettuce cups.

PORK-SAUSAGE-AND-SPINACH ORBS WITH CHEDDAR CHEESE .... Makes about 12

250g pork sausage filling
100g spinach, blanched, all the water
  squeezed out and chopped
1 tablespoon chopped parsley
½ cup (50g) grated Cheddar
2 tablespoons butter for frying

- Preheat the oven to 200°C.
- Mix together all the ingredients except the butter. Wet your hands and roll the mixture into 12 balls.
- Heat the butter in a frying pan and fry the balls until golden brown. Pop on a baking tray and bake for about 8 minutes to make sure they are cooked through.
- These are perfect cooked the night before.

HOMEMADE HUMMUS WITH VEGGIE DIPPERS .... Makes 2 cups

1 x 400g tin chickpeas, drained
the juice of 1 lemon
1 clove garlic
2 tablespoons olive oil
2 tablespoons tahini
½ teaspoon ground cumin
salt and pepper
smoked paprika (optional)

- Blend together all the ingredients in a food processor until smooth. Season to taste with salt and pepper. If the hummus is too thick, thin it down with a little water or the liquid that was drained off the chickpeas. Sprinkle with a little smoked paprika if you like.
- Serve with crunchy veg to dip, such as cucumber and blanched broccoli.

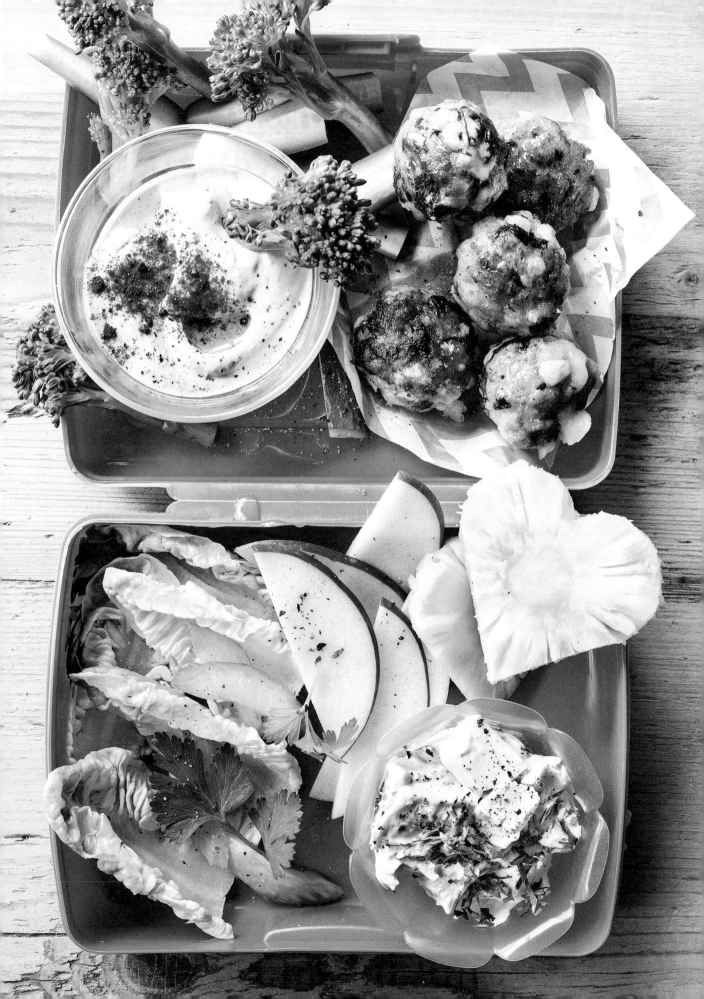

QUINOA CHICKEN POPS
Makes 3 portions

⅓ cup (30g) chickpea flour
salt and pepper
2 chicken breasts, cubed into
  8 pieces each
2 eggs, beaten
1 ½ cups (275g) cooked and well-
  drained quinoa
coconut oil for frying

- Season the chickpea flour with salt and pepper.
- Dip the chicken pieces into the seasoned chickpea flour, then into the egg and finally into the quinoa. Use your hands to make sure the chicken is completely covered.
- Heat the coconut oil in a pan and fry the chicken pops until golden on both sides and cooked through. Serve with homemade ketchup (p294).

HAM AND CHEESE MAKI
Makes 2 portions

4 slices ham (non-processed)
2 tablespoons cream cheese
8 slices Cheddar

- Lay the ham on a board and spread with the cream cheese. Lay out the Cheddar cheese on top of the cream cheese.
- Roll the ham into a cigar and cut into slices about 3cm thick.

AVO-AND-CUCUMBER SUSHI
Makes 2 portions

1 sheet nori, cut in half
½ avo, cut into wedges
¼ cucumber, cut into wedges
4 tablespoons cream cheese
1 carrot, julienned or shredded

- Place a piece of nori on a sushi mat and position some avo, cucumber, cream cheese and carrot in a horizontal line at the bottom of the nori.
- Roll it tightly in the mat to make a sausage. Wet the edge of the nori to make it stick. Slice into 2 centimetre pieces. Repeat with the other nori sheet and remaining filling.

BANANA MILK
Makes 1 portion

1 cup (250ml) milk
1 banana, peeled and roughly chopped
1 teaspoon vanilla extract

- Blend all the ingredients together and pour into a water bottle. This is best chilled overnight.

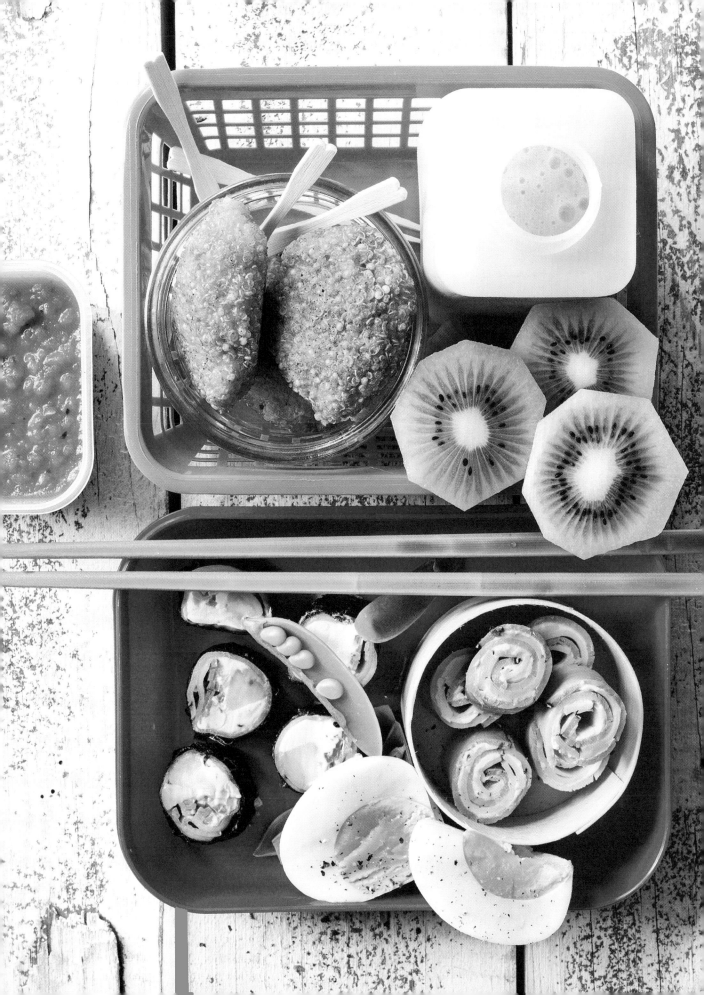

TUNA BITES .... Makes 8-10

2 x 170g tins tuna in spring water,
  well drained
2 tablespoons chickpea flour
2 eggs
1 teaspoon lemon zest
2 spring onions, chopped
1 teaspoon chopped parsley
1 teaspoon chopped chives
2 tablespoons butter for frying

- Mix together all the ingredients except the butter, and season with a little salt and pepper.
- Roll the mixture into mini cakes.
- Heat the butter in a pan and fry the tuna bites until golden on each side. Allow to cool and serve with homemade mayo (p301).

BACON-AND-BANANA ROLLS .... Makes 10 rolls

2 bananas, peeled and sliced
  into 5 pieces
250g streaky bacon

- Preheat the oven to 200°C.
- Roll each piece of banana in a slice of bacon and place on an oven tray. Use a toothpick to secure the bacon if necessary.
- Bake for 20 minutes, until the bacon is crispy. These can also be fried in a pan or cooked on the barbecue.

QUICK BEETROOT-AND-ORANGE SALAD .... Makes 2 portions

3 cooked beetroots, peeled and cut
  into wedges
1 orange, peeled and segmented
  – reserve the juice
¼ red onion, thinly sliced and rinsed
a drizzle of olive oil

- Mix together all the ingredients, including the orange juice, and drizzle with a little olive oil.

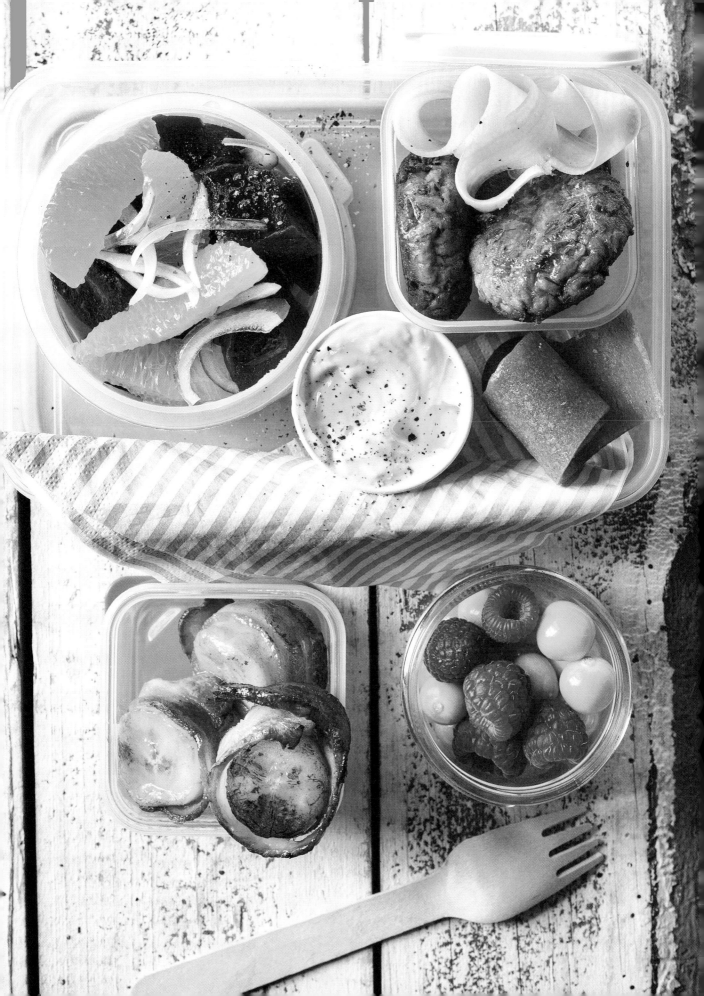

HERB-GRILLED CHICKEN STRIPS

Makes 2 portions

1 tablespoon herb rub
1 teaspoon melted coconut oil
1 chicken breast, sliced into strips
salt and pepper

- Heat a grill pan until smoking hot.
- Mix the coconut oil and herb rub and massage into the chicken. Season with salt and pepper.
- Cook the chicken strips on the grill pan until golden and cooked through.

CUCUMBER-AND-YOGHURT DIP

Makes ³⁄₄ cup dip

½ cup (75g) finely diced cucumber
1 teaspoon chopped mint
¼ cup (70g) Greek yoghurt
salt and pepper

- Mix together all the ingredients and seal in an airtight container.
- Goes well with chicken strips or any crunchy vegetables.

GREEN EGGS AND HAM FRITTATA

Makes 6 frittata

75g ham, roughly chopped
¼ cup (25g) grated cheese
6 eggs, beaten
2 tablespoons milk
salt and pepper
50g cooked spinach

- Preheat the oven to 180°C and grease a 6-cup muffin pan.
- Divide the ham and cheese between the 6 cups of the muffin pan.
- Beat together the eggs, milk, salt and pepper.
- Pour the egg mixture into the muffin pans, leaving about 50ml behind. Blend the spinach into the remaining egg using a hand-blender and pour a little bit of the green egg into each frittata.
- Bake for 25 minutes, until the egg has set.

CARROT-AND-PINEAPPLE SALAD

Makes 2 portions

1 cup (90g) grated carrot
¼ cup (40g) sultanas
½ cup (110g) chopped pineapple
2 tablespoons toasted sunflower seeds
the juice of half an orange
salt and pepper

- Mix together all the ingredients. Season with a little salt and pepper.

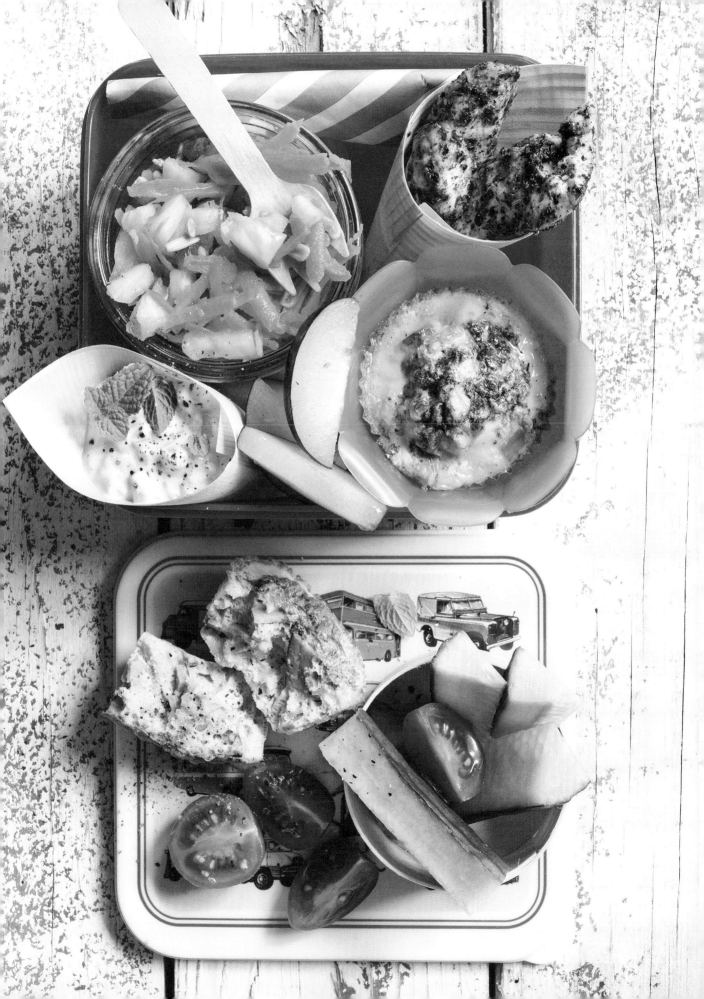

COURGETTE-AND-MOZZARELLA FRITTERS .... Makes about 12 fritters

4 courgettes, grated and squeezed
out in a cloth
1 tablespoon chopped mint
2 teaspoons arrowroot powder
2 eggs, beaten
⅓ cup (40g) grated mozzarella
2 tablespoons butter for frying
salt and pepper
Greek yoghurt to serve

- In a bowl, mix together all the ingredients except the butter, and season well with salt and pepper.
- Heat the butter in a frying pan and spoon the courgette mixture, about a tablespoon for each fritter, into the pan. Fry until golden on the one side and repeat on the other side.
- Serve with a little Greek yoghurt.

REUBEN SARNIE STICKS .... Make 2 skewers

4 slices pastrami
6 cubes Cheddar
3 mini gherkins, halved

- Divide the ingredients in half and skewer onto a kebab stick. Repeat with the remaining ingredients.
- Serve with a little mustard. Add some cherry tomatoes too if your kids enjoy them.

EGG, BACON AND AVO SANDWICH .... Makes 1 sandwich

2 thin slices low-carb bread (p296)
3 slices bacon, cooked until crispy
1 hard-boiled egg, peeled and sliced
½ an avo, peeled and sliced, with
a little lemon juice squeezed over it
soft butter for spreading

- Make a sandwich!

Some other sandwich fillings:
- Chicken and mayo with apple
- Tuna mayo salad
- Egg mayo salad
- Ham, cheese and gherkin with mayo
- Salami, cheese and mayo
- Crispy bacon and fried banana
- Pastrami, gherkin, cheese and coleslaw
- Leftover lamb, mint, cream cheese and tomato

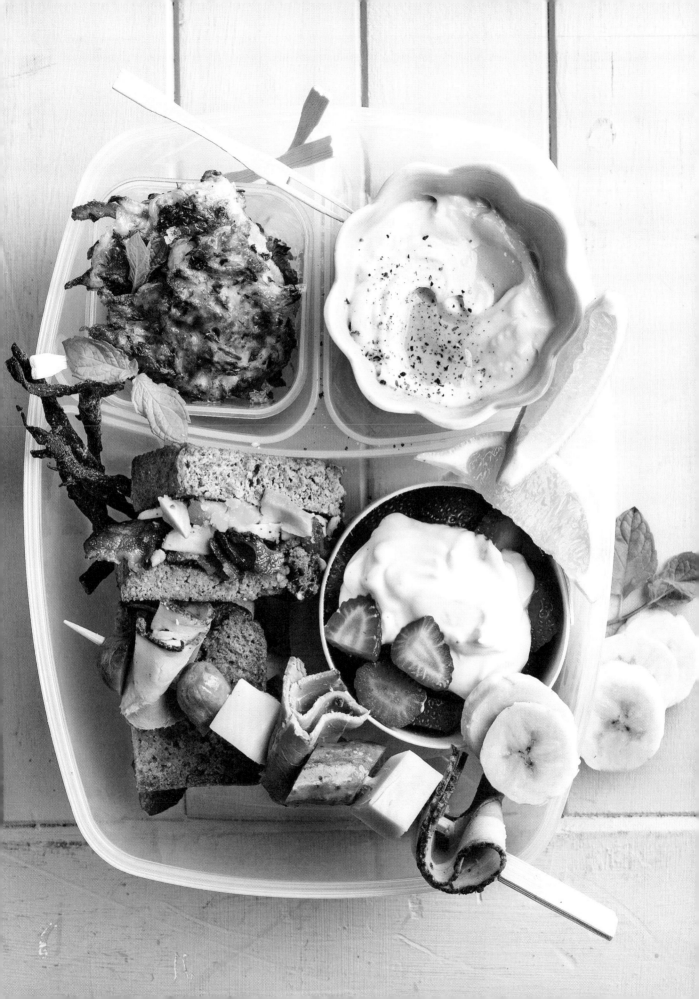

CHEESE-AND-HERB MUFFINS .... Makes 12 muffins

1 ½ cups (150g) almond flour
½ cup (60g) coconut flour
2 teaspoons baking powder
2 tablespoons chopped fresh herbs
  like parsley, basil, thyme or chives
1½-2 cups (150-200g) grated Cheddar
2 spring onions, sliced
3 eggs
¾ cup (90g) Greek yoghurt
⅓ cup (75g) melted butter

- Preheat the oven to 180°C.
- Line a muffin pan with 12 paper muffin cups.
- Sieve the almond four, coconut flour and baking powder into a bowl and stir in the herbs, cheese and spring onions.
- In a separate bowl whisk together the eggs, yoghurt and melted butter.
- Mix the wet and dry ingredients together.
- Spoon the mixture into the muffin cups and bake for 30 minutes until cooked.
- These muffins will freeze like a dream, so serve what you need and freeze the rest.

QUICK CAULI TABBOULEH .... Makes 2 portions

1 cup (100g) cauliflower, blitzed in the
  food processor
¼ cucumber, diced
a handful of cherry tomatoes, halved
1 tablespoon chopped parsley
juice and zest of 1 lemon
a drizzle of olive oil
salt and pepper

- Mix together all the ingredients, and season with salt and pepper.
- Add a little leftover chicken, if you have any, or whatever else your kids might fancy.
- Pop it all in an airtight container, and don't forget to pack a fork.

GRILLED AUBERGINE, TOMATO, BASIL AND MOZZARELLA ROLL-UPS .... Makes 6 rolls

1 large aubergine sliced lengthways
  into 6 pieces
a drizzle of olive oil
salt and pepper
6 slices mozzarella
2 tomatoes, thinly sliced
a few basil leaves

- Heat a griddle pan until smoking hot and grill the aubergine slices until they have grill lines on both sides. Take out of the pan, drizzle with a little olive oil, and season with salt and pepper.
- Roll up each aubergine slice with the mozzarella, tomato and basil inside. Secure with a skewer or toothpick.

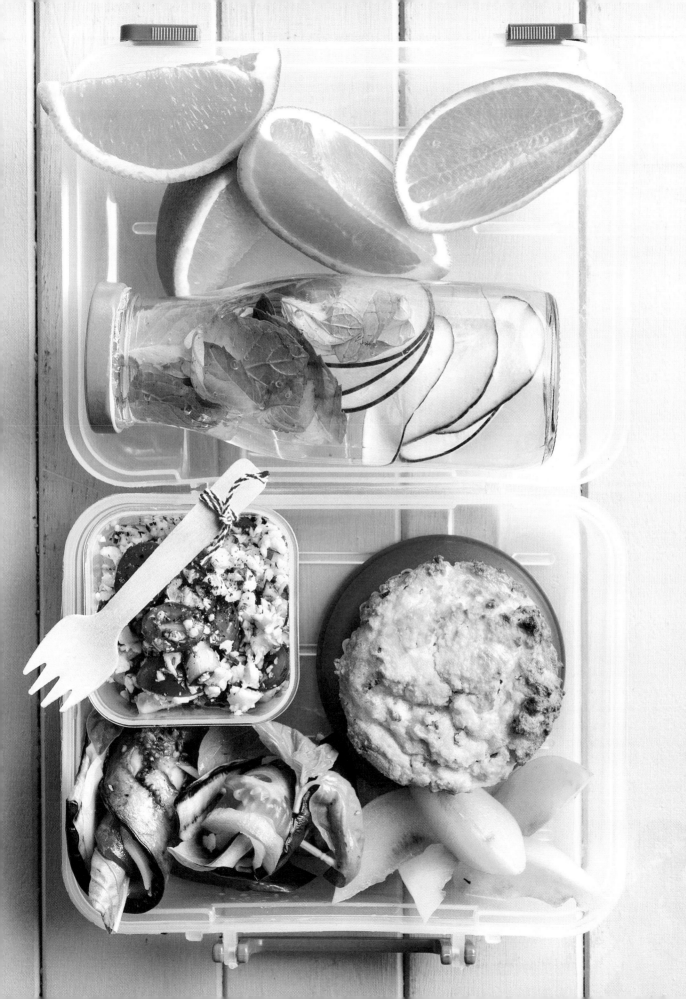

QUICK SCOTCH EGGS .... Makes 2

100g pork sausage meat (2 pork
   sausages)
2 tablespoons chopped parsley
salt and pepper
2 medium eggs, cooked in boiling
   water for 8 minutes and peeled
a little butter for frying

- Preheat the oven to 180°C and grease 2 small sheets of tin foil.
- Mix the sausage meat with the parsley and some salt and pepper.
- Wet your hands and carefully cover the boiled eggs with a thin layer of the pork mixture. Pop the eggs on to the greased tin foil and roll into a Christmas-cracker shape. Bake for 10-12 minutes.
- Heat the butter in a frying pan and fry the eggs until lightly golden. Serve with homemade mayo (p301).

CHICKEN CAESAR LETTUCE WRAPS WITH AVO .... Makes 4 salad wraps

8 baby gem lettuce leaves
150g cooked chicken
8 slices streaky bacon, cooked
30g parmesan shavings
1 avocado, sliced with a little lemon
   juice drizzled on top
homemade mayo (p301)

- Make a cup for each wrap using 2 lettuce leaves, and fill with the various fillings. Roll and secure using a strip of silicone paper.

CHICKPEA SALAD JAR .... Makes 2 medium-sized salads

100g cooked chickpeas
olive oil
salt and pepper
4 courgettes, sliced and roasted –
   or any leftover cooked veggies
a handful of sugar snaps, blanched
20g feta
a handful of fresh spinach leaves
salt and pepper

- Drizzle a little olive oil at the bottom of two glass jars with some salt and pepper.
- Layer the ingredients into the jar, finishing off with the spinach leaves.
- To eat, just give the jar a shake and it's good to go. Salad jars are a great way to use up leftover ingredients. Just remember to keep the lettuce at the top and the dressing at the bottom.

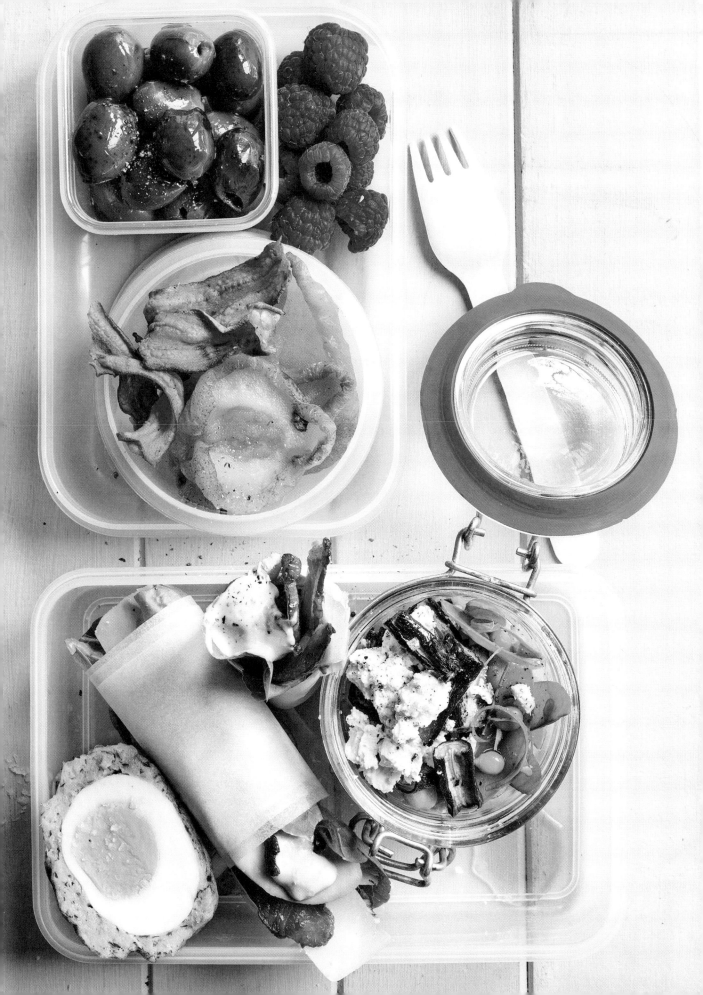

LANCASHIRE HOT POT WITH CRISPY SWEET POTATO TOPPING

Makes 4 portions
Prep time: 25 mins
Cooking time: 2 ½ hours

This rich and delicious creation is our answer to a warming winter pie. You can't rush it, so let it quietly bubble away while you get on with the day. Kidneys are a highly recommended super food for growing kids, but aren't to everyone's taste; leave them out if you prefer.

1.2kg lamb neck, sliced

salt and pepper

4 tablespoons butter and/or lard

4 lamb kidneys, cored, skinned and chopped quite small (optional)

500g onions, peeled and quartered

850ml beef stock

2 teaspoons Worcestershire sauce

1 bay leaf

3 sprigs fresh thyme

500g sweet potato, peeled and thinly sliced

melted butter for brushing

- Preheat the oven to 160°C.
- Season the lamb neck well with salt and pepper.
- Heat the butter and/or lard in a large, deep frying pan and brown the meat, a few pieces at a time, until golden on all sides. Set aside. Do the same with the kidneys.
- Heat a wide, flat casserole pot. Add a little more butter and/or lard, and slowly fry the onions until golden brown and soft.
- Add the meat and give everything a good stir to combine.
- Slowly pour in the stock and the Worcestershire sauce. Add the bay leaf and the fresh thyme and bring everything to a simmer. Simmer very gently for about 1 ½ hours until the meat starts to soften and the sauce thickens. Season with salt and pepper.
- Arrange the sweet potato slices in a circular pattern on top of the meat, overlapping each one as you go. Brush with the melted butter and season with salt and pepper.
- Cover the casserole dish with a tight-fitting lid and place in the oven for 30 minutes.
- Take the lid off, turn the oven up to 190°C and cook for a further 20 minutes.
- Turn on the oven grill and grill the casserole for a minute or two to crisp up the potatoes.
- Serve hot.

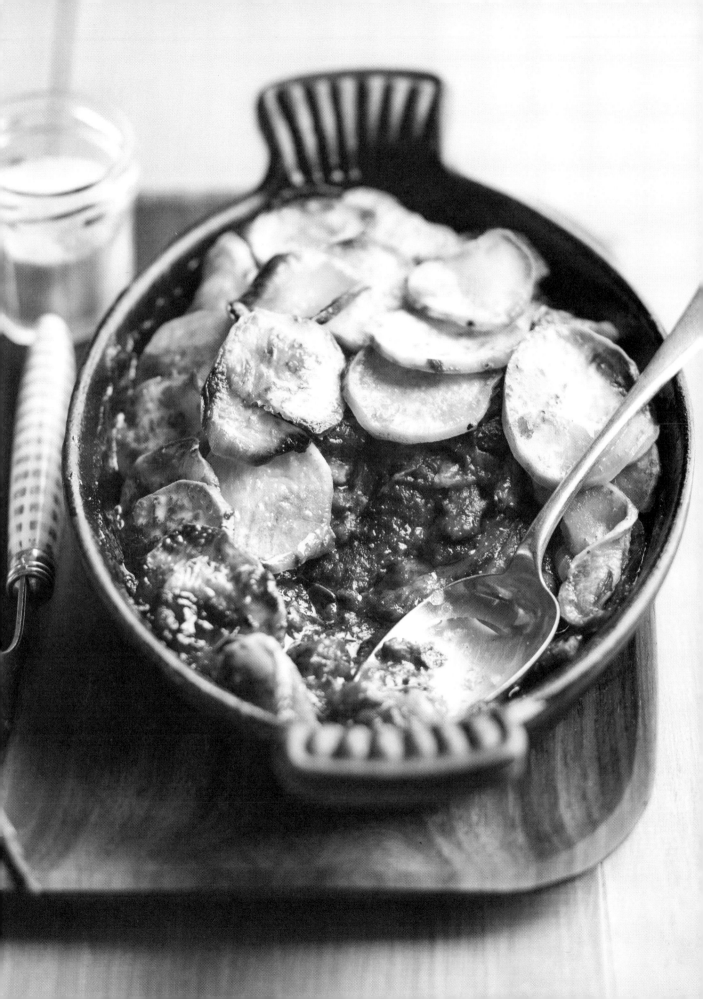

VEGGIE-PACKED BOBOTIE

Makes 6 to 8 servings
Prep time: 20 mins
Cooking time: 45 mins

This South African classic is a family favourite and a brilliant vessel for secret vegetables. We've kept our version quite mild in flavour; add a little more curry powder to spice it up for more adventurous kids.

5 tablespoons butter
1 onion, chopped
2 carrots, peeled and chopped
1 red pepper, seeded and chopped
1 cup (225g) grated courgette
1 tablespoon grated fresh ginger
3 cloves garlic, crushed
1 tablespoon mild curry powder
1 teaspoon turmeric
2 teaspoons ground cumin
2 teaspoons ground coriander
3 whole cloves
5 whole allspice
2 tablespoons honey (optional)
1 tablespoon red wine vinegar
1 x 400g tin whole peeled tomatoes, blended
800g beef mince
1 teaspoon dried mixed herbs
salt and pepper

For the custard:
1 cup (250ml) milk
2 eggs, beaten
8 bay leaves

- Preheat the oven to 180°C.
- Melt the butter in a wide-based pot and gently fry the onion, carrots, red pepper and courgette until soft. Stir in the ginger and the garlic and fry for a minute or so. Add the spices and fry for another minute to release their flavour.
- Pour in the honey, vinegar and tomato, and bring to the boil.
- Mix in the remaining ingredients, ensuring that everything is combined well; you don't want meatballs in your mince.
- Cook for about 15 minutes, stirring all the time. When it's done, season well with salt and pepper.
- Spread the mixture in a greased ovenproof dish.
- To make the custard, lightly beat together the milk and the eggs.
- Press the bay leaves into the bobotie mixture and carefully pour over the custard.
- Bake for about 30 minutes, until the egg topping has set.

ONCE COOKED, THIS BOBOTIE FREEZES LIKE A BOMB. YOU CAN EASILY DOUBLE THE RECIPE SO YOU HAVE LEFTOVERS TO FREEZE

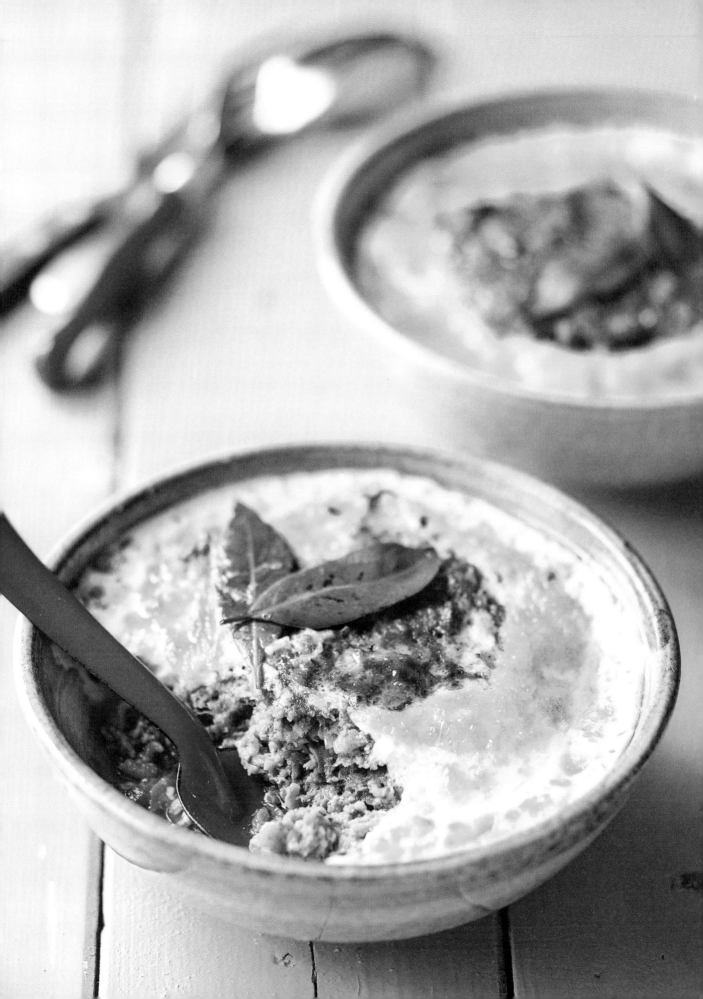

ONION AND FENNEL PORK CHOPS WITH APPLE

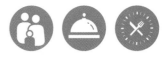

Makes 4 portions
Prep time: 15 mins
Cooking time: 20 mins

Everybody loves a pork chop, and this recipe will be a hit with the whole family. We make no excuses for the predictable (read: classic) flavours; they just work so well. Use the biggest, deepest frying pan you have and keep the heat high.

4 thick-cut pork chops
salt and pepper
3 tablespoons butter
1 onion, thinly sliced
2 fennel bulbs, thinly sliced
1 unpeeled Granny Smith apple,
  cored and sliced
1 cup (250ml) chicken stock
a handful of sage leaves

- Season the pork chops with salt and pepper.
- Melt the butter in a heavy-based frying pan on a high heat until it starts foaming.
- Fry the pork chops in the pan for about 4 minutes on each side until golden; they should be cooked medium at this point.
- Remove the chops from the pan, wrap in foil to keep warm, and set aside.
- Add the onion and fennel to the pan and fry until they start to soften. Add the apple and fry for a further minute or two. Pour the chicken stock into the pan and cook on very high heat until the liquid is reduced by half. This should take about 5 minutes. Stir in most of the sage leaves and season with a little salt and pepper.
- Place the chops on a platter, pour over the fennel and onion with the sauce, and top with the remaining fresh sage leaves.
- Serve with creamy cauli-mash, some pan-fried baby leeks and a fresh salad.

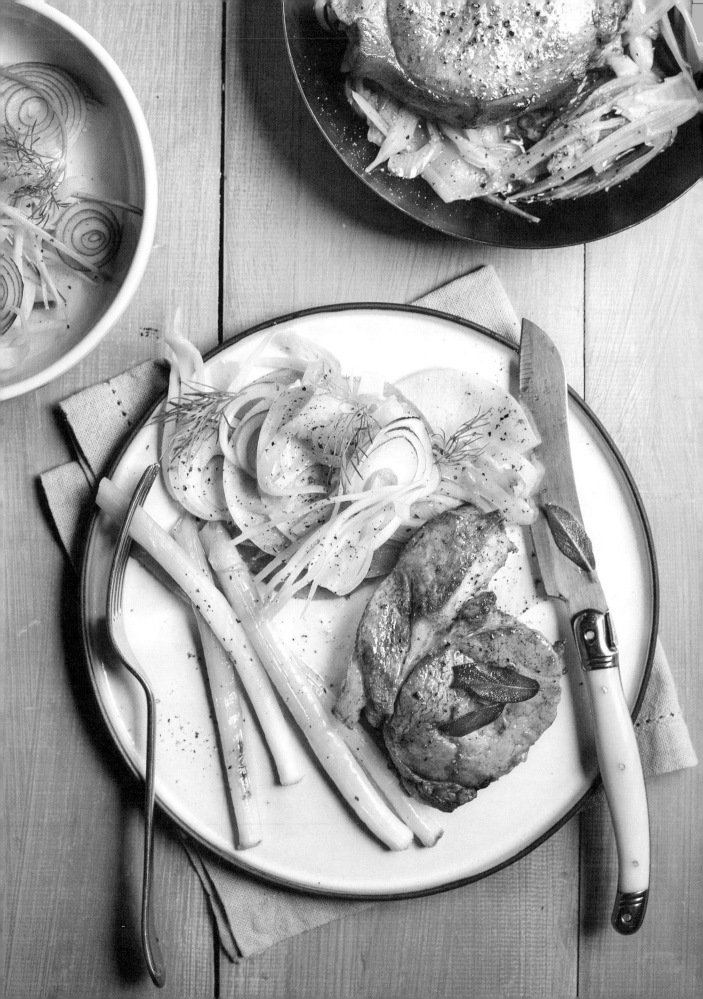

CREAMY BEEF STROGANOFF ON BUTTERED CABBAGE

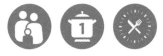

Makes 4 portions
Prep time: 15 mins
Cooking time: 15 mins

This is an old-fashioned recipe that gets a bump up to the next level when it's made with sour cream. If you're worried your kids may not be too keen on the mustard, halve the suggested amount and add more to taste at the end.

700g beef fillet, cut into strips about 1cm wide
salt and pepper
4 tablespoons butter
1 large onion, thinly sliced
1 tablespoon sweet paprika
350g button mushrooms, thinly sliced
300ml sour cream
2 tablespoon mild mustard (like Dijon)
the juice of half a lemon
2 tablespoons chopped fresh parsley

For the buttered cabbage:
3 cups (350g) finely shredded cabbage
3 tablespoons butter
salt and pepper

- Season the beef strips with salt and pepper.
- In a large frying pan, melt 2 tablespoons butter until hot, then fry the beef strips in batches until just browned. This should take literally a minute or two. Remove from the pan and set aside.
- Add the remaining butter to the pan and fry the onion until soft and sweet. Add the paprika and fry for a minute.
- Add the mushrooms and fry for a further 3 minutes until just soft. Add the sour cream and simmer for 2 minutes until thickened.
- Stir in the seared beef and mustard and warm through.
- Stir in the lemon juice and the chopped parsley and season with a little salt and pepper.
- To make the cabbage, fry it in a hot pan with the butter until soft. Season with a little salt and pepper.

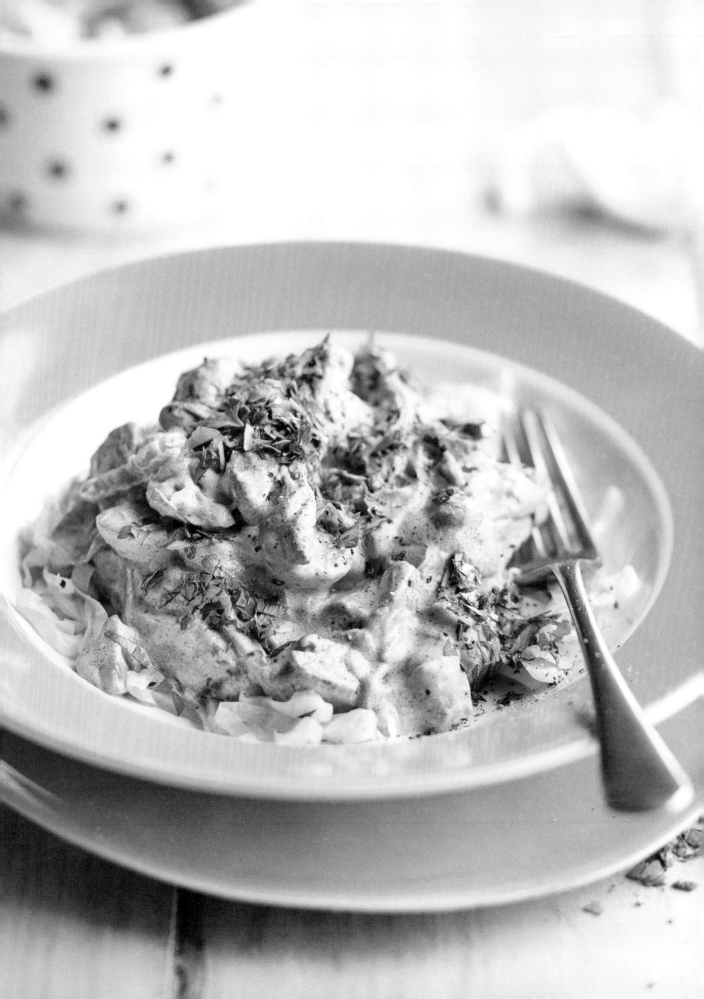

BEEFY PANCAKE CANNELLONI WITH MOZZARELLA

Makes 6 portions
Prep time: 45 mins
Cooking time: 1 ½ hours

This dish may sound like something of a mission to make, but it's perfect for special occasions and it'll be worth it when you see your family digging in. You can also ease the burden with good preparation; the pancakes, beef mince and tomato sauce can all be made in advance.

12 low-carb pancakes (p300)

For the filling:
2 tablespoons butter
1 onion, chopped
2 cloves garlic, chopped
2 carrots, grated
1 celery stalk, chopped
800g beef mince
250g button mushrooms, sliced
1 x 400g tin whole peeled tomatoes, blended
2 tablespoons tomato paste
1 cup (250ml) red wine
1 cup (250ml) beef stock
1 bay leaf
1 tablespoon dried mixed herbs
salt and pepper

For the tomato sauce:
2 cups (500ml) secret vegetable tomato sauce (p292)

For the topping:
a few basil leaves
2 x 125g balls mozzarella, sliced

- Preheat the oven to 180°C.

TO MAKE THE FILLING:
- Heat the butter in a medium-sized pot until hot and gently fry the onion, garlic, carrot and celery until soft.
- Crumble the mince and add it to the pot, using a spatula to make sure there aren't any lumps. Cook until browned.
- Add the remaining ingredients, except the salt and pepper, and bring to the boil. Reduce the heat to medium and simmer for about 45 minutes. Stir every now and then to make sure it doesn't stick.
- Once the sauce has reduced and thickened sufficiently, take it off the heat and season with salt and pepper.

TO ASSEMBLE THE DISH:
- Spread a few tablespoons of tomato sauce at the bottom of a greased lasagne dish.
- Spoon a few tablespoons of the mince mixture into a pancake and roll it up into a tube. Lay the pancake in the lasagne dish and repeat with the remaining pancakes to cover the bottom of the dish.
- Spoon the remaining tomato sauce over the pancakes and spread it out evenly. Tear a few basil leaves over the top of the sauce.
- Arrange the sliced mozzarella over the top of the tomato and basil.
- Bake for 35-40 minutes, until golden brown and bubbling.

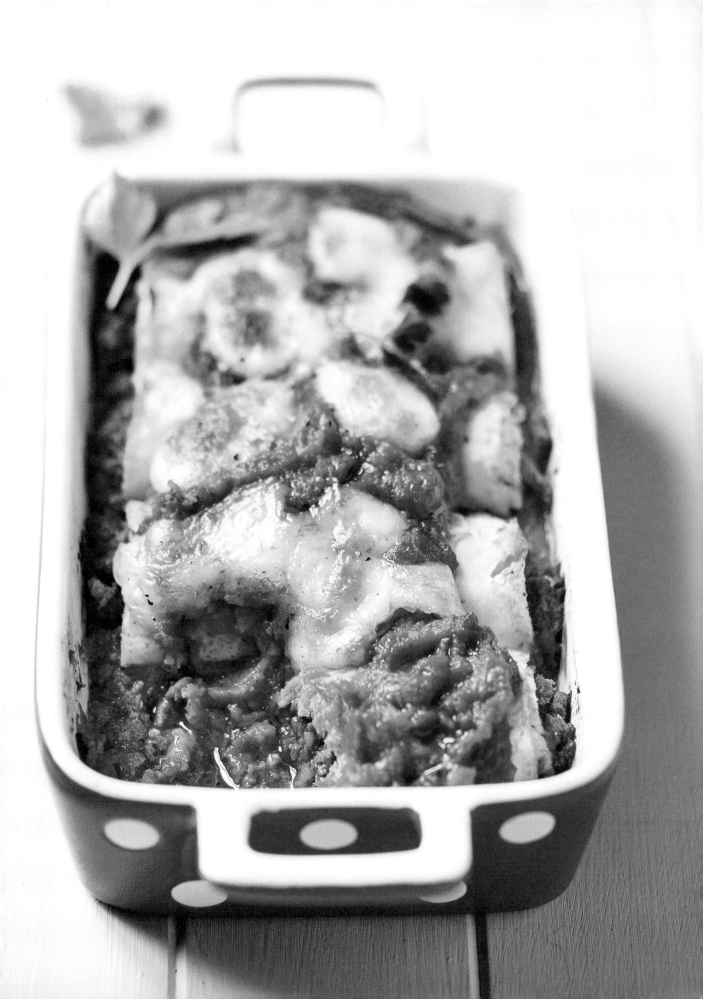

CAULI 'MAC-N-CHEESE' WITH THE WORKS

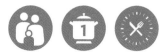

Makes 4 portions
Prep time: 15 mins
Cooking time: 40 mins

Here's another cheesy recipe but, unlike the previous one, it's quick and easy to make – a perfect midweek supper. It's also great with broccoli, though broccoli doesn't give it quite the same mac-n-cheese look...

salt and pepper
2 large heads cauliflower, cut into florets (about 700g)
500ml heavy cream
125ml cream cheese
2 teaspoons Dijon mustard
3 cups (300g) grated cheese
1 tablespoon butter
250g bacon, sliced
250g cherry tomatoes, halved

- Preheat the oven to 180°C.
- Fill a large pot with water and bring it to the boil. Add a little bit of salt to the water and add the cauliflower. Simmer the cauliflower for 5-7 minutes until just soft. Drain well and set aside.
- Pour the cream into a small pot and bring it to the boil. Simmer for 5 minutes. Remove from the heat and stir in the cream cheese, mustard and 2 cups (200g) grated cheese. Season with a little salt and pepper.
- While the cream is cooking, heat the butter in a frying pan and gently fry the bacon until crispy. Remove from the frying pan and set aside. Be sure to leave the bacon fat in the pan.
- Add the tomatoes to the hot pan and fry them in the bacon fat until they start to soften. Season well with salt and pepper and set aside.
- Place the cauliflower in an ovenproof dish and sprinkle with the bacon and fried tomato. Stir well and season with salt and pepper.
- Pour the cream mixture over the cauliflower, ensuring it's all covered. Top with the remaining grated cheese.
- Bake for about 20 minutes, until the cheese is melted and golden and the sauce is bubbling.
- Serve with a green salad.

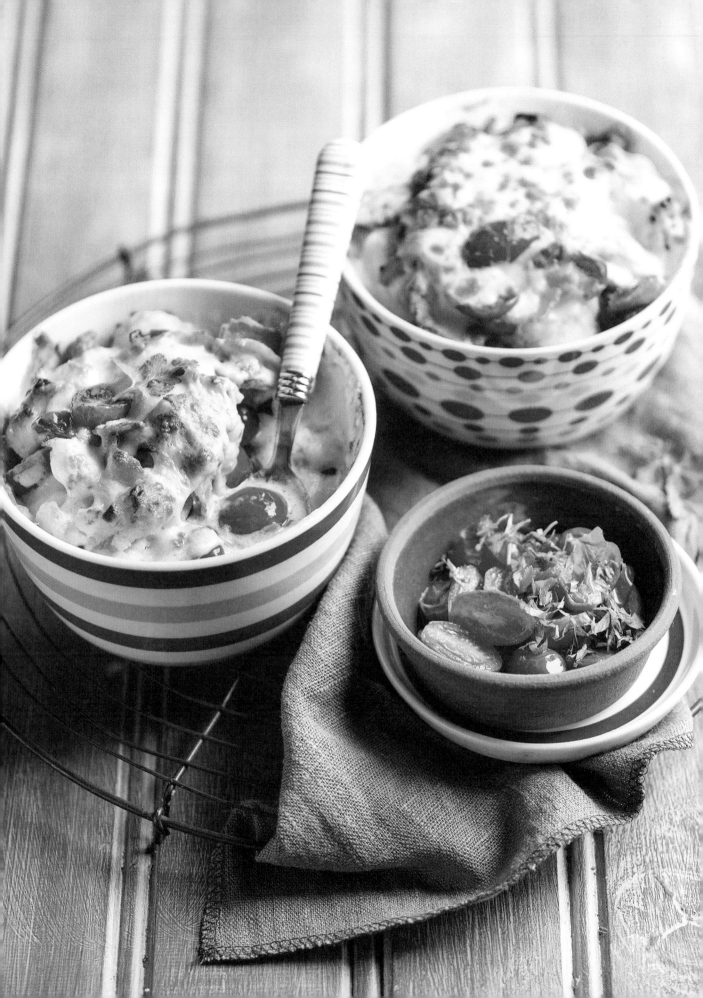

BATTERED FISH WITH SWEET POTATO CRISPS

Makes 4 portions
Prep time: 20 mins
Cooking time: 45 mins

Our yummy take on fish and chips calls for a lot of coconut oil, but you can strain it when you're finished and use it again if you like. Coconut oil gets very hot very quickly so keep an eye on the temperature. All the frying must be done over a moderate heat.

For the crisps:
4 sweet potatoes, washed and
  thinly sliced (use a potato peeler
  or a mandolin)
2 cups (400g) coconut oil for frying
salt and pepper
a sprinkle of paprika

For the fish:
750g-1kg fresh hake fillets, skin and
  bones removed and cut into strips
2 cups (200g) almond flour
4 eggs
1 cup (250ml) fresh milk
salt and pepper
homemade mayo (p301) to serve

TO MAKE THE CRISPS:
- Dry the sweet potato slices well.
- Heat the coconut oil in a deep frying pan over a medium heat, then fry the sweet potato slices in small batches until crispy. Keep a close eye on them so they don't burn.
- Drain on paper towel and season with salt, pepper and paprika. Set aside. (Once cold, these crisps can be kept in an airtight container and used for lunchboxes.)

TO MAKE THE FISH:
- Pat the fish dry with paper towel.
- In a bowl, mix together the almond flour, eggs, milk, salt and pepper, and give it a good blend with a hand-blender.
- In a pan, reheat the coconut oil on a medium heat.
- Dip the fish strips into the batter in batches so that they're completely covered. Allow the excess batter to drip off and pop the fish strips into the hot coconut oil.
- Fry until golden on both sides and drain on paper towel. Repeat with the remaining fish.
- Serve hot with the sweet potato crisps, a few wedges of lemon and homemade mayo. Add some chopped gherkins and capers to the mayo if you like.

MAKE MORE SWEET POTATO CRISPS THAN YOU THINK YOU NEED; THEY ARE VERY MORE-ISH! THE CRISPS ARE SERVED COLD AND CAN ALSO BE MADE FROM THINLY SLICED BEETROOT OR BUTTERNUT

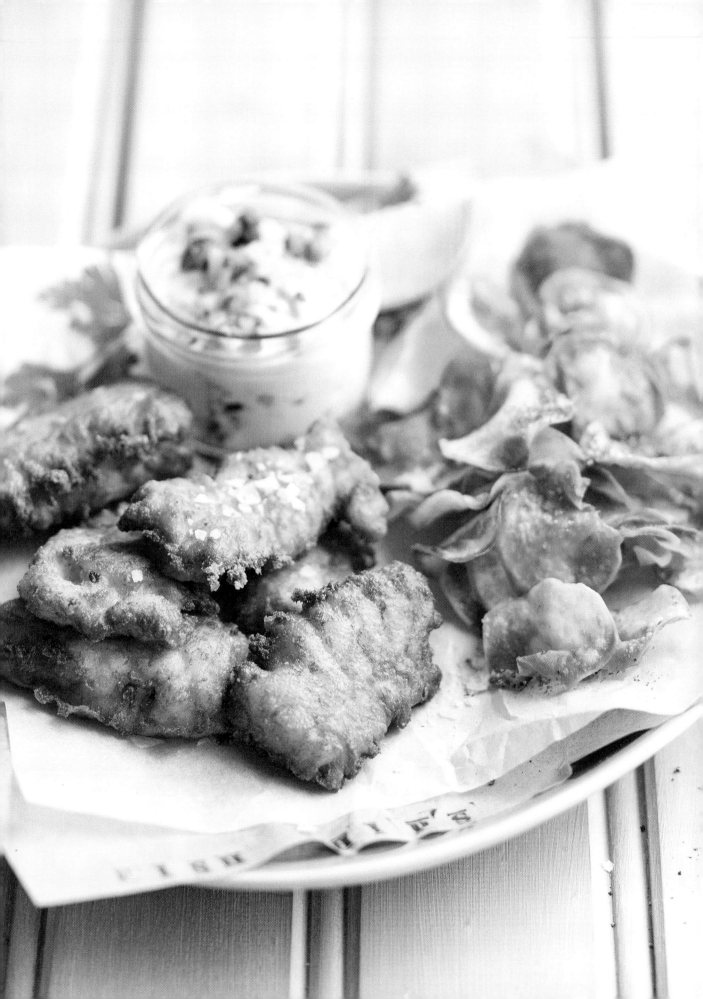

CHICKEN YAKITORI SKEWERS WITH CUCUMBER SPAGHETTI SALAD

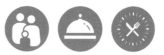

Makes 4 portions
Prep time: 45 mins
Cooking time: 20 mins

This is a great marinade for chicken that can be used on pieces and skewers, and is perfect for the barbecue. The cucumber salad may be a little advanced for some youngsters, but will be great for older kids. Leave the spring onion off the kebabs if your family isn't ready for them.

For the chicken:

3 tablespoons sake mirin

$^2/_3$ cup (170ml) tamari soya sauce

2 tablespoons honey

800g deboned chicken thighs,
   cut into thirds

8 spring onions, cut into 3cm lengths

For the salad:

1 English cucumber, julienned or cut
   into noodles

125g mangetout, shredded

1 cup (100g) bean sprouts

1 teaspoon salt

2 tablespoons white wine vinegar

2 tablespoons sesame oil

$^1/_2$ teaspoon honey

1 teaspoon lemon juice

1 tablespoon grated fresh ginger

1 clove garlic, crushed

2 tablespoons toasted sesame seeds

TO MAKE THE CHICKEN:

- In a bowl, mix together the mirin, soya sauce and honey. Add the chicken to the marinade and leave it to stand for 30 minutes.
- Soak 8 wooden kebab sticks in water and make the skewers, alternating the chicken and the spring onion.
- Heat a heavy-based frying pan to a medium heat and grill the kebabs for 10 minutes on each side until golden and cooked through. These are fantastic cooked on the barbecue too, or you can fry them for 2 minutes on either side, then bake them at 200°C for 12 minutes until cooked.

TO MAKE THE SALAD:

- In a large bowl, mix together the cucumber, mangetout and bean sprouts.
- In a separate bowl, whisk together the remaining salad ingredients to make a dressing. Toss the cucumber mix in the dressing and serve immediately with the chicken skewers. Garnish with a little fresh coriander.

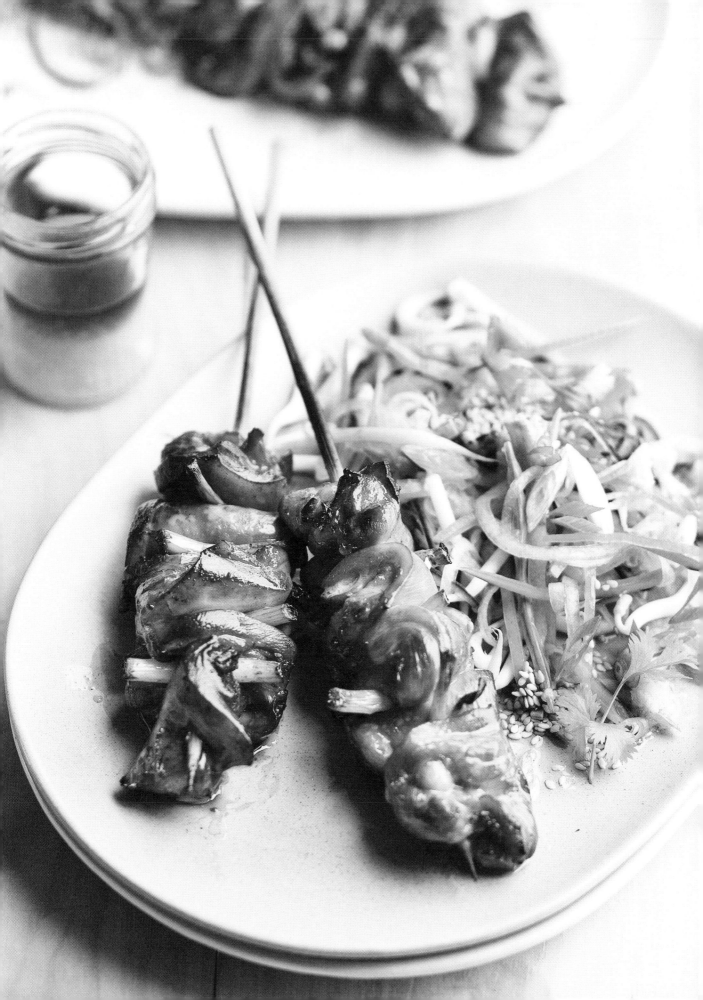

CREAMY CHICKEN AND MUSHROOM CASSEROLE WITH BACON AND SPINACH

Makes 4 portions
Prep time: 10 mins
Cooking time: 50 mins

This is another time-consuming dish, but it's the type you can play around with – and it ends up being wonderful comfort food for the whole family. Feel free to add any veggies you think your kids may enjoy.

8 chicken thighs, on the bone
salt and pepper
2 tablespoons butter for frying
100g bacon, diced
1 onion, finely chopped
2 leeks, finely chopped
1 stalk celery, finely chopped
2 cloves garlic, crushed
250g button mushrooms, halved
2 cups (500ml) chicken stock
1 bay leaf
2 teaspoons chopped fresh thyme
250ml cream
the juice and zest of 1 lemon
3 cups (90g) baby spinach

- Season the chicken thighs well with salt and pepper.
- Melt the butter in a medium-sized casserole dish, and brown the chicken pieces in the butter, a few at a time, until they are golden on both sides. Remove from the casserole dish and set aside.
- Add the bacon, and fry until crispy.
- Add the onion, leeks, celery, garlic and mushrooms, and fry until soft.
- Return the chicken to the casserole pot and add the chicken stock, bay leaf and thyme. There should be enough stock to just cover the chicken. If using a wider casserole dish, you may need to add some more stock.
- Reduce the heat to a simmer, and simmer the chicken with the lid off for 40 minutes until cooked. Keep an eye on it and give it a stir every now and then.
- Add the cream and simmer for a further 10 minutes. Finally stir in the lemon juice, lemon zest and spinach.
- Season well with salt and pepper and serve with creamy cauli-mash and some green veggies.

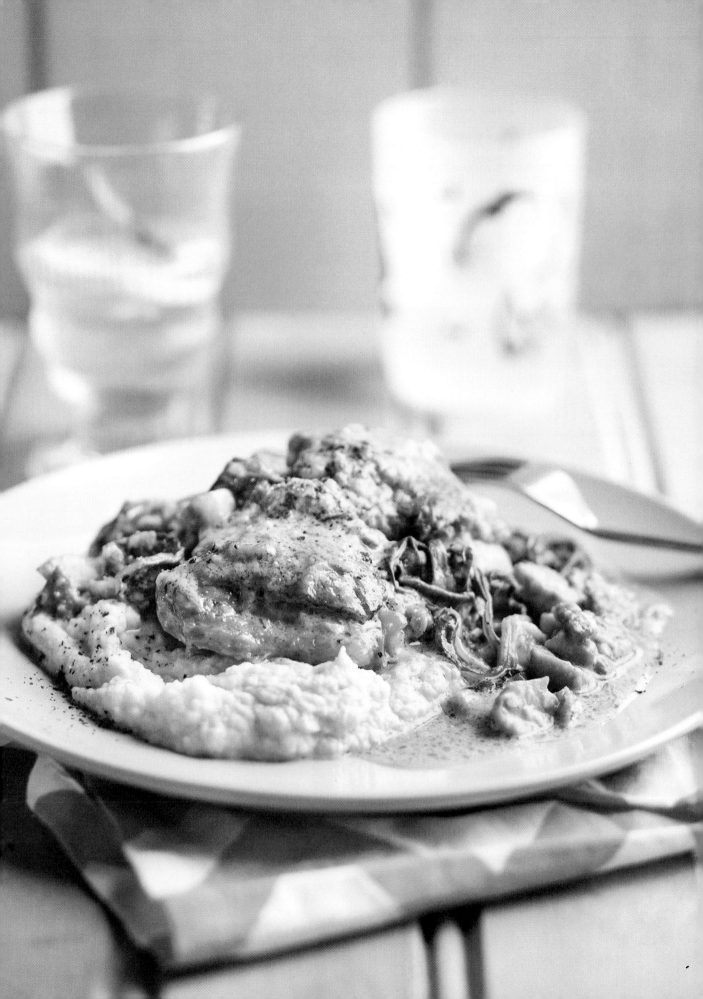

TRAINING-WHEELS LAMB CURRY

Makes 4 portions
Prep time: 20 mins
Cooking time: 1 ¾ hrs

This is a delicious curry that you could whip out at a dinner party if needs be, while the sweetness from the fruit makes it fantastic for a young palate's introduction to spicy food. If you're wary of the chilli powder, remove it and serve chopped fresh chilli on the side.

2 tablespoons ghee or butter
2 onions, finely chopped
4 cloves garlic, crushed
2 tablespoons grated fresh ginger
2 teaspoons ground coriander
2 teaspoons ground cumin
1 teaspoon ground turmeric
½ teaspoon cayenne pepper
5 cardamom pods, lightly crushed
2 tablespoons tomato paste
800g lamb shoulder, cubed
1 x 400g tin whole peeled tomatoes, blended
200ml water
1 mango, peeled and roughly chopped
1 x 400g can coconut milk
salt and pepper
2 tablespoons garam masala
fresh coriander to garnish

- Heat the ghee in a casserole dish on the stove and gently fry the onions until soft.
- Add the garlic and the ginger and fry for 1 minute.
- Stir in the spices and fry for a minute to release their flavour.
- Add the tomato paste and also fry for a minute or so. Toss the lamb cubes through the pot so that the meat is well coated.
- Pour in the blended tinned tomatoes and the water and leave the curry to simmer gently with the lid on for about an hour.
- Remove the lid from the casserole pot and stir in the mango and coconut milk. Leave the curry to simmer with the lid off for a further 45 minutes or so, until the lamb is soft.
- Remove from the heat, season with salt and pepper, and stir through the garam masala.
- Garnish with the fresh coriander and serve with cauli-rice or low-carb coconut pancakes (p300).

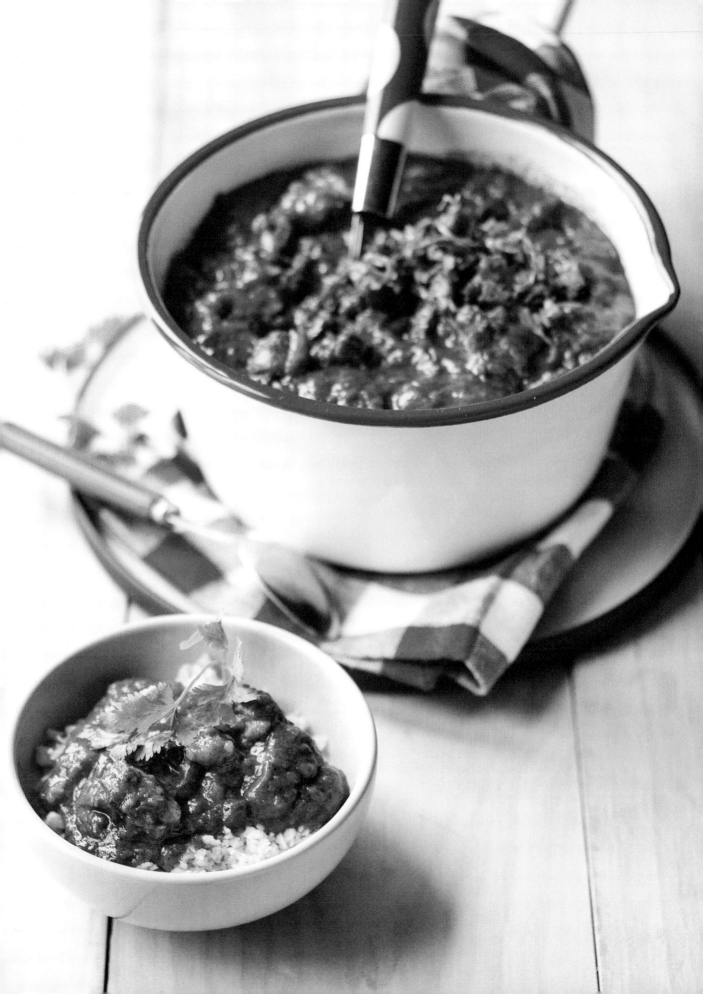

DIPPY CHIPPIES

Makes 4 portions
Prep time: 10 mins
Cooking time: 20 mins

These dippy chippies are our answer to corn chips. They're not quite Doritos, but they're equally delicious – and, of course, far healthier. We serve these with a little tomato salsa or some cream cheese as a dip, but they're also the base of our delicious nachos.

$^3/_4$ **cup (75g) almond flour**
$^1/_4$ **cup (45g) golden flax seeds**
$^1/_4$ **cup (90g) coconut flour**
30g butter
1 large egg
$^1/_2$ **teaspoon paprika**
$^1/_2$ **teaspoon dried thyme**
$^1/_2$ **teaspoon cumin**

- Preheat the oven to 180°C.
- Place all the ingredients in the bowl of a food processor and blitz until a dough is formed. Scoop out the dough and divide into two balls.
- Roll out one of the balls of dough between two sheets of silicone baking paper on a flat surface so that the dough is as thin as you can make it. Lift off the top sheet of paper, and use a pizza cutter or knife to slice the dough into triangles. Try not to cut the paper, though it isn't a train smash if you do; you can just peel it off after baking.
- Lift up the sheet of paper and place it on a flat baking tray.
- Bake for 8-10 minutes until the chips are light brown and crispy.
- Repeat the process with the second ball of dough.

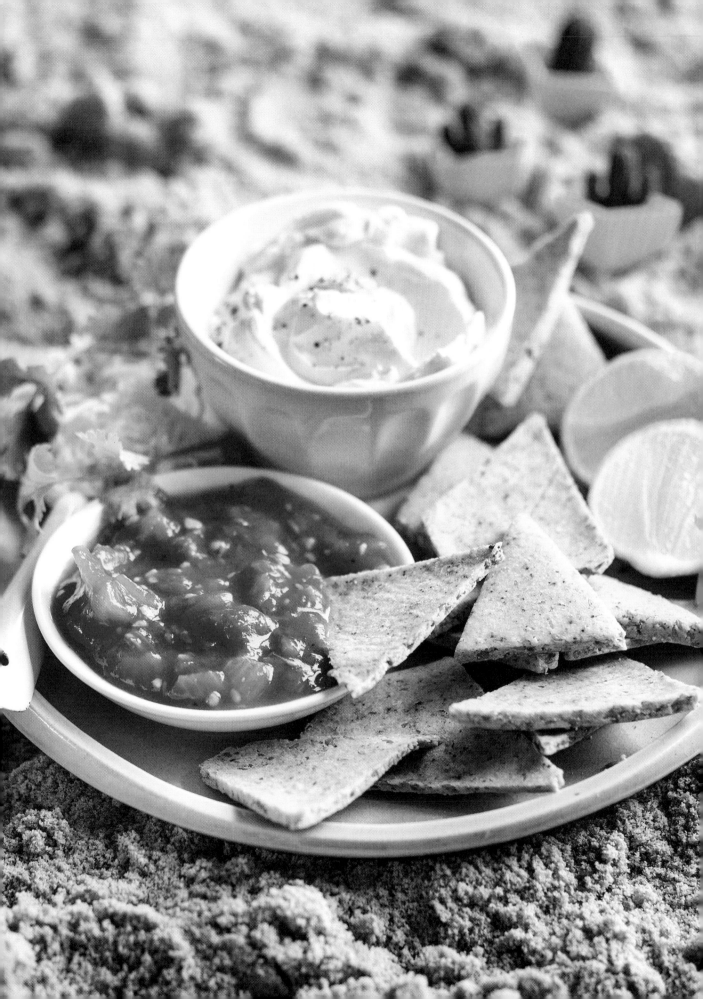

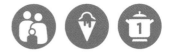

FUN FRUIT LEATHERS

Makes 2 sheets
Prep time: 15 mins
Cooking time: 8 hrs

Fruit leathers may sound like a bit of a tricky proposition, but they take just minutes to prepare and the real process happens in the oven overnight. Try them with mango or strawberry – or whatever you prefer. They're a great treat for a lunchbox, too.

3 cups (750ml) fresh fruit pulp
  (peeled and seeded), such as
  strawberry or mango
2 tablespoons honey

- Preheat the oven to 60°C.
- Line a baking sheet with silicone baking paper or use a silicone baking mat.
- Blend the ingredients together very well, and strain out any unwanted seeds. Remember to peel and seed the fruit before you blend it.
- Pour the mixture onto the baking tray and spread it thinly, to about 2mm thick.
- Place in the oven and leave it to dry out for about 8 hours. The fruit is ready when it's no longer sticky and can peel off the sheet.
- Peel the fruit leather off the baking paper it was cooked on and place it on a clean sheet. Cut it into 5cm-wide strips on the paper and roll it up to store it. It will last in an airtight container in the cupboard for up to a week, and it's perfect kept in the freezer.

THE EASIEST WAY TO SLICE FRUIT LEATHER IS WITH A CRAFT KNIFE AND A RULER. OTHERWISE JUST USE YOUR SHARPEST CARVING KNIFE

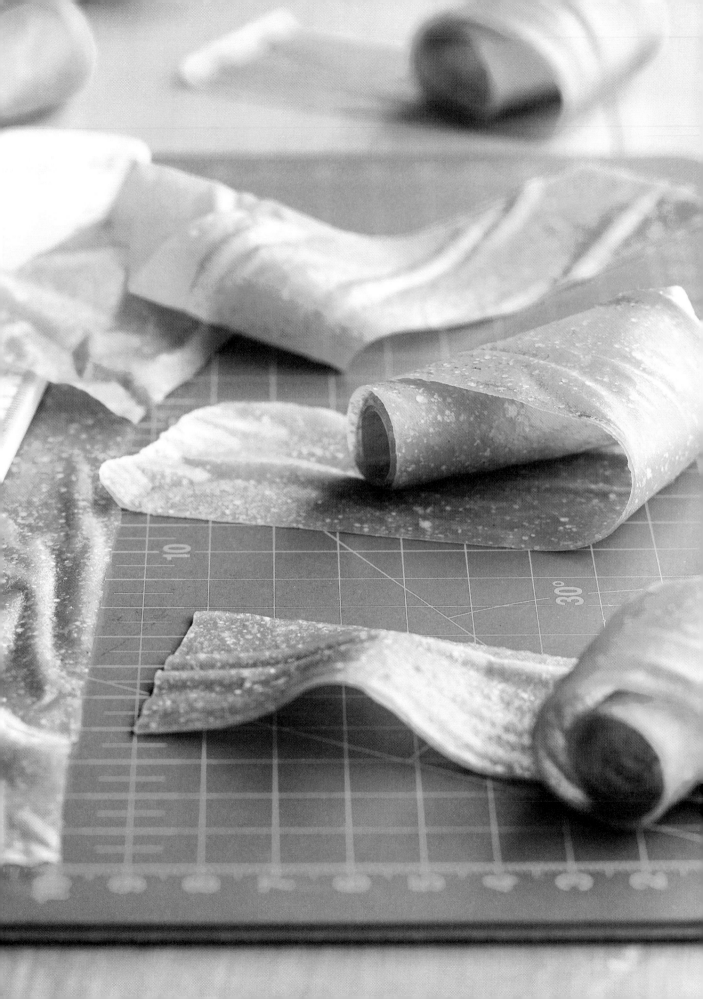

DELICIOUS RUSKS

Rusks are a South African classic – a treat that you don't have to be a grandma to make! These beauties will need longer to dry out than traditional rusks.

NOTE TO MUM: DO YOUR BEST TO KEEP TREATS AS EXACTLY THAT - TREATS! SERVE THEM AT PARTIES AND ON SPECIAL OCCASIONS, NOT AS EVERYDAY FOODS

NUTTY RUSKS

50g slivered almonds
50g pecan nuts
50g macadamia nuts
½ cup (60g) coconut flour
1 cup (100g) almond flour
1 tablespoon bicarbonate of soda
50g pumpkin seeds
3 tablespoons golden linseeds
3 tablespoons sunflower seeds
1 tablespoon psyllium husks
1 teaspoon xanthan gum
a pinch of salt
125g melted butter
⅓ cup (80ml) honey
3 eggs
1 cup (270g) Greek yoghurt

- Preheat the oven to 180°C.
- Chop the nuts, then mix together with all the dry ingredients in a large bowl.
- In a saucepan, melt the butter and honey and let it cool.
- Whisk together the eggs and yoghurt, then add them, with the cooled butter and honey, to the dry ingredients. Mix well to form a doughy consistency that isn't too crumbly. Add a little water if it's dry.
- Pour the dough into a baking tray lined with silicone paper, and spread it until it's 2-3cm thick.
- Bake for 35-40 minutes until golden brown and firm.
- Remove the baking tray from the oven and allow the giant rusk to cool for at least 10 minutes, then cut the rusk into fingers. Take care because they'll be crumbly.
- Turn the oven down to 50°C and dry out the rusks overnight. Store in an airtight container once cooled.

SEEDED BUTTERMILK AND ALMOND RUSKS

½ cup (90g) flax seeds
½ cup (75g) sesame seeds
½ cup (70g) pumpkin seeds
1 cup (140g) sunflower seeds
2 cups (200g) almond flour
1 cup (120g) coconut flour
1 teaspoon xanthan gum
1 tablespoon psyllium husks
½ cup (40g) desiccated coconut
4 teaspoons baking powder
3 eggs
2 cups (500g) buttermilk
300g soft butter
½ cup (125g) honey (or stevia)

- Preheat the oven to 180°C.
- In a large bowl mix together all the seeds. Grind 1 cup of the mixed seeds in a coffee grinder or blender until fine. Add the ground seed mix back into the other seed mix and add in the rest of the dry ingredients.
- Whisk together the eggs and buttermilk.
- In a mixer, cream together the butter and the honey (or stevia) until it is light in colour and fluffy. Add the dry ingredients to the butter mixture. Finally add the buttermilk mixture. Mix well to form a soft dough.
- Pour the dough into a baking tray lined with silicone paper and spread until it's 2-3cm thick.
- Bake for 45-50 minutes until lightly golden and firm.
- Continue as per the previous recipe: remove the baking tray from the oven; cool and cut the giant rusk; dry out in the oven overnight at 50°C.

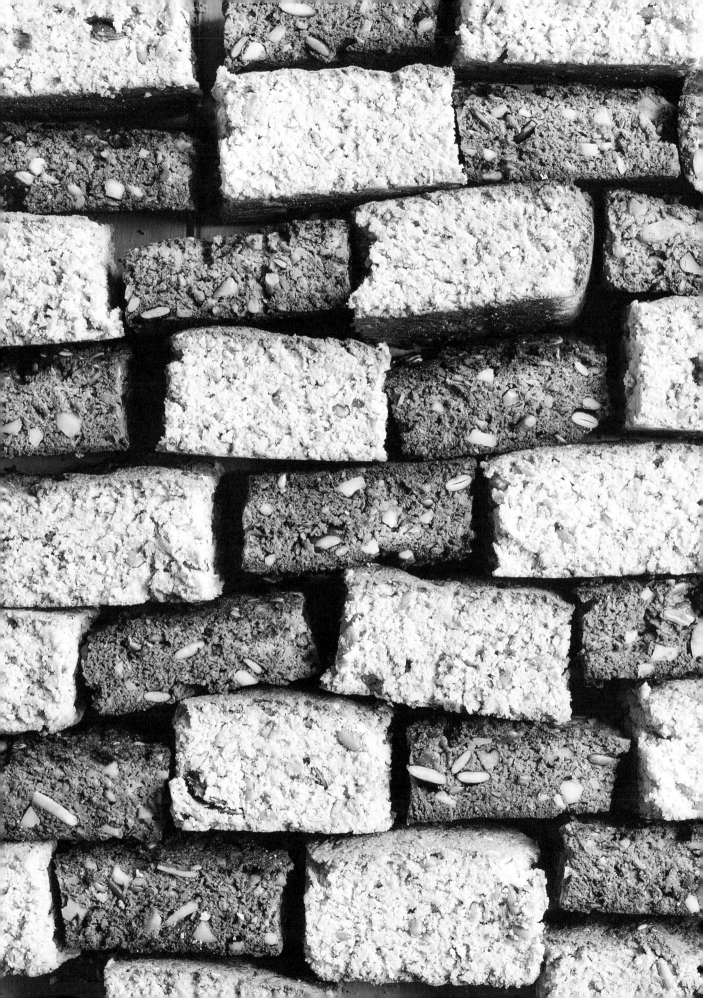

COOL COOKIES

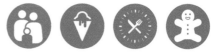

Prep time: 20 mins
Cooking time: 15 mins

These cookies are two of our favourite recipes in the book. To sweeten them we've used, respectively, honey and erythritol, which adds a minty flavour as well.

ROSEMARY AND APRICOT ALMOND COOKIES

½ cup (125g) butter
⅓ cup (80g) honey
½ teaspoon chopped rosemary
100g almond flour
45g coconut flour
1 teaspoon bicarbonate of soda
50g dried apricots, chopped
a pinch of salt

- Preheat the oven to 180°C.
- In a small saucepan, gently melt together the honey and butter. Take off the heat and add the rosemary.
- In a bowl, mix together the flours, bicarbonate of soda, dried apricots and salt.
- Pour in the melted butter mixture and mix very well.
- Cover the dough and place in the refrigerator for at least 10 minutes for the coconut flour to absorb any excess liquid.
- Cover a baking tray with silicone baking paper and spoon the dough onto it in mounds. Be sure to leave space between each mound for the cookies to spread. Use about 2 tablespoons of dough for each cookie.
- Bake the cookies for about 12 minutes, until golden brown.
- Allow to cool on a rack until they're firm, then serve.

MINTY DARK CHOCOLATE-CHIP COOKIES

1½ cups (150g) almond flour
½ cup (62g) cocoa
½ teaspoon bicarbonate of soda
½ teaspoon salt
1 cup (225g) erythritol granules
115g butter, cubed
1 teaspoon vanilla extract
115g dark chocolate, melted
2 large eggs
115g dark chocolate, roughly chopped

- Preheat the oven to 180°C.
- Line a baking tray with silicone baking paper.
- Place the almond flour, cocoa, bicarbonate of soda, salt and erythritol into the bowl of a food processor and blitz together.
- Add the butter and vanilla and pulse until it is all combined and the dough looks like breadcrumbs. Add the melted chocolate and eggs and give the mixture another good blitz.
- Finally stir in the chopped chocolate.
- Spoon the dough onto the baking tray, several centimetres apart, and bake for 10-12 minutes.
- Remove the tray from the oven and allow the cookies to cool completely.
- Wait for the cookies to set before peeling them off the paper to serve.

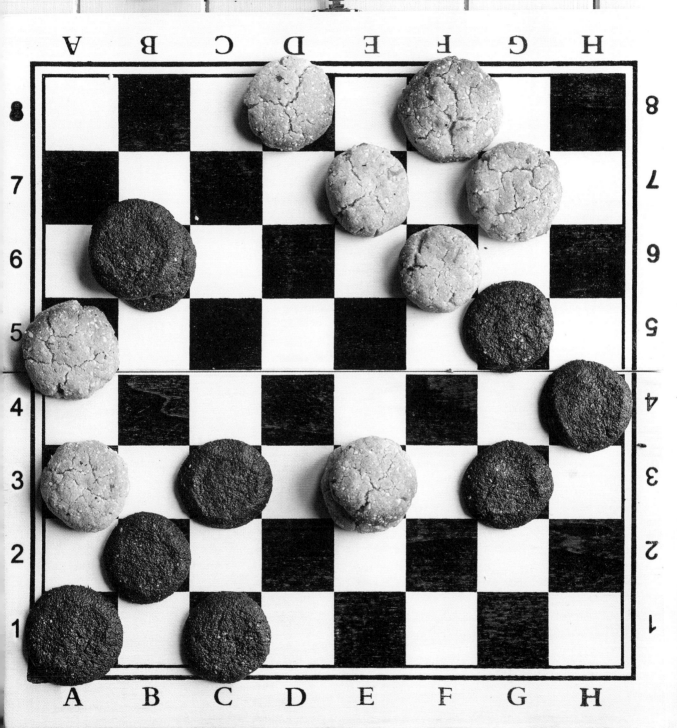

YOGHURT AND RASPBERRY-RIPPLE ICE-CREAM POTS

Makes 6 frozen pots
Prep time: 5 mins
Freeze overnight

These ice-cream pots literally take 5 minutes to make, followed by a night in the freezer. Conveniently, they don't need popsicle moulds; you can just use the plastic container that the yoghurt comes in to freeze them.

6 x 100g sugar-free vanilla-flavoured yoghurt (ideally full-cream)
160g fresh raspberries, blended

- Remove the foil from all six yoghurt tubs.
- Blend the raspberries and spoon them into the yoghurt tubs to fill them to the top.
- Stick a wooden sucker stick into each yoghurt pot and freeze overnight.
- Remove from the pots and serve.

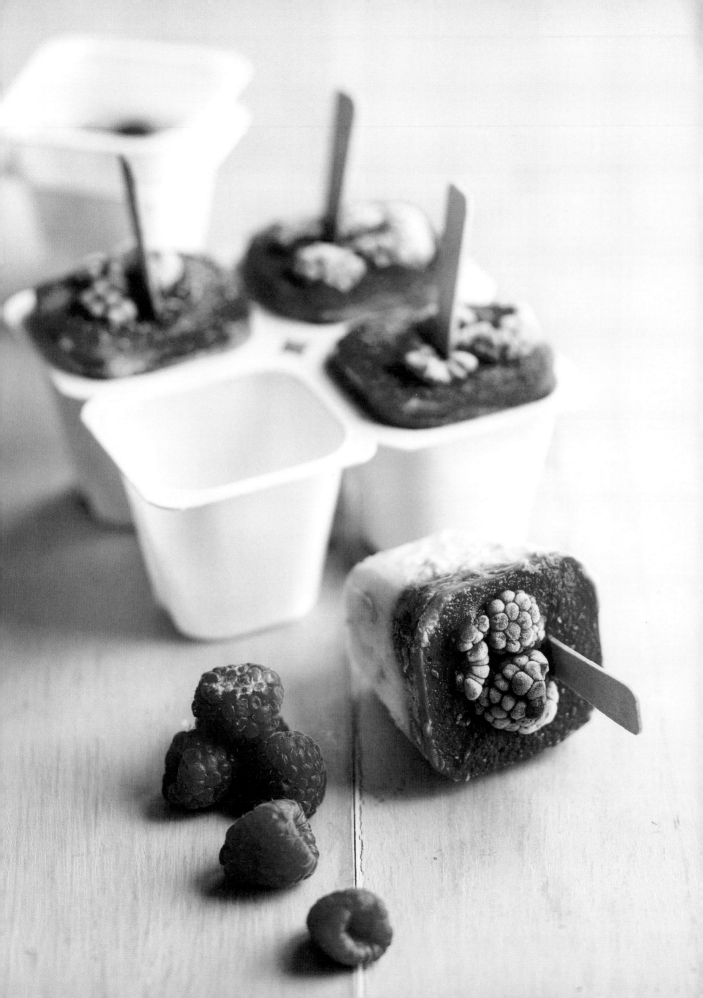

BANANA-AND-BUTTERMILK ICE LOLLIES WITH CHOCOLATE CRUNCH

Makes 5 popsicles
Prep time: 10 mins
Freeze overnight

Ice lollies are great fun to make with your kids. You can play around with different types of fruit, and try them with yoghurt as well.

5 large bananas, peeled, diced and frozen

1 cup (250ml) buttermilk or coconut milk, chilled

200g chocolate, melted

100g macadamia nuts, toasted and roughly chopped

30g coconut shavings, toasted

- Place the frozen bananas in the blender and add the buttermilk or coconut milk.
- Blend until smooth and pour into ice-lolly moulds. Freeze overnight.
- Remove the lollies from their moulds and dip in the melted chocolate. Sprinkle with the toasted nuts and coconut, and they're ready.

IF YOUR KIDS LOVE MAKING THESE WITH YOU, MIX THINGS UP FROM WEEK TO WEEK WITH DIFFERENT TOPPINGS

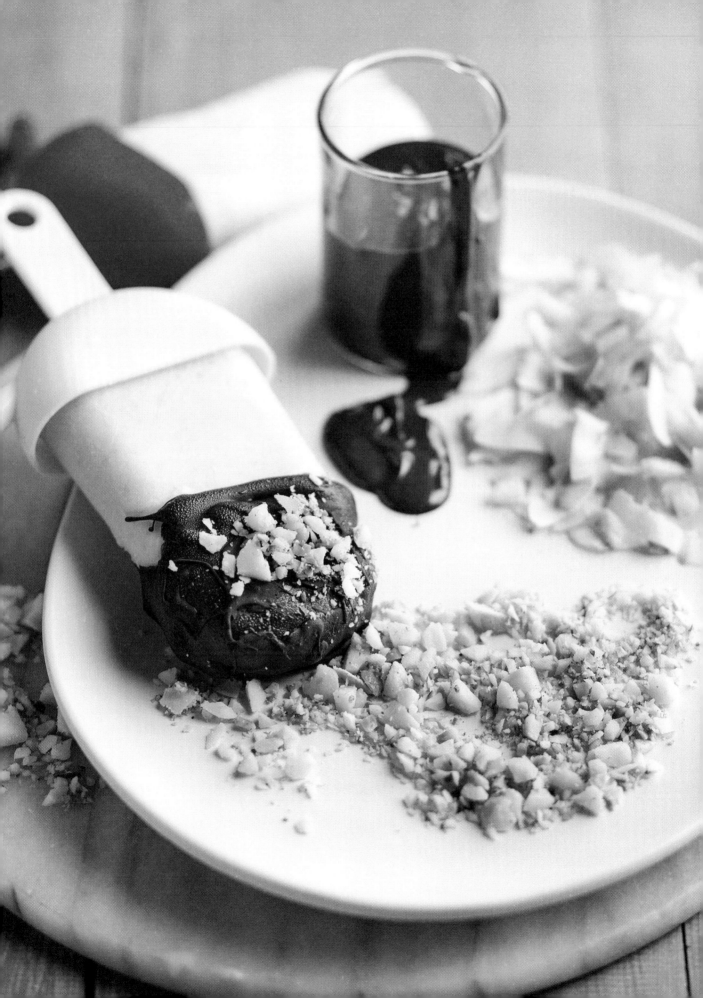

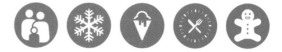

CHOCOLATE BARK

Makes 1 sheet
Prep time: 10 mins
Cooking time: 30 mins

This is a great recipe to make with your kids. They can sprinkle the toppings on the bark and choose their own combinations. You can also set the bark quickly in the freezer for almost instant gratification.

200g dark chocolate (at least 70%)
2 teaspoons coconut oil
2 tablespoons butter
¼ cup (35g) macadamia nuts, toasted and chopped
¼ cup (35g) assorted seeds, toasted
a sprinkle of dried and toasted coconut flakes

- In a heat-proof bowl over a pan of simmering water, gently melt the chocolate, coconut oil and butter.
- While the chocolate is melting, line a flat baking sheet with silicone baking paper.
- Pour the chocolate onto the lined baking sheet and smooth it out to just less than half a centimetre thick.
- Sprinkle the nuts, seeds and toasted coconut flakes over the chocolate, making sure that they stick into the melted chocolate.
- Either leave the bark in the fridge for a few hours to set, or freeze it to set quickly.
- Break into pieces and serve.

STORE CHOCOLATE BARK IN THE FRIDGE OR EVEN THE FREEZER, AS THE CHOCOLATE WILL MELT EASILY

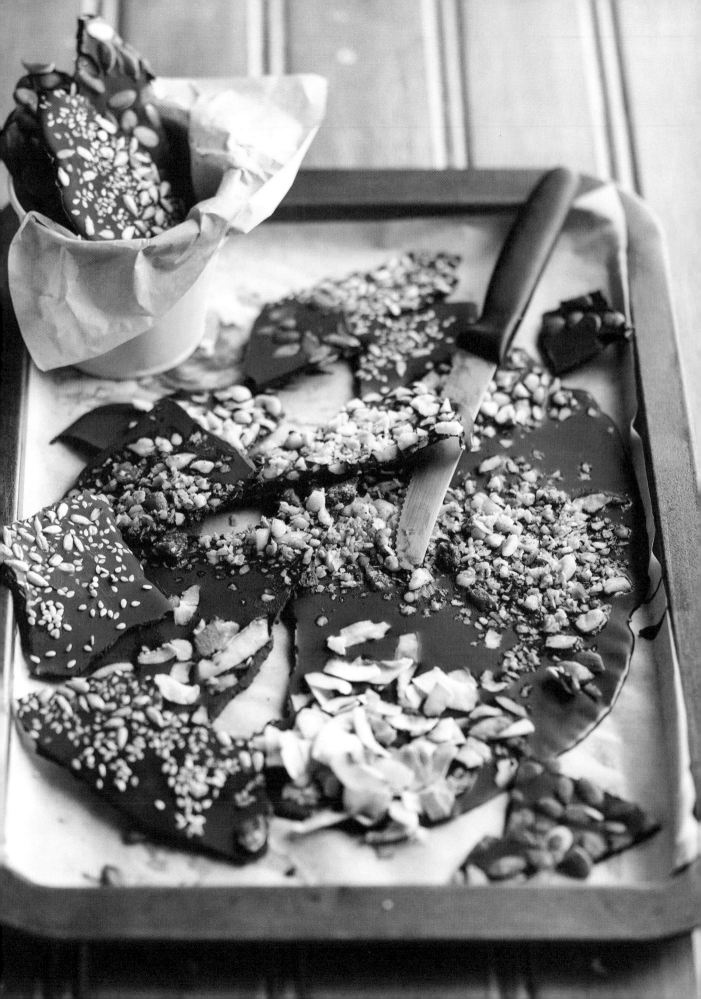

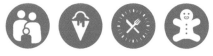

CHOCOLATE DATE BITES

Makes about 25
Prep time: 20 mins
Cooking time: 5 mins

Chocolate date bites are a superb 'emergency treat' because you can make a load at a time and store them in the freezer. This is another fun dish to make with your kids, who will enjoy the rolling and coating process.

350g pitted dates, finely chopped
50g butter
1 egg, lightly beaten
1 tablespoon cocoa powder
a pinch of salt
125g almonds, roughly chopped

Choose one of the following for the coating:
toasted desiccated coconut
toasted sesame seeds
chopped nuts
cocoa powder

- Heat the dates and butter in a saucepan until the dates are soft.
- Pour the mixture into a bowl and allow it to cool until it's just warm to the touch.
- Slowly add the egg to the mixture and stir it in well. If the mixture is too hot you'll end up with scrambled egg, so be careful!
- Mix in the cocoa powder, salt and nuts.
- Roll the mixture into balls about 3cm wide, then into your coating of choice.
- Allow the date bites to cool in little pastry cases (mini muffin cups). They will keep well for a few days in a sealed container or they can be frozen if you'd like to keep them longer.

TO GIVE THESE BITES MORE OF A CHOCOLATE-TRUFFLE FEEL, DIP THEM IN MELTED CHOCOLATE AND ALLOW TO SET. ADD DIFFERENT KINDS OF NUTS TO MIX THINGS UP

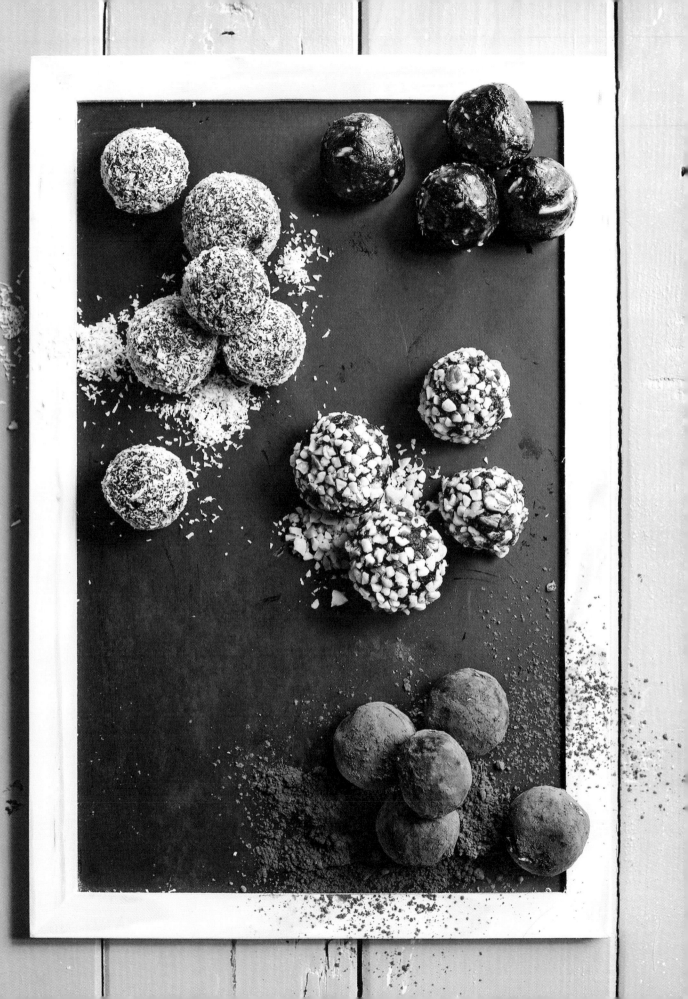

CHOCOLATE ALMOND BUTTER CUPS

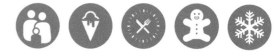

Makes about 25
Prep time: 20 mins
Cooking time: 30 mins

These babies are so delicious there may not be any left for your kids by the time you've finished 'sampling' them. We've used almond butter in this recipe, but feel free to play around with the many other nut butters available.

½ cup (125g) almond butter
1 tablespoon honey
2 tablespoons coconut flour
2½ tablespoons arrowroot powder
350g dark chocolate (at least 70%)

- Line a mini-muffin pan with mini-muffin cups.
- In a bowl, stir together the almond butter, honey, coconut flour and arrowroot until well combined.
- Gently melt the chocolate in a double-boiler.
- Spoon a teaspoon or two of chocolate into each muffin cup and swirl it around so that the bottom and three-quarters of the sides of the muffin cup are lined with chocolate. Allow the chocolate to set in the cup.
- Spoon the almond butter mixture into the little cups so that they are a third full.
- Drizzle another tablespoon of chocolate over the top of the almond mixture so that it's completely covered.
- Allow the butter cups to set in the fridge. When they're set, peel off the paper and serve. They can be dusted in a little cocoa to stop them getting too melty on the fingers.

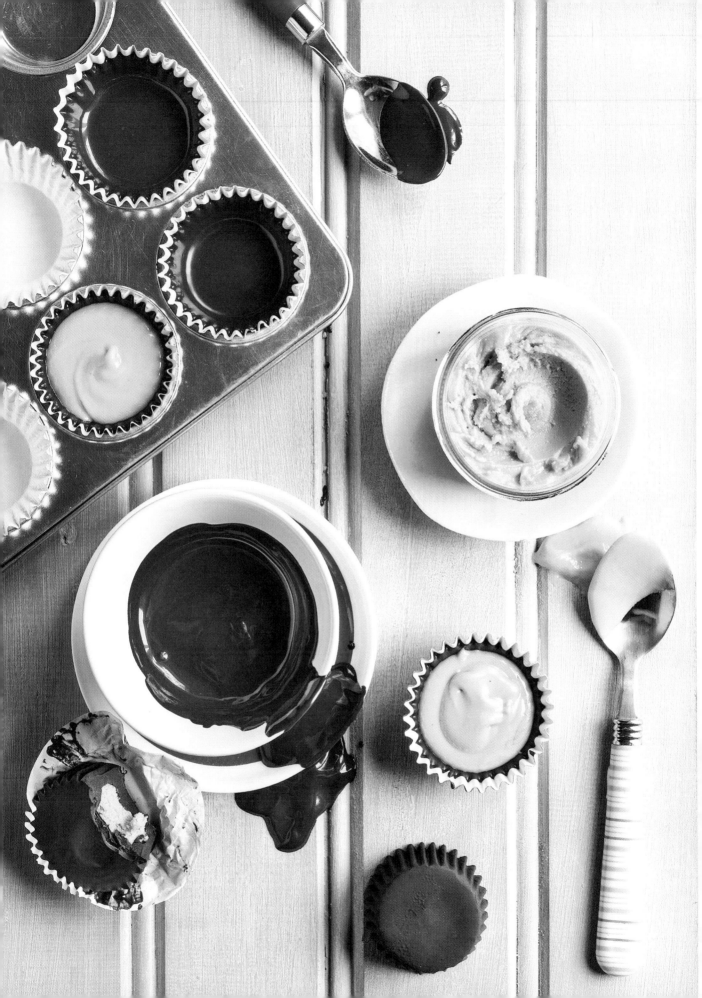

STRAWBERRY-AND-VANILLA FROZEN-YOGHURT CAKE

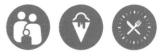

Makes 10 portions
Prep time: 1 ½ hours
Total: 2 days (on and off!)

Our version of an ice-cream cake looks spectacular when you get it right. You'll need an ice-cream maker for the frozen yoghurt; alternatively you could buy it (NB: sugar-free and full-cream) from a reputable purveyor and just put the cake together yourself.

For the strawberry frozen yoghurt:
600g strawberries, washed and
    quartered
½ cup (125ml) honey
2 teaspoons lemon juice
3 cups (800g) Greek yoghurt
a pinch of salt

For the vanilla frozen yoghurt:
1ℓ Greek yoghurt
½ cup honey
1 teaspoon vanilla extract
2 teaspoons lemon juice
a pinch of salt

TO MAKE THE STRAWBERRY FROZEN YOGHURT:
- Drizzle the strawberries with the honey and allow to stand for an hour.
- Blend all the ingredients together until smooth and pass through a sieve to remove any seeds and bits. Freeze in an ice-cream maker. Spoon into a freezer container and freeze overnight or until needed.

TO MAKE THE VANILLA FROZEN YOGHURT:
- In a bowl, mix together all the ingredients until they're combined. Freeze in an ice-cream maker. Spoon into a freezer container and freeze overnight or until needed.

TO ASSEMBLE THE CAKE:
- When the frozen yoghurt is properly set in the freezer, you're ready to make the cake.
- Line the sides of a 20cm springform cake tin with a sheet of plastic acetate. Secure the acetate with some sticky tape, ensuring that it's on the inside of the cake tin. Place it all on the plate that you wish to make the cake on, then pop it into the freezer to chill for a few hours.
- When you're ready to make the cake, remove the frozen yoghurt from the freezer and allow it to soften slightly. Spoon it into the prepared cake tin, starting with the strawberry and finishing with the vanilla.
- Pop the cake back into the freezer overnight. The longer you freeze it for, the longer it will take to melt when it comes out.
- When you're ready to serve, remove the cake tin and peel away the acetate.
- Top with berries or dark-chocolate shavings, or simply make it beautiful and girly with rose petals.

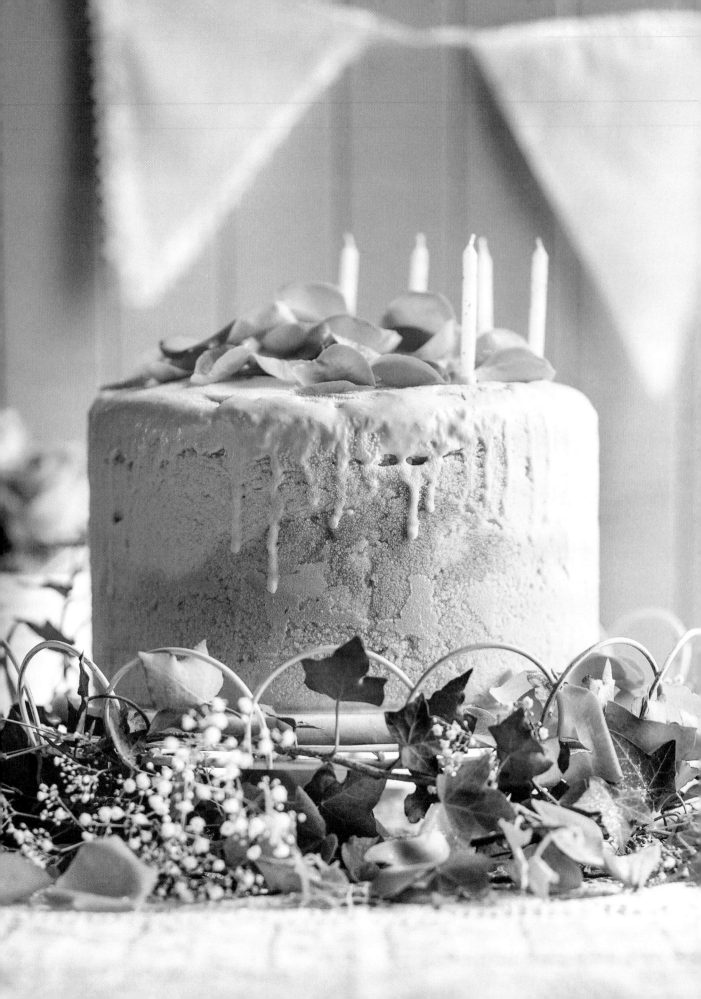

VANILLA CHOC-CHIP ICE-CREAM-CUP CAKE

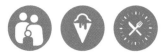

Makes 1 litre
Prep time: 30 minutes
Freeze overnight

It can be tricky to make a regular cake interesting if you don't want to include sugar and flour – you can't make icing, for instance. So ice-cream cakes are a clever alternative. For this invention, we've used ice cream and incorporated colours and party themes to add a bit more fun.

For the ice cream:
10 egg yolks
500ml milk
500ml double cream
1 teaspoon vanilla paste
4 teaspoons liquid stevia or
   ½ cup (125ml) honey (sweeten
   to your taste)
100g dark chocolate, chopped

For the chocolate sauce:
200ml cream
100g dark chocolate, chopped

Topping ideas:
Assorted fruit and berries
Toasted nuts
Toasted coconut shavings

TO MAKE THE ICE CREAM:
- Using an electric mixer with the whisk attachment, whisk the egg yolks until they're light and fluffy.
- Pour the milk and cream into a saucepan with the vanilla paste, and bring the mixture to the boil. Remove from the heat.
- Add a little of the hot cream mixture to the egg yolks, then pour the yolk mixture into the cream mixture in the saucepan. Stir well to combine.
- If you'd like a sweeter ice cream, add sweetener or honey to taste at this stage.
- Return the saucepan to a very low heat. Stirring constantly with a wooden spoon, let the mixture cook until it has thickened enough to coat the back of a spoon. Allow it to cool completely. Stir in the chopped chocolate and place in an ice-cream maker to freeze.
- Spoon the churned ice cream into ice-cream cups and return to the freezer for party day.

TO MAKE THE CHOCOLATE SAUCE:
- Bring the cream to the boil in a pot on the stove then remove from the heat. Mix in the chopped chocolate and stir until completely melted.

TO SERVE:
- Pile the ice-cream cups on top of each other and serve with the chocolate sauce and toppings.

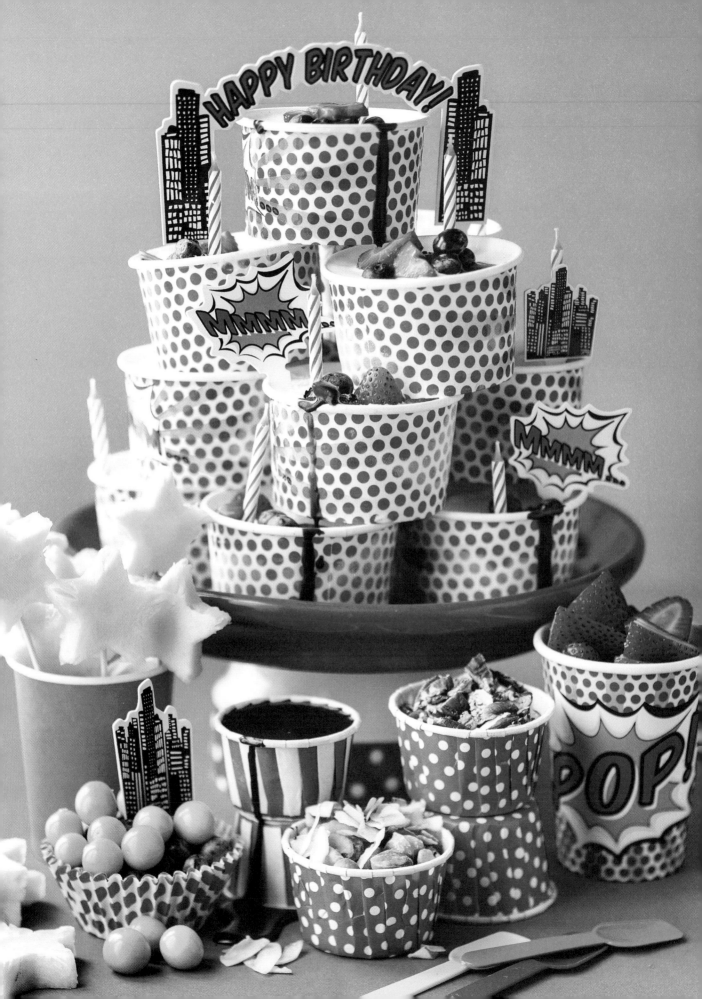

FROZEN CHOCOLATE BANANA ROCKETS

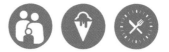

Makes 10 frozen popsicles
Prep time: 10 minutes
Freeze overnight

This is so easy it's like cheating on a test... For best results, make the frozen bananas yourself but let the kids do the dipping and sprinkling with nuts. They taste better that way! If you *do* want to complicate things just a tad, serve the rockets with a chocolate fountain.

10 small bananas, peeled
400g dark chocolate, melted
200g chopped almonds, toasted

- Pop each banana on a popsicle stick. Place on a baking tray and freeze overnight.
- Just before serving, dip the bananas into the melted chocolate and sprinkle with toasted nuts.

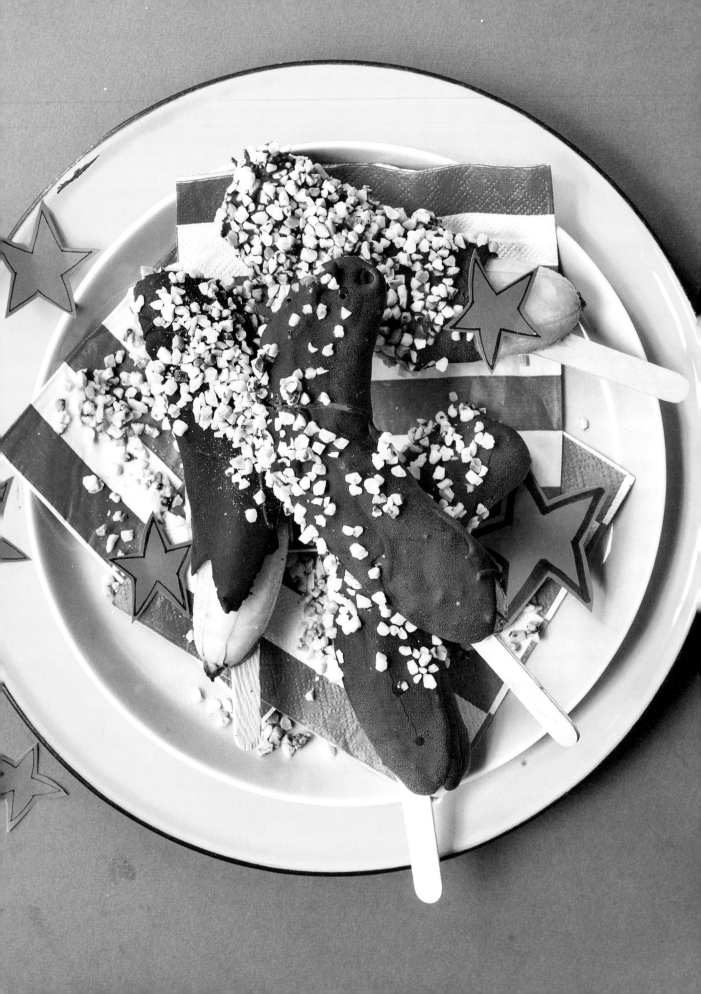

LEMON-AND-VANILLA CHEESECAKE

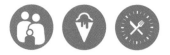

Makes 10 portions
Prep time: 30 mins
Chill: 4 hours

This is a lovely recipe to use as a basic fridge cheesecake. Spoon sliced berries through the mixture or add some melted chocolate to make it interesting. It can be made in jars or in a springform cake tin.

For the base:
½ cup (40g) desiccated coconut
½ cup (50g) almond flour
60g melted butter

For the cheesecake:
½ cup (125ml) water
20g gelatine
1 cup (250ml) cream
1 cup (225g) cream cheese
2 cups (500ml) buttermilk
⅓ cup (80ml) honey
the zest of 1 lemon
1 teaspoon vanilla extract
fresh gooseberries to serve

TO MAKE THE BASE:
- Mix together the ingredients for the base and press into 12 little glass jars.

TO MAKE THE CHEESECAKE:
- Pour the water into a heat-resistant bowl and sprinkle with the gelatine. Allow to stand for 5 minutes.
- Pour the remaining ingredients into the bowl of an electric mixer and whisk until they've thickened.
- Melt the gelatine mixture over a little boiling water until it's clear. Spoon a few tablespoons of the cheesecake mixture into the gelatine and mix well. Pour the gelatine mixture into the bowl with the cream cheese and mix until well combined.
- Pour the cheesecake filling into the glass jars and chill in the fridge for at least 4 hours to set.
- Serve with fresh gooseberries.

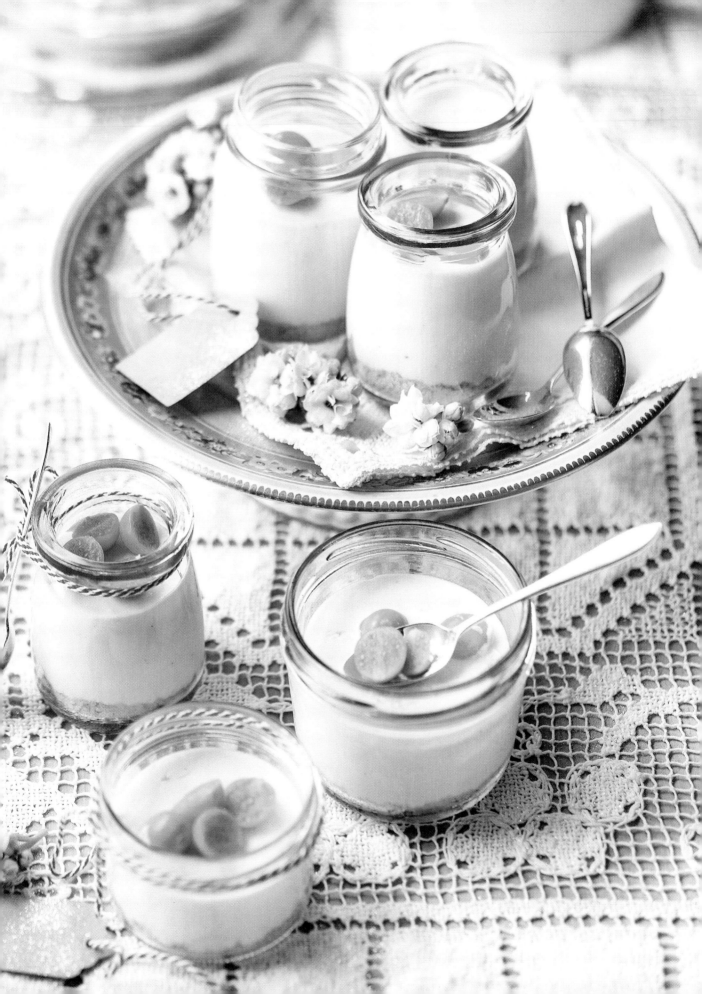

PARTY DRINKS 1

We've said it before; we'll say it again: sugary soft drinks and fruit juices are sweet kryptonite to kids. It takes just a little bit of effort to make a cool, tasty – and healthy - beverage.

RASPBERRY-AND-ROSE SMOOTHIE .... Makes 2-3 smoothies

These can be made in advance and popped in the freezer. Just make sure you take them out in time to defrost. Besides parties, use this recipe for breakfasts, lunches and packed lunches.

1 cup (250g) vanilla yoghurt
(sugar-free, full fat)
2 cups (210g) ice cubes
125g fresh or frozen raspberries
1 teaspoon rosewater
a little honey to sweeten if you'd like

- Blend all the ingredients until smooth and pour into little bottles. Keep in the fridge or freezer until ready to serve.

BERRY ICED TEA .... Makes 2 litres

This iced tea works a treat at girls' parties – it's full of fruity yumminess but it's oh-so grown-up!

10 berry tea bags
6 rooibos tea bags
2ℓ boiling water
a little honey or stevia for sweetness
1 lemon, sliced
150g fresh berries, sliced
10g mint leaves

- Make a big jug of tea with all the tea bags. Remove the bags, and sweeten the brew with a little honey or stevia to taste. Chill in the fridge overnight.
- When you're ready to serve, add the lemon slices, berries and mint.

FLAVOURED WATERS ....

Flavoured waters are fantastic drinks that are exciting for kids but not jampacked with the sugar of commercial soft drinks. They're visually lovely and taste more interesting than plain old water. We've gone with a classic here – orange and mint – but play around with different fruits, vegetables and herbs.

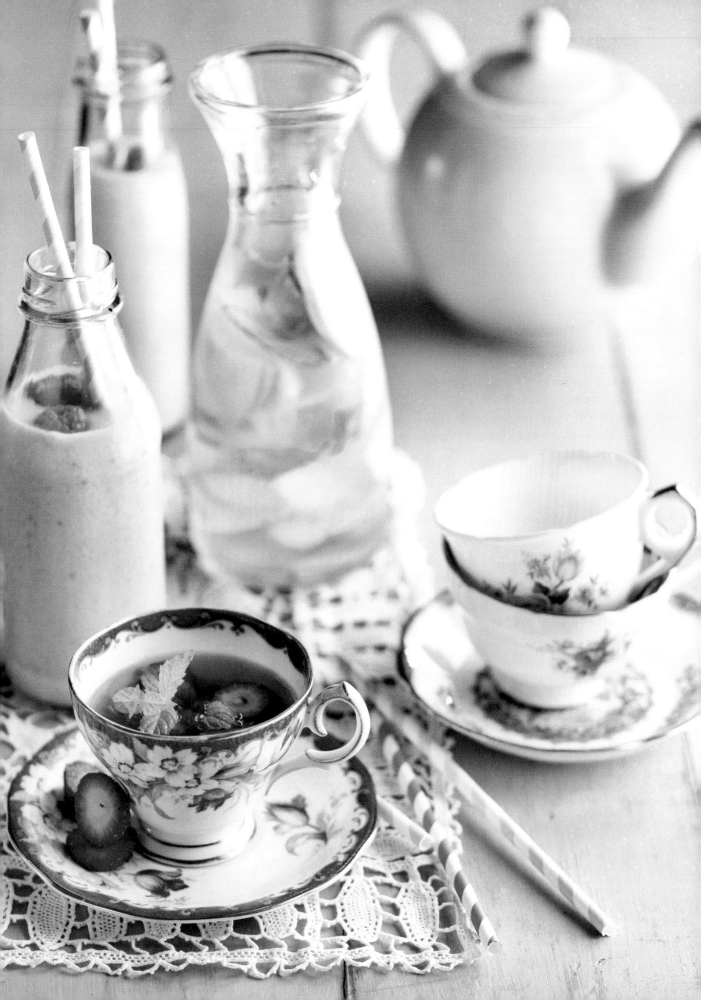

PARTY DRINKS 2

Yes, we know we've said it before but here it is again: steer clear of soft drinks and fruit juices. It's worth the effort to create healthy party drinks for your kids.

STRAWBERRY SLUSHY .... Makes 2-4 slushies

We made these with strawberries to suit the colour scheme of the party, but you can make them with any fruit that blends well. Try peeled mango, watermelon or frozen banana.

3 cups (315g) ice cubes
2 teaspoons lemon juice
½ cup (125ml) honey
  or 3 teaspoons stevia
200g fresh or frozen strawberries

- Place all the ingredients in a smoothie blender and blend until smooth. Pour into cups and keep in the freezer until ready to serve.

ORANGE-AND-GRANADILLA COOLER .... Makes 2 litres

This cooler is effectively a maxed-out flavoured water, but remember: it's a treat, not an everyday drink. The sparkling water gives it a little extra excitement – just make sure it's cold. If you can't get hold of granadillas, use passion fruits instead.

1ℓ freshly squeezed orange juice
1ℓ sparkling water
the pulp of 4 fresh granadillas
a few fresh mint leaves

- Mix the ingredients and serve in a big jug with ice.

FLAVOURED WATERS ....

As mentioned on the previous page, flavoured waters are a fantastic way of providing drinks that aren't full of the sugar of commercial soft drinks. We've gone with a simple pineapple-in-water mix here, and added some cool shapes for kicks – but play around with different fruits, vegetables and herbs.

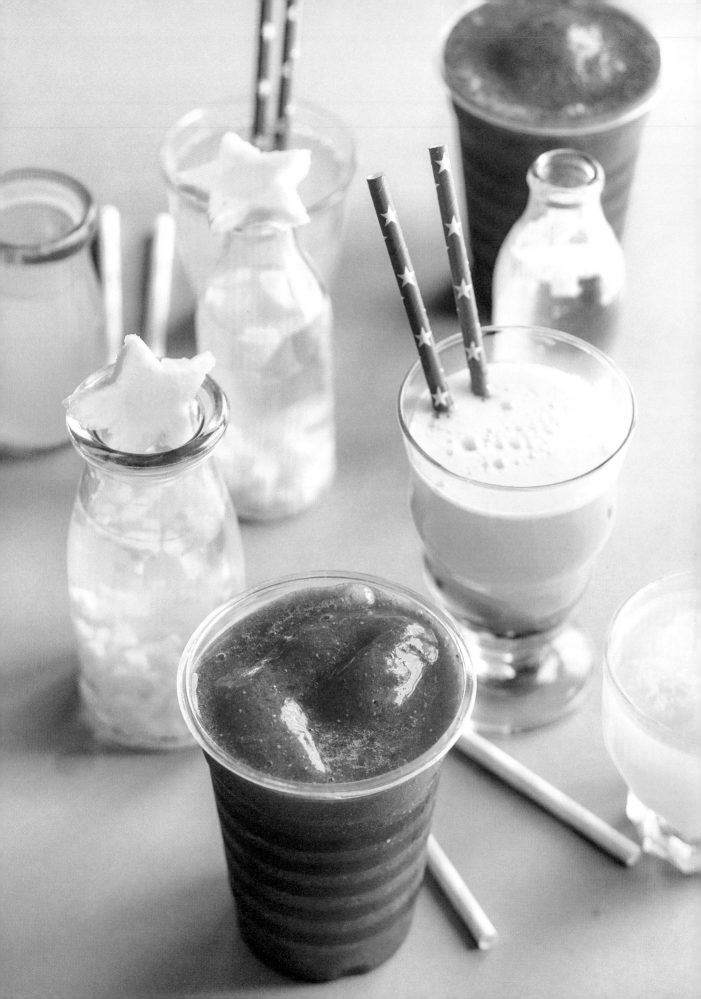

BUTTER BEAN DIP WITH CRUDITÉS

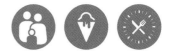

Makes 8-10 portions
Prep time: 30 minutes

Crudités aren't just healthy; they're a great way to incorporate some fun, or even a theme, into a dish by cutting vegetables into shapes. Use a variety of cooked and raw veggies to make the spread even more enticing, and add some fruit to the mix if you'd like.

2 x 400g tins butter beans, drained
1 clove garlic, crushed
$\frac{1}{2}$ teaspoon ground cumin
1 $\frac{1}{2}$ tablespoons lemon juice
$\frac{1}{3}$ cup (80ml) olive oil
2 tablespoons chopped parsley
salt and pepper
a large pinch of paprika

- Pop all the ingredients except the paprika into the bowl of a food processor and purée until smooth.
- Pour into a bowl and sprinkle with the paprika.
- Serve with crunchy crudités. We've used melon balls, carrot flashes, red-pepper stars, celery batons and sugar snaps.

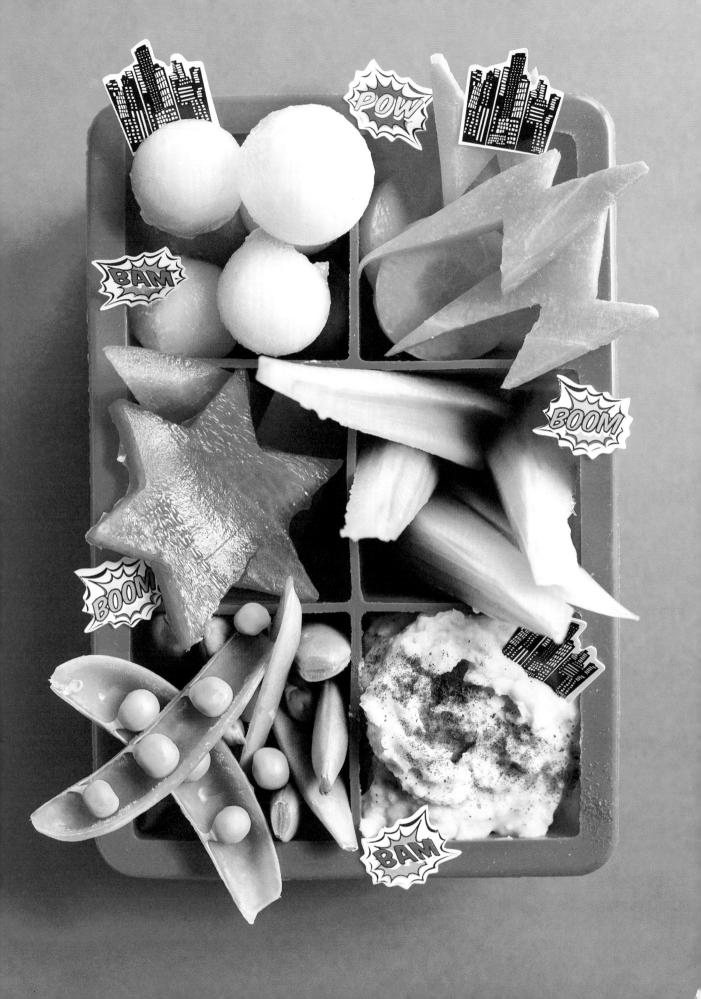

PARMESAN CHICKEN STRIPS

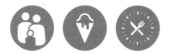

Makes 8 portions
Prep time: 10 mins
Cooking time: 20 mins

These chicken strips are a little more grown-up than the others in the book, so are great to do as a family snack. You could also use the coating on a flattened chicken breast to make a delicious schnitzel.

120g Parmesan, finely grated
120g ground almonds
salt and pepper
4 chicken breasts, cut into strips
2 eggs, beaten
2 tablespoons coconut oil for frying
2 tablespoons butter for frying
homemade mayo (p301), lemon
   wedges and chopped chives to serve

- Mix the Parmesan and almonds in a bowl and season with a little salt and pepper.
- Dip the chicken strips into the egg then coat with the Parmesan mix.
- Heat the coconut oil and butter in a pan and fry the chicken strips until golden on both sides.
- Serve in little cups with homemade mayo to dip, lemon wedges and chopped chives. If you're feeling creative, flavour the mayo for extra interest.

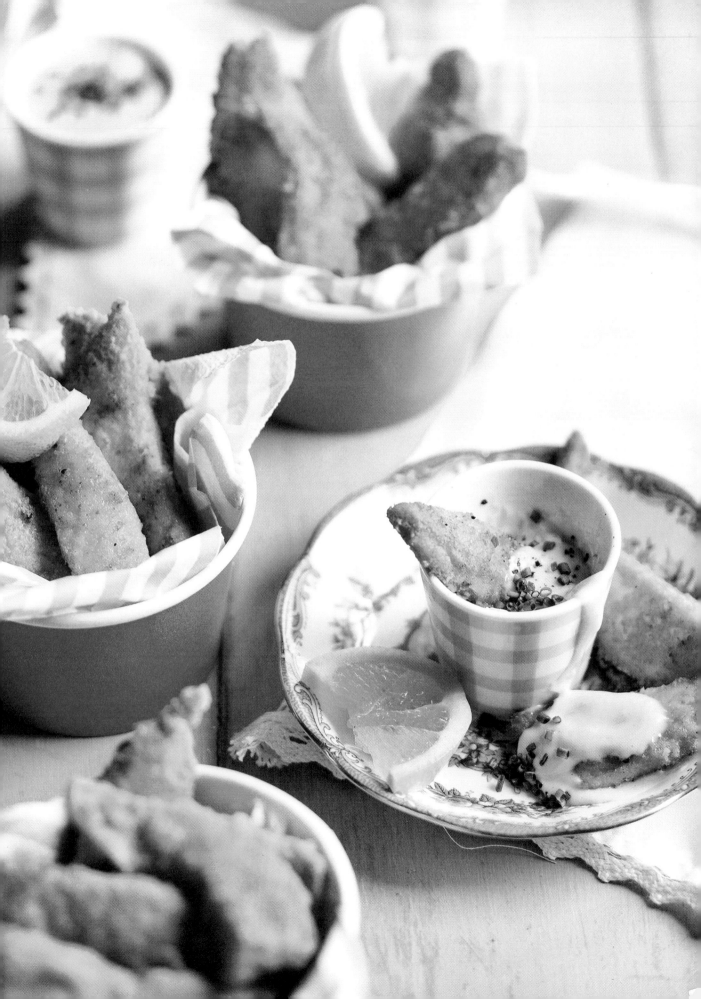

PRINCESS RITZ

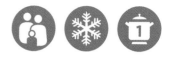

Makes 6 portions
Prep time: 30 minutes

Little girls love to act sophisticated and grown-up, and this dish is the perfect thing to make them feel like real princesses.

250g cream cheese
200g smoked salmon
⅓ cup (80ml) homemade mayo (p301)
the juice and zest of 1 lemon
2 heads baby gem lettuce
2 avocados

- Roll the cream cheese into 24 small balls then wrap the balls in the smoked salmon.
- Mix the mayo and the lemon juice and zest in a bowl.
- Use a few old-fashioned champagne glasses to serve the ritz. Put 2 pieces of lettuce, some sliced avocado and the smoked salmon balls into each glass.
- Top with a little lemony mayo and serve with a small fork.

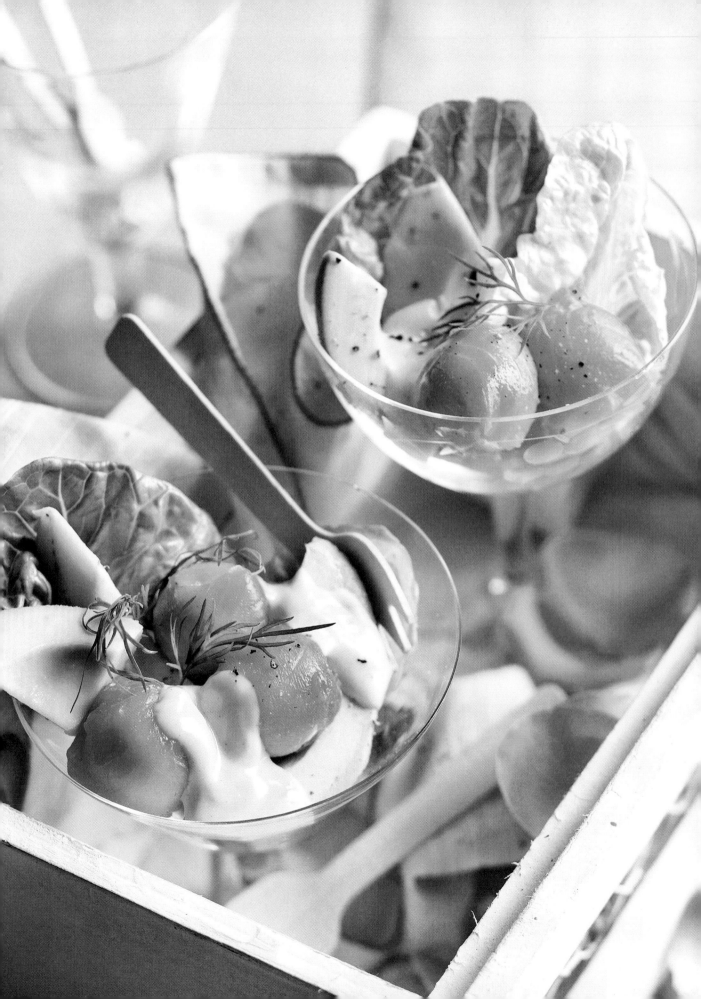

NOSHY NIBBLES

At the cake-and-jellybean jols of yore, there would be – besides the cake and jellybeans – piles of mini chocolates and miscellaneous sweeties. Here are some modern (healthier) equivalents.

APPLE PIE BITES .... Makes 12 bites

½ cup (90g) pitted dates
1 cup (80g) dried apple, chopped
½ cup (45g) oats
½ teaspoon ground cinnamon
½ teaspoon vanilla extract
2 tablespoons chopped pecans
(optional)

- Place all the ingredients in a food processor and blitz until they come together.
- Roll the mixture into balls and they're good to go.

COCOA-AND-COCONUT GRANOLA BARS .... Makes 12 bites

⅓ cup (80ml) honey
⅓ cup (80g) butter
1 teaspoon vanilla extract
¼ cup (30g) cocoa powder
100g chopped dark chocolate
1 cup (25g) organic puffed brown rice cereal
½ cup (45g) rolled oats
½ cup (40g) desiccated coconut
¼ cup (35g) sunflower seeds
¼ cup (30g) ground almonds

- Line a small square baking tray with silicone paper.
- In a small saucepan melt the honey, butter and vanilla. Bring it to the boil and cook for one minute. Take off the heat and add the cocoa and the chocolate and stir until it's all melted together.
- Mix the remaining ingredients in a bowl and pour the chocolate mix over them. Give everything a good stir so that they combine well.
- Using a spatula, press the mixture tightly into the lined baking tray.
- Place the tray in the fridge for at least an hour to set.
- Remove from the fridge and cut into bars or squares with a bread knife. The mixture is fragile so be gentle.

CHEWY HONEY-AND-COCONUT COOKIES .... Makes 12-15

3 tablespoons honey
90g butter
1 egg
¼ cup (60ml) milk
1 teaspoon vanilla extract
1 ½ cups (150g) almond flour
½ cup (40g) desiccated coconut

- Preheat the oven to 180°C.
- In a mixer, cream together the honey and butter until light and fluffy.
- Add the egg, milk and vanilla and mix until combined.
- Mix in the remaining ingredients to form a soft dough.
- Chill the dough in the fridge for an hour.
- Line a cookie sheet with silicone baking paper and roll the dough into 15 balls. Place them on the baking sheet with enough space for them to spread.
- Bake for 12-15 minutes until golden. Allow to cool before serving.

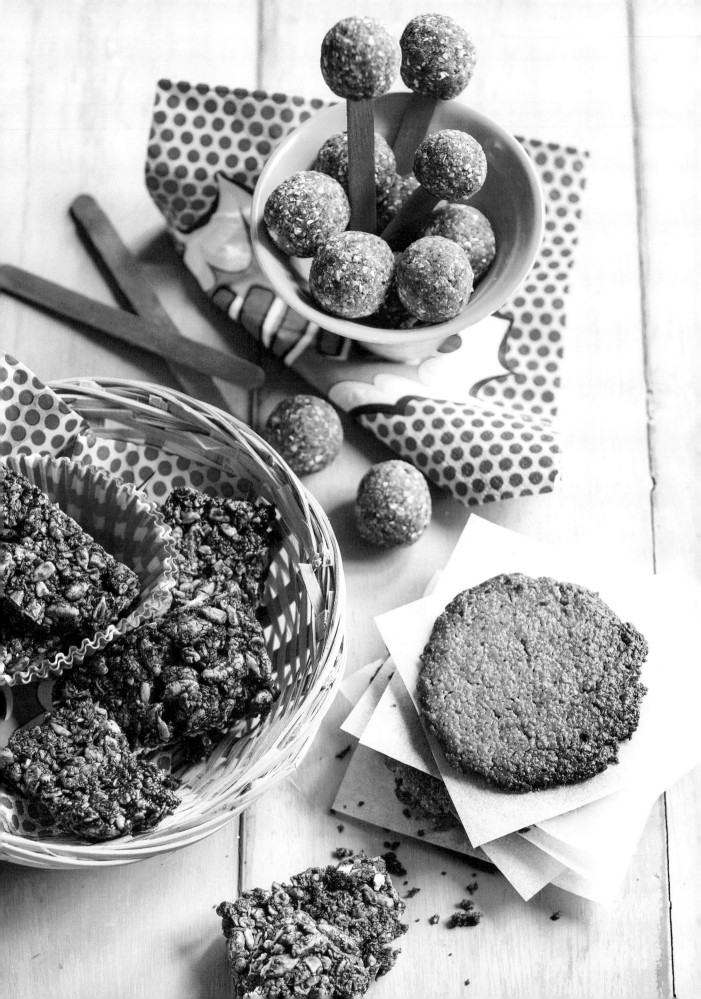

MINI CHEESE-AND-TOMATO PIZZAS

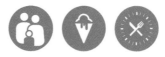

Makes 3 mini pizzas
Prep time: 30 mins (+ 1-2 hours' rest)
Cooking time: 20 mins

Everybody loves pizza! These cauli-pizzas take a bit of effort to make, but they're well worth it, and the recipe can be doubled quite easily. If you don't have a pizza stone for your oven (let alone a pizza oven), never fear: a heavy baking tray works just fine.

For the bases:
1 large head cauliflower, cooked
a pinch of salt
1 teaspoon dried mixed herbs
½ teaspoon garlic powder
¼ cup (22g) grated Parmesan
¼ cup (30g) grated mozzarella cheese
1 egg
almond flour if the mixture needs
   to be a little drier

For the topping:
3 tablespoons tomato purée
a handful of grated cheese (try a mix
   of mozzarella and cheddar)
100g cherry tomatoes, halved
salt and pepper
a little basil to garnish (optional)

TO MAKE THE BASE:

- Blitz the cauliflower in a food processor until it's very fine. Pour onto a clean kitchen towel to get rid of any excess water and to cool. Wring it out in the towel if necessary. There should be about 2 ½ cups (250g) of cauliflower.
- Pour the cauliflower into a bowl with the remaining ingredients (for the bases) and mix very well with your hands.
- Grease 3 small squares of silicone paper and press the dough tightly into 3 rounds on the paper. Allow to stand for an hour or two before you bake them.
- Preheat the oven to 240°C – probably as hot as your oven goes – along with a heavy baking tray or pizza stone.
- Pop the pizza bases onto the tray or stone and bake for 8-10 minutes until they start to darken. Remove from the oven.

TO COMPLETE THE PIZZAS:

- Top your pizzas with the tomato purée, cheese and cherry tomatoes and season with salt and pepper. Return the pizzas to the oven and cook until the cheese melts and starts to bubble.
- Remove from the oven and allow to cool slightly.
- Feel free to serve them on the silicone paper – cool and casual!

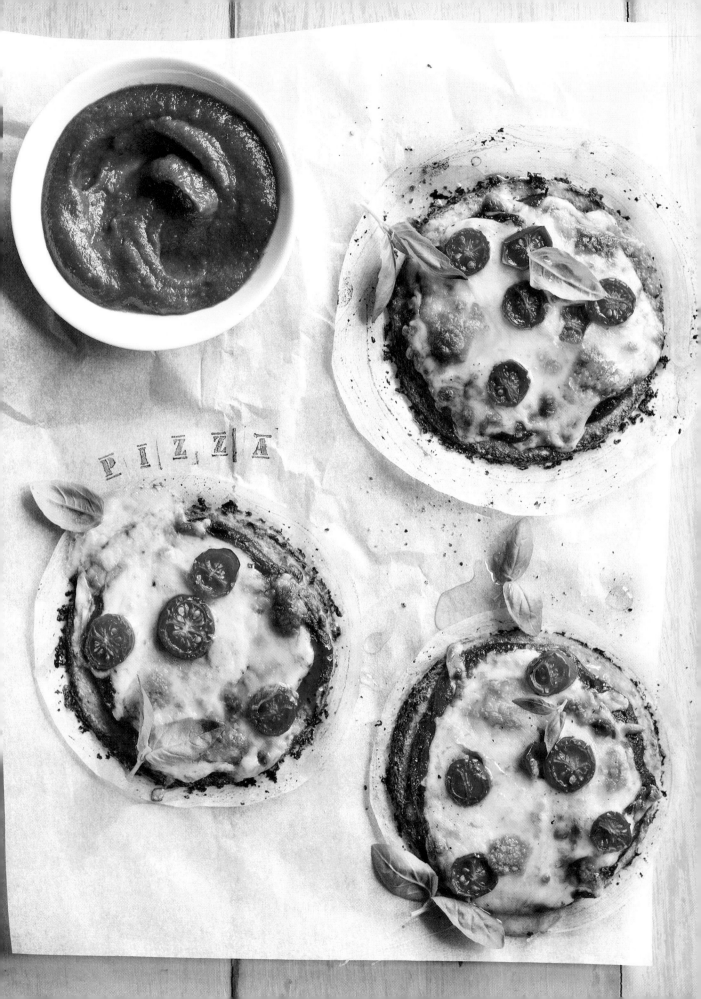

TREMENDOUS TEENS

Super food for ages

13 years +

From ages 5 to 12 or thereabouts, there's an outside chance your children will be mature enough to entertain themselves and be reasoned with, but happy enough to defer to your better judgement. A joyous time! Then comes high school – and one day your sweet girl is exchanged for a surly, catty teenager. Or your wide-eyed boy disappears and there's a gawky, spotty wastrel in his place. With this change – the arrival of puberty! – comes a change in eating habits and dietary requirements. For a number of reasons – read on – it can be a tricky time to keep your children on the right dietary track at this age. Teenagers are hard-wired to take the easy option whenever possible, so the dangers of convenience foods are multiplied. It's up to you to use this trait to your advantage: put the right foods under a teenager's nose and he won't bother looking elsewhere. Meanwhile, the good news is your teens are now old enough to cook for themselves and understand exactly why good nutrition is so important, so pass this book over and let them learn for themselves. You never know; they might even cook *you* a meal sometime...

WHAT'S GROWING ON?

What's growing on? *Everything*, that's what. Your little child is not so little any more, and will be becoming less so day by day. Teenage growth spurts start from 8-12 years in girls and 10-14 years in boys, and propel them skywards respectively at 9cm and 10.3cm on average per year at their peak. Girls gain around 25cm during the pubertal growth period until age 15, and boys 28cm – almost a full ruler length – until age 17. [1]

To fuel this hormone-induced body metamorphosis, teenagers need food, and lots of it. Girls of 14-18 need around 2,000 calories per day, while boys at that age need 20-40% more – up to 2,800 calories per day. (Wondering where all the food in your house is going? We'll give you a clue: it's your teenage son.) Throw in the raging hormones, exhausting school schedules, possible love interests, temper tantrums and sulk sessions, and it's enough to leave any parent at a loss for what to do. The kiddie honeymoon is over – what you've got now is a young adult in the making. (Enjoy it; next thing she'll be all grown up.)

CHANGING BODIES

To meet their growing needs, teens need *more*, and if yours is a son you may suddenly notice your food bills escalating while your fridge supplies vanish. Boys often seem almost impossible to satisfy, which can be strenuous on both you and your bank account. You may be tempted to drop the ball now and opt for the convenience of processed foods. Don't. Rather fill your kitchen and your fridge with accessible snacks for your teenager to help himself to. Think boiled eggs, roast chicken, a variety of fruit, nuts and so on. Teenagers are generally more open to experimenting than younger kids, so be aware that his menu is probably expanding. Just remember that if you buy a bulk bag of macadamias he may just eat the entire thing in one go. So think smart and plan ahead! As ever, protein helps with satiety and healthy fats are essential for energy, so make sure they're included at every meal. Offer energy-dense tubers (like sweet potato) and high-fibre foods (vegetables, fruits, nuts) to help him feel fuller for longer.

For girls, the beginning of adolescence can be some of the most turbulent years of their (and your) lives. With the onset of menstruation, their bodies begin to change rapidly, a process that can be more traumatic to deal with than it is for boys, and one that can come with a whole host of problems, both physical (like anaemia) and mental (like eating disorders). As usual, refined carbs exacerbate most of these difficulties, so teach your daughter to avoid them and to eat REAL food. This will also help neutralise those yo-yo-ing blood-sugar levels that can make a difficult time even harder.

SLOTH OR HUMAN?

Oh, the irony. You once spent *hours* trying to convince your toddler to go to sleep and now you cannot, for love or bribery, get your teenager out of bed. How is it possible for a human to sleep for 12 hours? Has it turned into a sloth?

You know what? Don't let it get to you. Teens need their sleep. Not 12 hours, perhaps – but between 9 and 10 hours a night is just fine. To help keep up the energy levels, make sure she's getting enough iron and vitamin B12.

TEEN TROUBLES

Acne

There's been a lot of research into the connection between diet and acne, though not much in scientific consensus. Because acne doesn't arise in traditional societies eating traditional foods, we believe it's directly linked to the modern industrial diet, and recommend removing sugar and wheat, in particular, from your teen's diet. There is strong evidence that certain foods exacerbate the problem, and the first suspects support our position: high-glycaemic foods[2]; in other words, foods packed with sugar and refined carbohydrates, such as white bread and cornflakes. The second suspect is milk, so we suggest dropping milk and possibly even dairy when the spots strike to see if that makes a difference. Note, however, that your teen will most likely require a calcium supplement for any extended spells off milk and dairy. [3]

An effective treatment for acne comes in the form of retinoids, a class of chemical compound found in vitamin A. A 2014 study has shown that vitamins A and E, along with zinc, are effective in both preventing and treating acne, so consider a multivitamin that includes high doses of these. [4]

Anaemia

Anaemia is a common complaint in teenage girls, usually as a result of menstruation in conjunction with poor eating choices. Adolescence is often a time of experimentation, and if your teenager gets her timing right/wrong, she may, for example, go vegan just as her period hits. (At the risk of sounding repetitive, we don't recommend vegetarianism, let alone veganism, for children.)

If your teen is diagnosed with anaemia, she will need to take an iron supplement for at least three months or as long as her doctor suggests. Animal protein will help to increase her iron levels, so fill her plate with red meat, eggs, chicken and fish. If she's decided to become a vegetarian, give her eggs, peas, beans and lentils, and ensure she eats foods high in vitamin C (tomatoes, citrus fruit, sweet potato), which is necessary to help the absorption of plant iron.

Eating disorders

Having a child suffer from an eating disorder ranks right up there on the parental-nightmares list. They are more likely to manifest in girls, but boys are also susceptible to them, so keep your wits about you and look out for any of the following warning signs:

- Obsession with body image/weight ▪ Fixation on calories, food and nutrition ▪ Relentless dieting even when thin ▪ Consumption of diet pills or laxatives ▪ Fast, unexplained weight loss or gain ▪ Obsessive (and unnecessary) exercising ▪ Making excuses not to eat ▪ Avoiding social events involving food ▪ Going to the bathroom straight after eating ▪ Eating alone or in secret ▪ Hoarding high-calorie food.

If you suspect your child may be suffering from an eating disorder, seek help from a professional immediately. The longer it's allowed to manifest, the worse it will become. And be gentle; many eating disorders are the result of anxiety and low self-esteem.

Mood swings

Was it something I said? Yes, almost certainly. Or not. You didn't say the right thing, or you did but in the wrong tone. The only thing more sensitive than a teenager's moods is a pumice massage on sunburnt skin. So what's the remedy? For you, deep breaths and the recognition of a passing phase. For them, there are some habits and foods that can help balance their moods.

- **Eat regularly – and don't miss breakfast.** Anyone who's experienced the symptoms of *hanger* (that's anger brought on by hunger, prevalent in pregnant women and teens alike) will know the importance of eating regularly. Breakfast is one of the most common meals missed by teenagers, especially late risers rushing to get to school, so make sure she starts the day with something more than a seed cracker.
- **Avoid caffeine.** It can cause irritability, sleeplessness and headaches.
- **Consider an essential fatty-acid supplement.** They have been known to aid in improving depressive symptoms.
- **Look out for nutrition deficiencies.** The following deficiencies can have negative effects on mood:

DEFICIENCY	MOOD-ALTERING EFFECT	FOOD TO EAT
B vitamins	Tiredness, irritability, feelings of depression	Animal proteins: eggs, meat, fish
Folic acid	A specific B vitamin to look out for; increases the chances of depression	Liver, green veg, citrus fruits
Iron	Tiredness, lethargy, chronic weakness	Red meat, poultry, fish. Avoid tea with meals; it can affect iron absorption.
Selenium	May increase feelings of depression	Fish, seeds, Brazil nuts, mushrooms

Other supplements to consider

Ideally, your teenager will be getting all her nutrient requirements from her diet and won't need any supplements. But teens can be hard-headed and short-sighted, and won't necessarily eat what you tell them to, especially when you're not around or if, for example, they're going through that vegetarian phase. As we've seen, there are also certain conditions, such as depression and acne, that may benefit from the addition of specific vitamins and minerals to their daily intake. Consider supplements if these important nutrients are not being consumed in sufficient quantities:

Iron: *Lots* needed. Daily requirements generally triple in adolescence due to increased blood volume and lean body mass, and this is exacerbated further in girls when their menstrual cycles begin. (See Anaemia on p269.) Found in red meat, seafood, green and leafy vegetables. [5]

Calcium: Half a person's adult strength is built during the teen years, and calcium is critical for this. 3-5 servings per day – found in milk, yoghurt, cheese.

Folic acid: An essential B vitamin for growth and development, it also aids in warding off depression (as above). Consume regularly – found in spinach, avocado, asparagus.

Vitamin D: Essential for bone health. 2-3 servings per week of oily fish – also found in liver, cheese and eggs.

Magnesium: Required for healthy nerve and muscle function. Consume regularly – found in dark green veg, fish, dairy, nuts.

Zinc: A powerful antioxidant for optimum health, and effective in treating acne (see Acne on p269). Consume regularly – found in meat, shellfish, dairy.

Fruit and vegetables: Generally good, especially the veg.

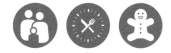

DIPPY CHIPPY NACHOS

Serves 2-4 as a snack
Prep time: 5 mins
Cooking time: 10 mins

As amazing as corn chips might taste, they're pure refined carbs – out of a bag they're about as unhealthy as can be, loaded with junk ingredients and cooked in seed oil. Make our dippy chippy nachos the delicious alternative for teen snacking.

2-3 handfuls homemade dippy chippies (p226)

1 cup (250g) cooked beef mince, warmed (p294)

2 tomatoes, chopped

1 cup (100g) grated Cheddar

1 avocado

the juice of ½ a lemon

salt and pepper

½ cup (125ml) sour cream

1 tablespoon chopped fresh coriander

1 pickled jalapeno, sliced

- Preheat the oven to 200°C.
- Place the dippy chippies onto a large ovenproof plate and spoon the mince mixture over them.
- Sprinkle the chopped tomato and the grated cheese over the mince.
- Bake the nachos uncovered in the oven for about 10 minutes, until the cheese has melted.
- While the nachos are cooking, mash the avocado and the lemon juice together with a fork to make a quick guacamole. Season with a little salt and pepper.
- Remove the nachos from the oven, top with the guacamole and sour cream, and serve with the fresh coriander and sliced chilli.

WE'VE MADE OUR DIPPY CHIPS WITH BEEF MINCE, BUT TRY THEM WITH SECRET VEGETABLE TOMATO SAUCE OR WITH GRILLED CHICKEN

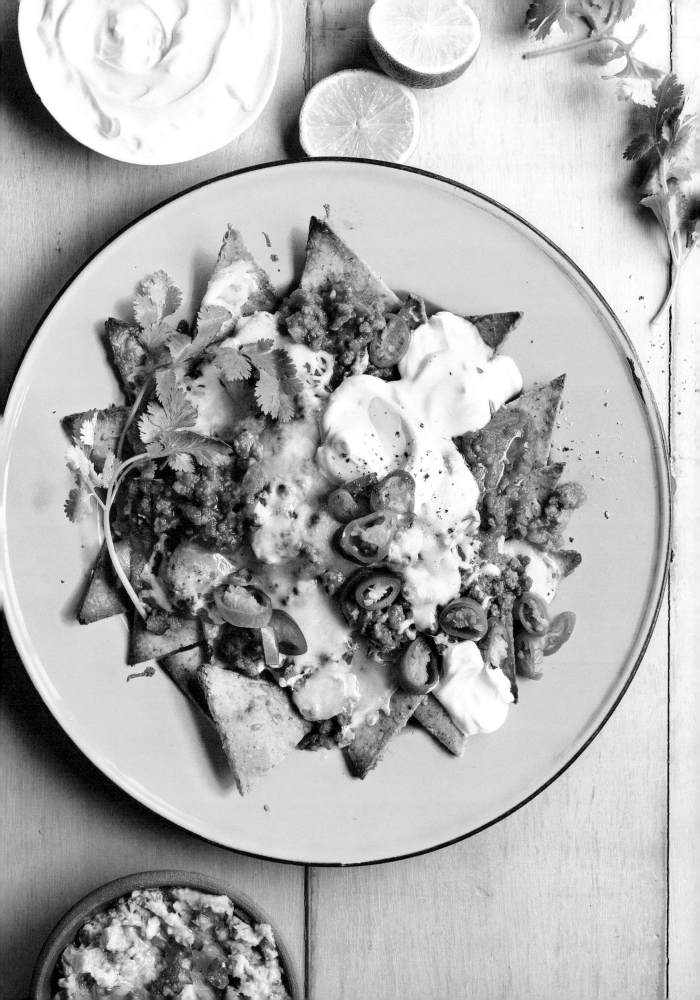

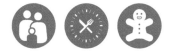

POWER POPPERS

Makes 14 poppers
Prep time: 20 mins
Cooking time: 20 mins

Chilli poppers are absolutely delicious and they're even better when they're not drenched in soggy batter and dripping in reheated seed oil. Try these bacon-wrapped flavour bombs on your teens – they won't ever want the restaurant version.

14 fresh large jalapeño chillies
250-300g streaky bacon

For the Mexican white sauce:
2 cups (500ml) homemade mayo (p301)
¾ cup (185ml) milk
¼ teaspoon smoked paprika
1 teaspoon ground cumin
½ teaspoon salt
1 ½ teaspoons garlic powder
1 ½ teaspoons dried oregano

For the filling:
70g grated mozzarella
70g grated Cheddar
70g cream cheese
1 clove garlic, crushed
1 tablespoon chopped parsley
salt and pepper

- Bring a small pot of water to the boil.
- While you're waiting, make a single lengthways slit in each chilli.
- Add the chillies to the water and boil for about 3 minutes. When the skin starts to peel, transfer them into a bowl of cold water. Using your fingers, scoop the seeds out and dry the chillies well.
- In a bowl, mix all the ingredients for the Mexican white sauce and set aside.
- To make the filling, mix all the ingredients in a bowl.
- Stuff each jalapeño with enough filling for the chilli to return to its original shape.
- Wrap one or two pieces of bacon around each chilli, ensuring the slit is completely covered, and lay the chillies on a baking tray.
- Preheat the grill, then place the chillies underneath it to cook. Grill until the bacon is crispy, turning as needed.

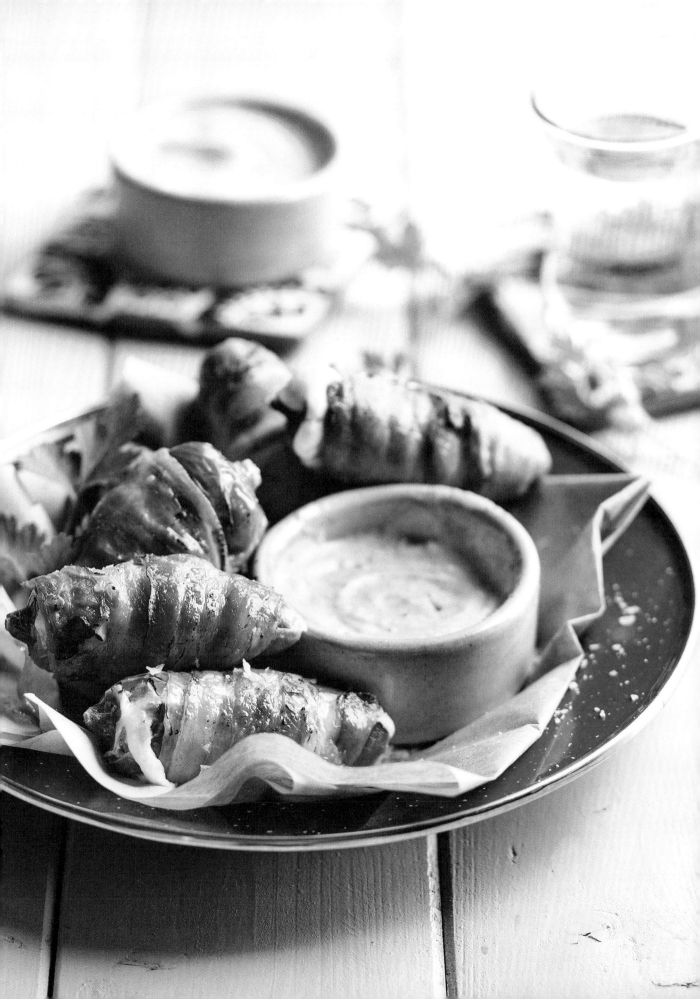

FUNKY FISH TACOS

Makes 6 small tacos
Prep time: 20 mins
Cooking time: 15 mins

This recipe uses our low-carb pancakes as the tacos. We cooked them in a slightly smaller pan this time and got 6 tacos from the recipe. Plop them on the table with bowls of fillings, and leave everyone to make their own. If your brood isn't into fish, try them with chicken.

6 low-carb pancakes (p300)

For the fish:
600g firm white fish, bones and skin
  removed
salt and pepper
2 tablespoons butter

For the salsa:
2 radishes, thinly sliced
½ cup (75g) finely diced cucumber
1 spring onion, finely sliced
a handful of cherry tomatoes,
  quartered
the juice of 2 limes
50ml olive oil
a handful of fresh coriander leaves
1 chopped chilli (optional)
salt and pepper
½ cup (125ml) sour cream or Mexican
  white sauce (previous page)

TO MAKE THE FISH:
▪ Cut the fish into thick fingers and season well with salt and pepper. Heat the butter in a frying pan and fry the fish for 2 minutes on each side, until cooked through. Remove from the heat and roughly flake.

TO MAKE THE SALSA:
▪ Mix together all the ingredients, except the sour cream or Mexican white sauce, and season well with salt and pepper. Leave out the chilli or serve it on the side, depending on preferences.

TO MAKE THE TACO:
▪ Hold the pancake in your hand and spoon in a little sour cream or white sauce. Top with the flaked fish and finally spoon in some salsa. Eat immediately – and don't even think about using a knife and fork!

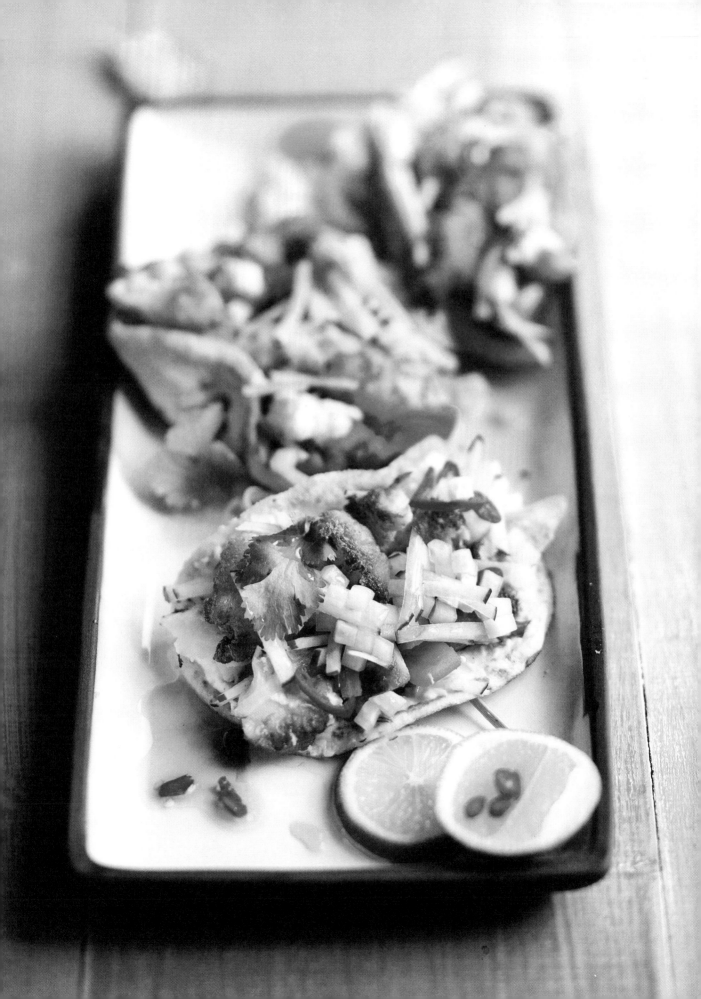

SUPER BEEF BURGERS

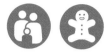

Makes 4 big burgers
Prep time: 20 mins
Cooking time: 10 mins

There are few meals more satisfying than a juicy, delicious, freshly made hamburger – another reason why commercial burger patties should be banned for all eternity. If you have a good relationship with your butcher, order your mince with 20% pork; it'll just melt in your mouth.

For the burger patties:
800g best-quality beef mince
1 onion, finely chopped
2 tablespoons barbecue spice
10g chopped parsley
2 eggs
salt and pepper
3 tablespoons butter, for frying

For the burger:
8 pieces crispy bacon
4 thick slices of Cheddar
4 pieces of lettuce
2 tomatoes, sliced
4 gherkins, sliced
1 red onion, halved and thinly sliced
homemade mayo (p301) and ketchup
   (p294)
a little butter for the rolls
4 sesame burger buns, halved
   (p297)

- In a bowl, mix together the burger patty ingredients, except the butter, using your hands.
- Heat a little butter in a frying pan and fry off a teaspoon of the mixture. Taste it for seasoning. Add a little more salt and pepper if necessary.
- Shape the prepared mince into 4 generous burger patties. Expect them to thicken as they cook, so make them a little thinner than the end size you want.
- Heat the butter in a frying pan and fry the patties for about 4 minutes per side. Make sure they are dark and golden. Lay the bacon and cheese over each patty and place a lid over the pan for a minute. This will heat the bacon through and melt the cheese.
- While the patties are cooking, construct your burgers. Start with lettuce, tomato, gherkin and sliced onion, layered with homemade ketchup and mayo. Top the pile with the cheesy beef patty and any other toppings that take your fancy. Finish off with the top of the burger bun, then prepare for burger bliss.

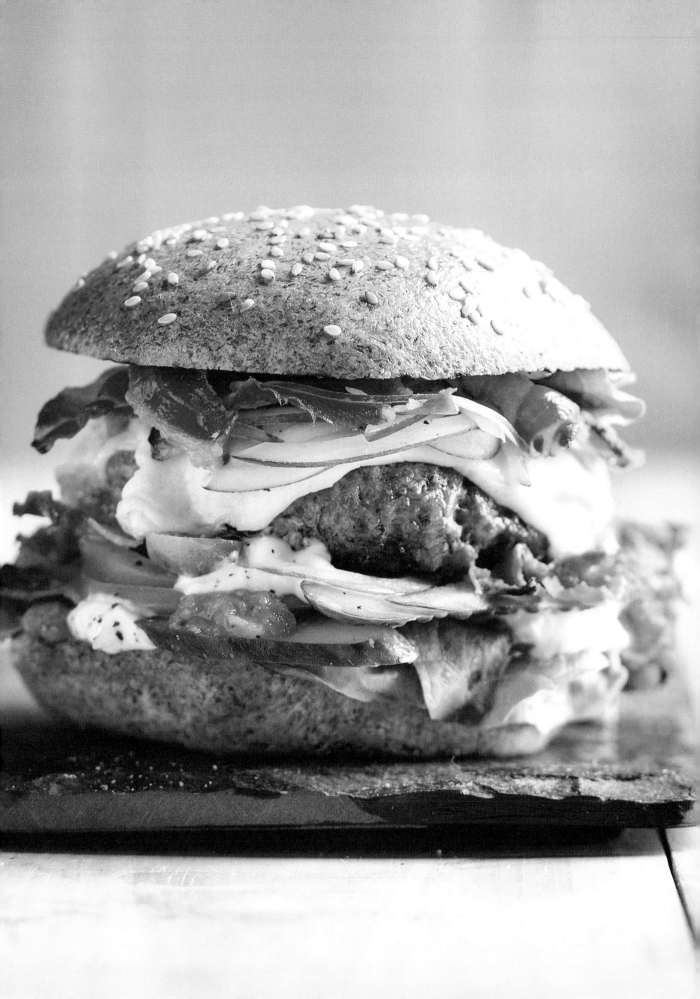

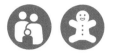

RADICAL RIBS

Makes 3-4 portions
Prep time: 2 hrs
Cooking time: 10 mins

Sticky ribs! It doesn't get much better than this. Yes, they may take a bit of time to make well, but the whole process is worth it in the end. Any teenagers in the vicinity – and your entire family – will love your efforts.

1 batch of homemade BBQ marinade (p295)
2 cups water
2 teaspoons grated ginger
2 large racks pork belly ribs

- Preheat the oven to 160°C.
- Mix together the BBQ sauce, water and ginger.
- Place the ribs in a deep oven tray so that they're lying flat, and pour the watery BBQ sauce over them. Cover the tray tightly with tin foil.
- Bake the ribs for 1 ½ hours until they just start to soften.
- When the ribs come out of the oven, pour the sauce into a pot. Place the pot on the stove and cook the sauce until it thickens to an almost sticky consistency. (You can get this step out of the way the day before eating if you'd prefer; simply store the ribs and sauce separately in the fridge and bring to room temperature the next day before the next step.)
- Baste the ribs with the reduced sticky BBQ sauce and place them on the barbecue or under the grill for a few minutes on each side until they're dark, sticky and crispy.
- Serve hot!

USE BELLY RIBS IF YOU CAN. THEY HAVE A BIT MORE FAT ON THEM AND ARE THE PERFECT SIZE

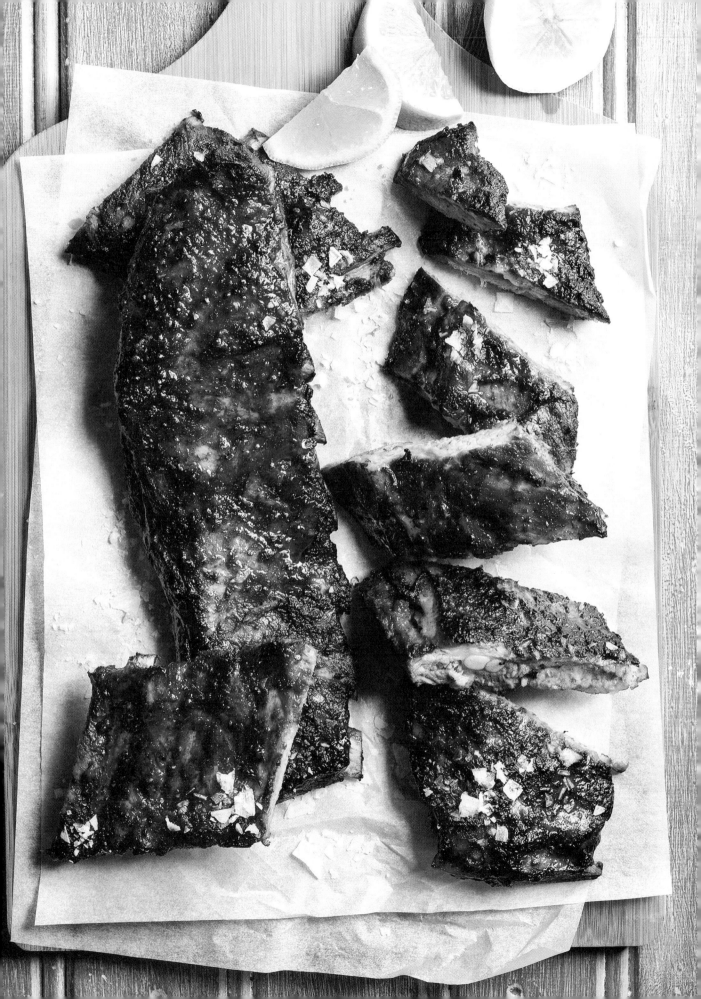

EGG-FRIED VEGETABLE 'CAULI-RICE'

Makes 2-4 portions
Prep time: 25 mins
Cooking time: 10 mins

What's more take-out than egg-fried rice? Try this version, which just happens to exclude the rice. Once you get into the swing of things, you can play around with different veggies and perhaps add some chicken or bacon.

4 tablespoons coconut oil
4 eggs, beaten
2 tablespoons grated ginger
4 cloves garlic, crushed
1 onion, finely chopped
1 red pepper, chopped
100g sliced mushrooms
4 courgettes, chopped
3 tablespoons mirin
3 cups (300g) raw cauli-rice (cauliflower blitzed to a rice texture in the food processor)
100g finely sliced spring onions
3 tablespoons tamari soya sauce
1 teaspoon sesame oil
fresh chilli or sugar-free chilli sauce to serve
fresh coriander to garnish

- Heat half the coconut oil in a hot wok.
- Pour the beaten eggs into the wok and cook for about a minute or so, until they're the consistency of a lightly scrambled omelette. Carefully remove them from the wok and set aside.
- Wipe out the wok with paper towel and add the remaining coconut oil.
- Fry the ginger and garlic for a minute or so, and add the onion, pepper, mushrooms and courgettes. Stir-fry everything until lightly browned and tender – about 2 minutes.
- Stir in the mirin and stir-fry for a further 30 seconds.
- Add the cauli-rice, egg, spring onion, soya sauce and sesame oil.
- Stir-fry everything together until it's heated through. Using a spatula, roughly chop the egg into smaller pieces as you stir.
- Garnish with fresh coriander and serve with chilli.

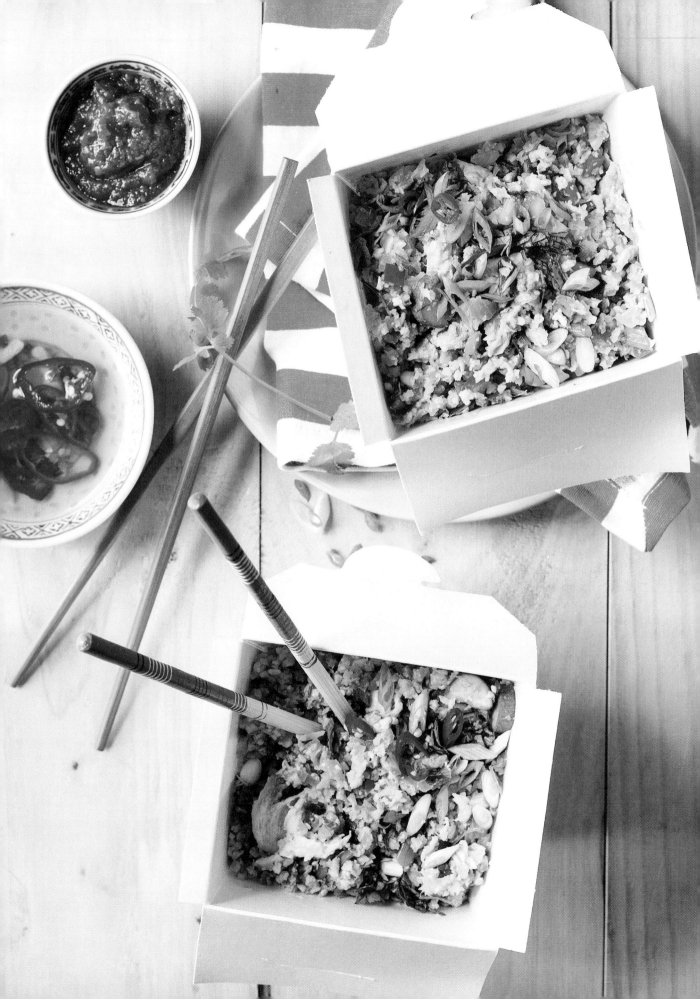

FANTASTIC FONDUE

Serves 6-8 people
Prep time: 30-60 mins
Cooking time: 10+ mins

Fondues may seem pretty passé, but they're great fun as long as you're not wearing chocolate-brown corduroy trousers... They're also a great way to keep teens entertained – by doing the cooking themselves while enjoying a selection of interesting new tastes.

For the cheese sauce:
1 ½ cups (375ml) white wine (optional)
500ml cream
2 heaped teaspoons Dijon mustard
3 cups (300g) grated cheese (mild
  gruyère, emmenthal or Cheddar)

Dipping suggestions:
fried mushrooms
slices of fried chorizo
meatballs (use the burger patty
  recipe on p278)
lightly cooked carrots
lightly cooked asparagus
lightly cooked radish
gherkins
pickled onions
cherry tomatoes
chunks of apple
lightly cooked broccoli or cauliflower
  florets
burger buns, cubed (p297)

- Pour the wine into a saucepan and bring it to the boil. Simmer until it has reduced by half.
- Add the cream and mustard and continue to simmer until the cream thickens slightly – about 5-10 minutes. Remove from the heat. (NB at this point: once the cheese is mixed into the sauce, you need to serve it immediately. If you want to finish it off later, allow the cream sauce to cool and reheat it just before serving.)
- Add the cheese to the hot sauce and stir until melted. Pour it into a fondue pot and serve immediately with a variety of bits and pieces for dipping.

DON'T STOP AT CHEESE FONDUES – GO CHOCOLATE FOR DESSERT!

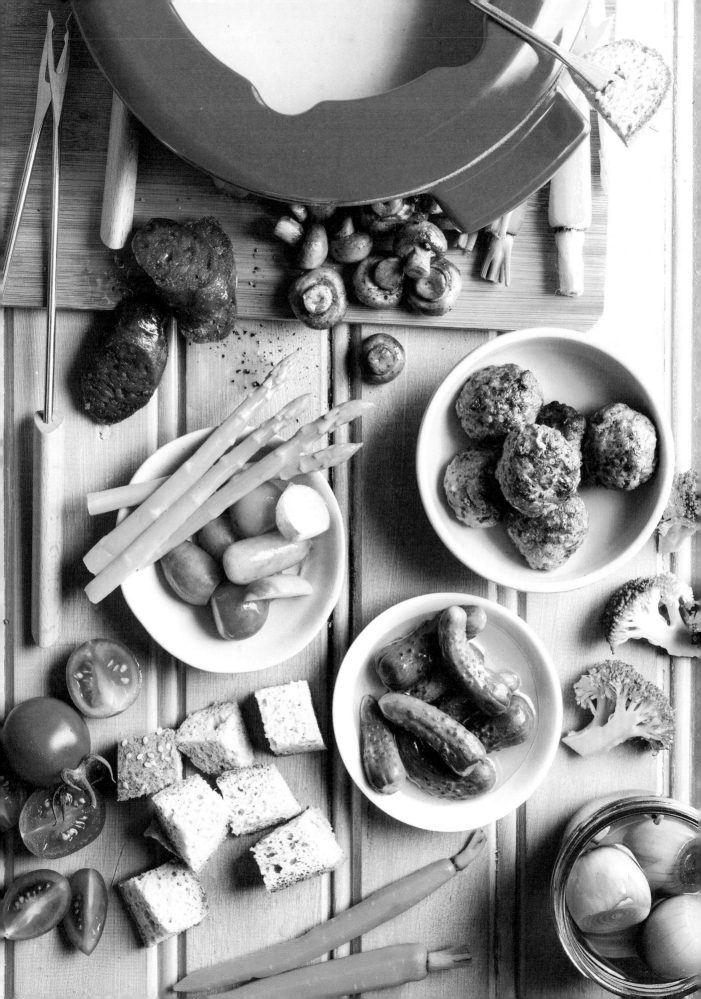

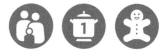

CRISPY CHICKEN

Makes 4-5 portions
Prep time: 10 mins
Cooking time: 1 hour

You'd never guess that these crispy chunks of chicken are baked, not fried – but they're scrumptious nonetheless. Make more than you think you need and keep the paper napkins handy, because there are going to be loads of sticky fingers to deal with!

2 ½ cups (250g) almond flour
salt and pepper
1 teaspoon cayenne pepper
2 teaspoons paprika
1 teaspoon dried oregano
1 teaspoon garlic powder
2 eggs, beaten
¼ cup (60ml) buttermilk
8-10 chicken pieces (we used legs and thighs)
¼ cup (60ml) melted butter

- Preheat the oven to 180°C.
- Line a baking tray with tin foil and place a greased oven rack on top of it.
- Sieve together the almond flour, salt, pepper, cayenne pepper, paprika, oregano and garlic powder into a bowl. Add a little extra almond flour if a lot is left behind in the sieve.
- In a separate bowl beat the eggs with the buttermilk.
- Dip each chicken piece into the almond flour mixture, then the egg mixture, and finally back into the almond flour. Use your hands to fill any gaps on the chicken pieces.
- Lay the crumbed chicken pieces on the greased rack, and sprinkle over any leftover almond flour.
- Carefully drizzle the melted butter over the chicken pieces, or use a pastry brush to dab it on.
- Bake for an hour until the chicken is golden and cooked through.
- Serve with some homemade coleslaw (p186).

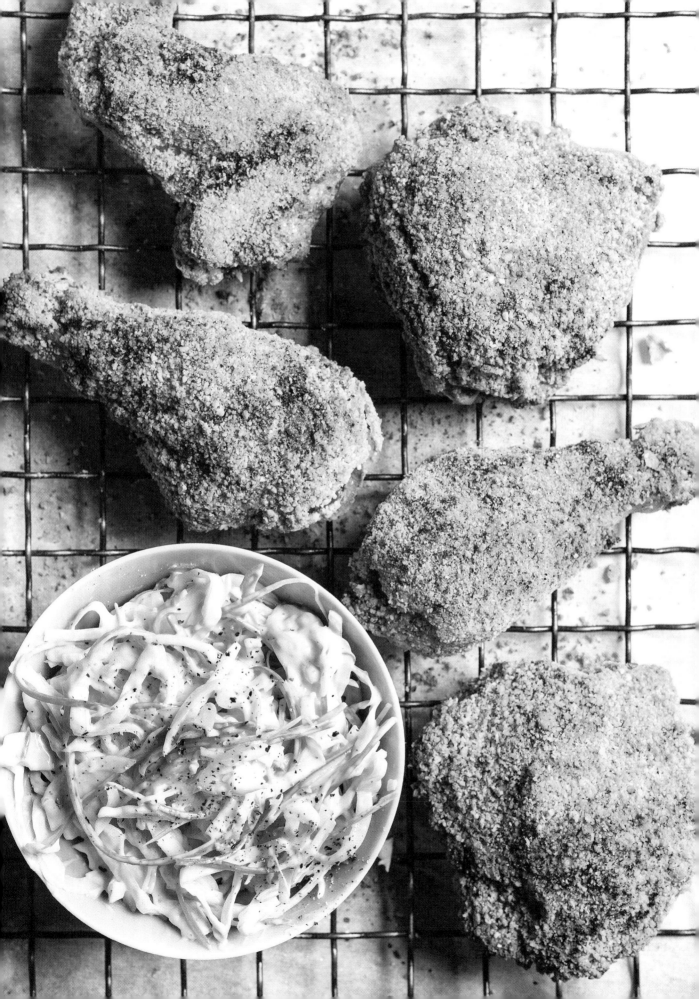

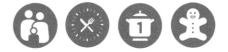

KILLER CALAMARI

Makes 4 portions
Prep time: 20 mins
Cooking time: 10 mins

For some reason, homemade calamari often comes out wrong. Here's the secret so that never happens again: get the pan smoking hot, flash fry the calamari, don't crowd the pan. Get that right and this recipe is a breeze. Don't forget the tentacles – they're the tastiest bit.

500g cleaned calamari tubes and tentacles
salt and pepper
3 tablespoons butter
lemon wedges and homemade mayo (p301) to serve

For the sauce:
½ cup (125g) melted butter
4 cloves garlic, crushed
10g chopped parsley
the juice of 2 lemons
1 teaspoon paprika
1 chopped green chilli (optional)
salt and pepper

- Slice the calamari tubes in half and lightly score the inside. Make sure they are very dry and season well with salt and pepper.
- To make the sauce, place the sauce ingredients in a small saucepan and bring to the boil. Remove from the heat and set aside.
- Heat a little butter in a heavy-based frying pan until very hot. Using more butter as needed, sear the calamari in batches for about 2 minutes and set aside. (If you fry it all together it will release liquid and boil.)
- Once you've seared all the calamari, return it to the pan and pour over the hot sauce. Let it cook in the sauce for a few minutes until soft.
- Serve the calamari with fresh lemon wedges and mayo; add some interesting flavours to the mayo to spice it up.

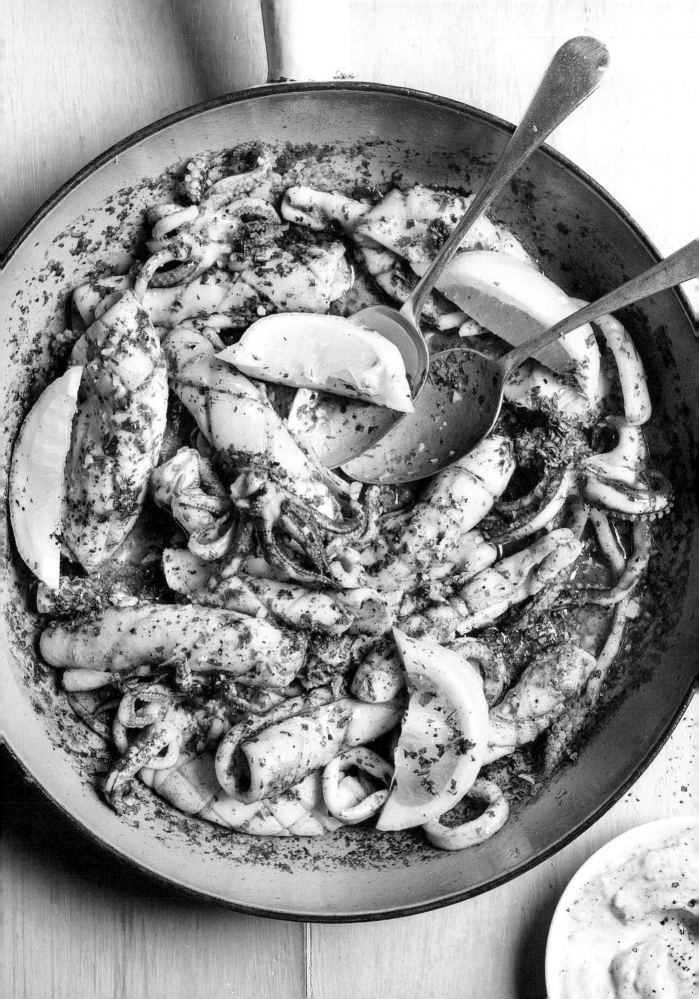

STOCK

TO COMPLEMENT THE AGE-GROUP-APPROPRIATE MEALS THROUGHOUT THE BOOK, HERE ARE THE BASIC KITCHEN STAPLES THAT WILL SET YOU AND YOUR FAMILY UP FOR LIFE – FROM CHICKEN STOCK TO BASIL PESTO.

CHICKEN STOCK
Makes about 1.5 litres

1 whole chicken or 1.5kg chicken bones
2.5 litres water
200g carrots, thickly sliced
2 leeks, thinly sliced
1 stalk celery, roughly sliced
2 onions, peeled, studded with 3 cloves
150g button mushrooms, sliced
4 sprigs parsley
2 sprigs thyme
1 bay leaf
5 peppercorns

- Place the chicken or chicken bones in a large pot and cover with the water.
- Bring to the boil, then turn down to a gentle simmer. Using a slotted spoon, skim off any scum that has risen to the surface.
- Add the remaining ingredients to the stock and simmer gently for 1½-2 hours.
- When it's ready, strain the stock through a fine sieve or muslin cloth. Allow to cool.
- Use immediately or freeze for later use.

SIMPLE FISH STOCK
Makes about 1 litre

1kg white fish bones and trimmings
2 tablespoons butter
1 onion, thinly sliced
2 leeks, thinly sliced
4 sprigs parsley
2 sprigs thyme
4 sprigs fennel
1 bay leaf
5 peppercorns
juice of ½ a lemon
1.5 litres cold water

- Rinse the fish bones under cold running water and drain.
- Melt the butter in a pot and gently fry the onions and the leeks until completely soft but not browned.
- Add the remaining ingredients to the pot and bring to the boil.
- Reduce the heat and gently simmer for 25 minutes. Skim off any foam that rises to the top of the liquid.
- When it's ready, strain the stock through a fine sieve or muslin cloth. Allow to cool.
- Use immediately or freeze for later use.

BEEF STOCK
Makes about 1 litre

1.5kg beef bones
200g carrots, roughly sliced
2 stalks celery, roughly sliced
1 onion, coarsely chopped
2 leeks, thinly sliced
2 litres water
6 tomatoes, seeded and chopped
150g button mushrooms, thinly sliced
2 cloves garlic, peeled
4 sprigs parsley
2 sprigs thyme
1 bay leaf
5 peppercorns

- Preheat the oven to 220°C.
- Place the bones on a roasting tray and roast for 30 minutes in the oven until well browned. Turn them occasionally.
- When the bones are brown, add the carrots, celery, onion and leeks to the pan and roast together for 5 minutes. Give everything a good stir before it goes into the oven.
- Transfer everything from the roasting tray into a large pot, ensuring you scrape out all the flavourful sticky bits.
- Add the water and the remaining ingredients to the pot and bring to the boil. Reduce the heat to a gentle simmer, and simmer uncovered for about 3 hours, skimming off any scum that rises to the surface.
- When it's ready, strain the stock through a fine sieve or muslin cloth. Allow to cool.
- Use immediately or freeze for later use.

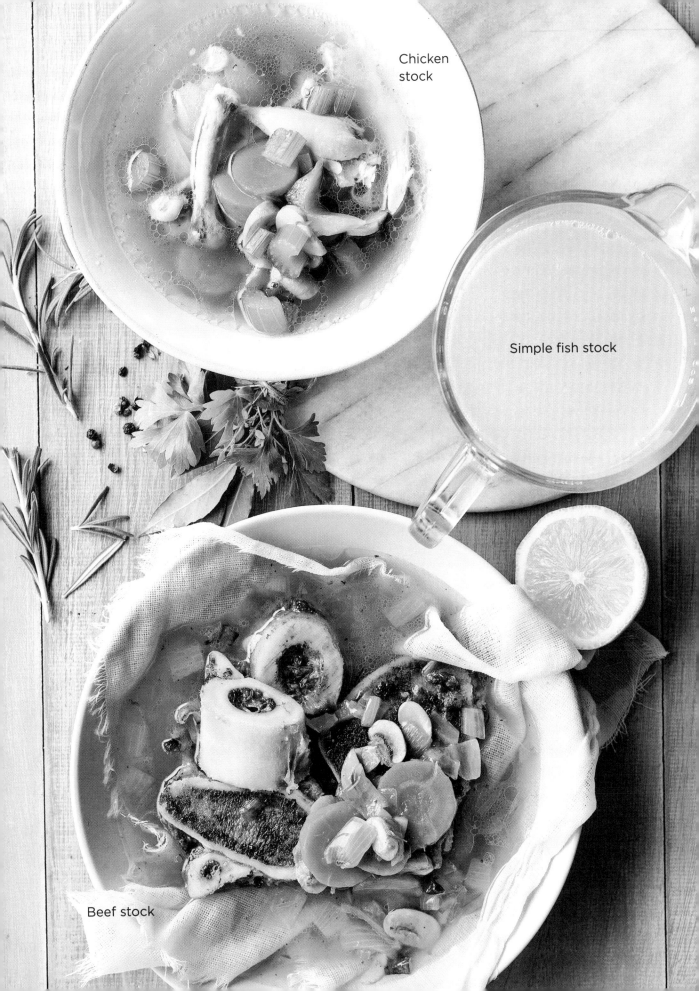

Chicken stock

Simple fish stock

Beef stock

SAUCES, KETCHUP AND DRESSING

Store-bought ketchup, sauces and dressings are absolutely packed with sugar and any number of flavourants, stabilisers and seed oils. These recipes are far healthier and really delicious. Turn the page for the meaty beef mince, and other sauces not pictured.

SECRET VEGETABLE TOMATO SAUCE .... Makes about 1 litre

This sauce is superb for kids who are iffy about veggies – they won't even know they're in there.

1 tablespoon butter

1 tablespoon coconut oil

1 onion, finely chopped

2 cloves garlic, chopped

4 courgettes, grated *(zucchini - use what we have)*

2 stalks celery, chopped

3 carrots, peeled and grated

50g tomato paste *(1 small can)*

4 x 400g tins whole peeled tomatoes

400ml water

1 teaspoon dried mixed herbs *(½t basil ½t oregano)*

salt and pepper to taste (optional)

- Heat the butter and coconut oil in a large pot. *medium heat* Add the onion, garlic, courgettes, celery and carrots and fry together until everything is soft.
- Add the tomato paste and cook for 1 minute.
- Blend together the tinned tomatoes, then add them to the pot with the water and herbs, and bring everything up to a simmer.
- Simmer for about 30-45 minutes until thick and reduced.
- Remove from the heat and blend well with a hand-blender.
- Season with salt and pepper.

RATATOUILLE .... Makes 4 portions

Keep the veggies chunky and ratatouille can be a meal on its own, or chop them finely for a sauce. This is another dish worth making in bulk and freezing for quick meals or as additions to others.

2 tablespoons butter

1 onion, chopped

1 aubergine, diced

1 yellow or red pepper, seeded and diced

4 courgettes, sliced or diced

125g button mushrooms, chopped

1 clove garlic, crushed

1 tablespoon tomato paste

1 x 400g tin chopped tomatoes, blended

½ cup water

a handful fresh basil, chopped (optional)

salt

- In a wide pan, melt the butter on a medium heat. Add the vegetables and gently fry until soft. Add the garlic and fry for a minute.
- Stir in the tomato paste and fry for another minute or so. Add the tinned tomatoes and water and simmer slowly for about 20 minutes until the sauce thickens.
- Add the chopped basil and a little salt. The ratatouille is now ready to serve as a vegetable option or as a delicious Mediterranean sauce. Or freeze it for future meals.

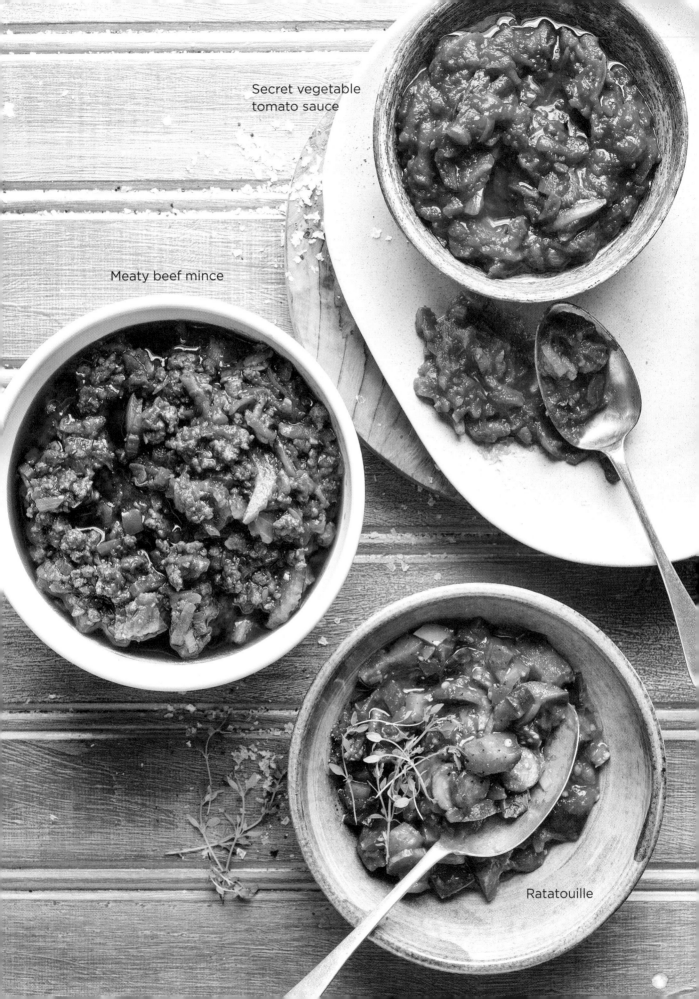

Secret vegetable
tomato sauce

Meaty beef mince

Ratatouille

MEATY BEEF MINCE (pictured on previous page) .... Makes 4 portions

An emergency supply of beef mince in the freezer can be a lifesaver, whether you need a quick breakfast, lunch or supper. We suggest making 4 times this recipe and freezing the rest in batches.

2 tablespoons butter
1 onion, finely chopped
2 celery stalks, finely chopped
1 carrot, peeled and grated
2 teaspoons rosemary, finely chopped
1 clove garlic, crushed
3 rashers bacon, chopped (optional)
400g beef mince
2 tablespoons tomato purée
1 x 400g tin chopped tomatoes,
   blended
½ cup (125ml) beef stock or water
1 bay leaf
salt and pepper

- Heat the butter in a saucepan and gently cook the onion, celery, carrot and rosemary until soft. Add the garlic and cook for a minute, then add the bacon and cook for a further 5 minutes.
- Sprinkle the beef mince into the saucepan and brown on a higher heat, using a wooden spoon to separate it.
- Stir in the tomato paste and fry for a few extra minutes.
- Add in the chopped tomatoes, stock and the bay leaf and simmer for 45 minutes or until the sauce has thickened and is a rich dark colour. Add a little salt and pepper to season.

HOMEMADE KETCHUP (pictured on p299) .... Makes 500ml

Homemade ketchup is a true winner; the only problem with this recipe is your kids will want you to make it over and over. It keeps in the fridge for at least two weeks so make a generous batch.

50g butter
1 onion, roughly chopped
2 cloves garlic, chopped
½ teaspoon ground ginger
¼ teaspoon ground cinnamon
½ teaspoon ground cloves
¼ teaspoon ground allspice
60g tomato purée
150ml water
200g grated Granny Smith apple,
   no skin or core
1 x 400g tin whole peeled tomatoes,
   blended
salt and pepper to taste
1 teaspoon honey
1 ½ tablespoons apple cider vinegar

- Heat the butter in a saucepan on medium heat, and gently fry the onion and the garlic until soft.
- Add the spices and fry for a minute to release their flavour.
- Add the tomato paste and cook for another minute.
- Add the water, apple and whole peeled tomatoes, and simmer gently on a low heat until the mixture has thickened. This will take at least an hour.
- Using a hand-blender, blend the sauce until smooth and season well with the salt, pepper and honey. Add the vinegar.
- Place in a glass jar and allow to cool. Keep refrigerated once cool.

BBQ MARINADE (not pictured) .... Makes about 400ml

This recipe is perfect as a marinade for chicken and beef or a BBQ sauce for burgers.

2 tablespoons tomato purée
1 x 400g tin whole peeled tomatoes
the juice of 1 orange
2 tablespoons Worcestershire sauce
2 tablespoons tamari soya sauce
1 tablespoon red wine vinegar
1 clove garlic, crushed
1 teaspoon grated ginger
½ cup (125ml) extra virgin olive oil
½ teaspoon smoked paprika
salt and pepper to taste

- Place all the ingredients in a bowl and blend until smooth using a hand-blender.
- Pop the blended ingredients into a pot on the stove and simmer for 10 minutes until the sauce thickens.

BASIC FRENCH DRESSING (not pictured) .... Makes about 600ml

This is a great basic dressing. It lasts in the fridge for ages and can be tweaked to suit your palate.

½ cup (125ml) red wine, brown spirit
 or cider vinegar
2 cups (250ml) extra virgin olive oil
3 tablespoons Dijon mustard
1 teaspoon honey
2 cloves fresh garlic, grated
 or crushed
salt and pepper to taste

- Whisk the ingredients together until well combined. (You can use a hand-blender to make it quick and easy.)
- Pour the dressing into a glass bottle with a lid and keep in the fridge until needed.

DRESSING TIPS:
- Add some freshly chopped Mediterranean herbs for a little more flavour.
- Try mixing the dressing with a little Greek yoghurt and some chopped chives.
- Instead of vinegar, use lemon juice and add some lemon zest with chopped dill – great for seafood! Replace the dill with fresh mint and it's great with lamb.

BREADS & BISCUITS

. . . .

One of the inconveniences of low-carb eating is the lack of easy bread for sandwiches – a particular problem when trying to feed kids. Happily, there are more and more excellent low-carb breads and biscuits becoming available in speciality shops and even supermarkets. Just try to steer clear of wheat, barley and rye if you go this route – and of, course, don't have anything to do with breads containing modified starches, stabilisers, 'conditioners' and any other suspect ingredients. Now check out the various bread, roll and cracker options you can make at home.

BANTING SEED BREAD (pictured on p299) .... Makes 1 small loaf

Our Banting seed bread can be kept for a few days and is perfect for freezing.

2 whole eggs
½ cup (125ml) water
5 tablespoons olive oil
1 teaspoon fennel seeds
250g golden flax seeds, ground
2 tablespoons sesame seeds
40g pumpkin seeds
25g whole brown flax seeds
1 teaspoon baking powder
1 teaspoon salt
1 teaspoon honey
½ teaspoon xanthan gum
5 egg whites, whisked to stiff peaks

- Preheat the oven to 180°C and grease a small loaf tin.
- In a small bowl, whisk together the whole eggs and the water with the olive oil.
- Bash the fennel seeds a bit using a pestle and mortar to release the flavours.
- In a large bowl, mix the dry ingredients together.
- Add the wet ingredients to the dry ingredients and mix until combined.
- Fold in the egg whites until completely incorporated.
- Pour the mixture into the loaf tin and bake for 45-50 minutes.
- Cool and serve, or freeze if desired.

ALMOND AND POPPY SEED BREAD (pictured on p298) .... Makes 1 small loaf

This loaf will last for a few days in the fridge. It's particularly good with lashings of butter and avo.

4 eggs
3 tablespoons water
1 cup (165g) dark flax meal
½ cup (60g) ground almonds
1 teaspoon baking powder
1 teaspoon salt
1 teaspoon caraway seeds
1 teaspoon honey
½ teaspoon xanthan gum
2 tablespoons poppy seeds
¼ cup (35g) sunflower seeds
¼ cup (20g) flaked almonds

- Preheat the oven to 180°C and grease a small loaf tin.
- Whisk together the eggs and water in a bowl until well combined.
- Place the rest of the ingredients in another bowl and stir to combine. (If you don't have flax meal, you can grind flax seeds yourself.)
- Mix the eggs into the dry ingredients and stir well.
- Pour the mixture into the greased loaf tin and bake for 35-40 minutes.
- Allow to cool and serve.

BURGER BUNS (pictured on p298) .... Makes 3 large or 4 medium-sized buns

Try these rolls when you're craving a burger or a hot dog. They can be shaped as you'd like them.

1 ½ cups (150g) almond flour or (190g) ground almonds

5 tablespoons psyllium husks

2 teaspoons baking powder

1 teaspoon salt

3 egg whites

1 ½ tablespoons white wine vinegar

⅞ cup (220ml) boiling water (quite specific!)

1 egg, beaten, for brushing

1 tablespoon sesame seeds (optional)

- Preheat the oven to 180°C.
- Combine the ground almonds, psyllium husks, baking powder and salt in a bowl. Sieve them well. If not enough ground almond gets through the sieve, replace it with some more.
- Add the egg whites and vinegar to the dry ingredients and mix well.
- Finally, add the boiling water, stirring until the mixture is a doughy consistency.
- Grease a baking tray and wet your hand to shape the dough into burger buns. Place them on the greased baking tray, brush each one with a little beaten egg and sprinkle a few sesame seeds on top, if you like.
- Bake the buns for about 55 minutes until they're golden and cooked through.
- Remove from the oven and allow to cool.

SEED CRACKERS (pictured on p298) .... Makes 30 biscuits

Crackers are good for a quick bite: instantly good to go. Play around with the seed proportions.

2 cups (500ml) water

3 tablespoons psyllium husks

200g pumpkin seeds

100g white sesame seeds

70g dark linseeds

10g black sesame seeds

2 teaspoons cumin seeds or fennel seeds (optional)

1 teaspoon salt

- Preheat the oven to 150°C.
- In a bowl, mix together the water and psyllium. Leave it to stand for about 10 minutes, at which point it should have thickened up to the texture of slime. (Don't panic, that's what you want.)
- In a separate bowl, mix together the other ingredients.
- Pour the gloopy psyllium water into the seed mixture and combine well.
- Line a baking tray with silicone paper or a silicone mat. (Wax paper doesn't work, so don't even go there.)
- Spoon tablespoons of the mixture onto the paper, spreading them into round shapes about 2mm thick. Make sure there are no holes or bubbles and that you leave about 2cm between the crackers.
- Bake for about 1 hour, until the crackers are crispy.

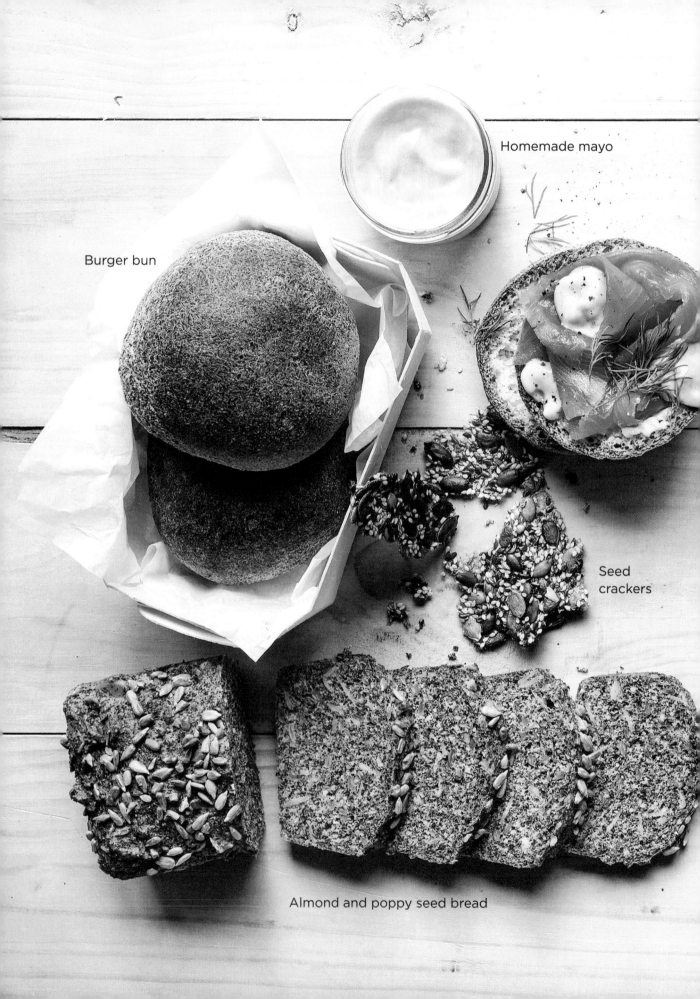

Homemade mayo

Burger bun

Seed
crackers

Almond and poppy seed bread

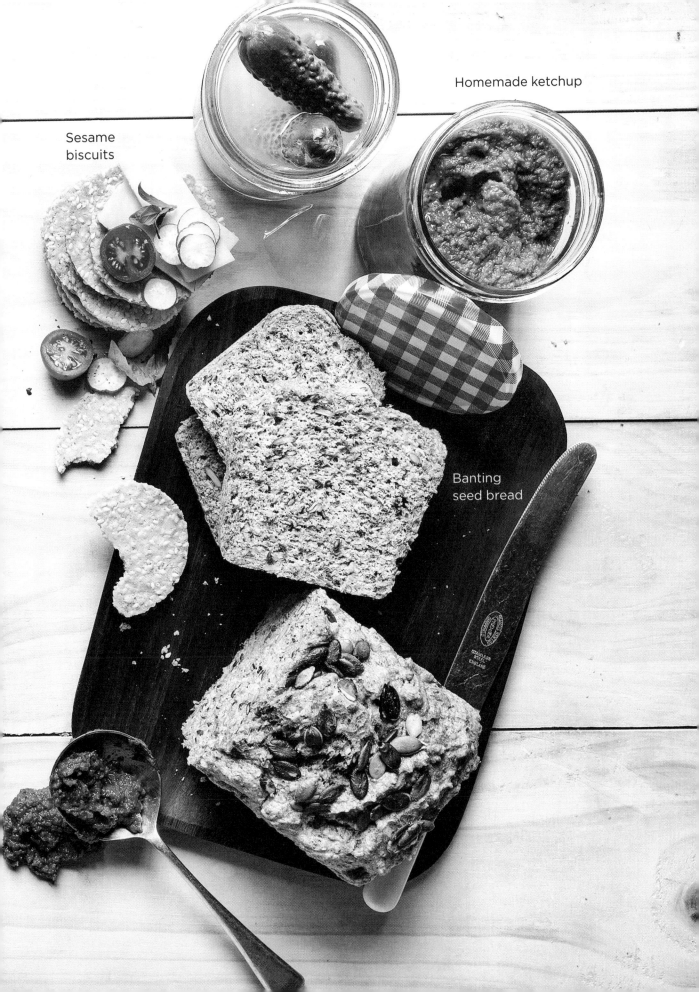

Sesame biscuits

Homemade ketchup

Banting seed bread

SESAME BISCUITS (pictured on p299) .... Makes 50 biscuits

These biscuits are delicious but they may need crisping in the oven if they lose their crunch.

3 cups (300g) almond flour or (375g)
  ground almonds
1 ½ teaspoons salt
1 cup (150g) sesame seeds
2 eggs, whisked until frothy
2 tablespoons olive oil

- Preheat the oven to 180°C, and grease a baking sheet well or line one with baking paper.
- In a large bowl, mix together the almond flour, salt, sesame seeds, eggs and oil. It will form a thick dough, and you may need to get stuck in with your hands to give it a good mix.
- Divide the dough in half.
- Place one half of the dough on a sheet of baking paper and place another sheet over the top. The paper will make it easier to roll out. Using a rolling pin, roll the dough (through the paper) until it's about 2-3mm thick. Remove the top layer of paper and slide it onto the baking tray.
- Using a knife or a pizza slicer, slice the dough into 6cm squares.
- Bake for 10-12 minutes, until the biscuits are golden brown.
- Repeat with the remaining dough.
- Cool and serve. Once cooled, store in an airtight container. If they soften over time, reheat them to crisp up.

LOW-CARB PANCAKES (not pictured) .... Makes 4

These pancakes are really multi-purpose. They can be used in lieu of pasta sheets in lasagne or cannelloni, as wraps with fillings, as tortillas or soft tacos, and as sweet or savoury pancakes.

⅓ cup (85ml) water
¼ cup (30g) coconut flour
½ teaspoon salt
¾ cup (190g) egg whites

- In a bowl, combine the water and the coconut flour. Add the salt and egg whites and blend well using a hand-blender. Allow the mixture to stand for a few minutes.
- Heat a greased frying pan to medium heat. Spoon a thin layer of the pancake batter into the frying pan, using the back of the spoon to spread it evenly. Allow it to gently brown. Carefully flip the pancake – remember, there is no gluten so it won't be as robust as a regular pancake – and brown it lightly on the other side. Repeat with the remaining batter.
- Serve immediately or freeze for later use.

HOMEMADE MAYO (pictured on p298) .... Makes 375ml

Homemade mayo isn't just (a lot) better for you than the store-bought stuff; it's better, period. The thing is to not let it terrify you! It's actually simple to make once you get the hang of it.

2 egg yolks
3 tablespoons apple cider vinegar
  (a little less if you want less bite)
1 tablespoon Dijon mustard
½ teaspoon salt
1 teaspoon honey
1 clove garlic, grated (optional)
150ml extra virgin olive oil (choose
  a mild one as the heavy ones can
  make the mayo bitter)
150ml macadamia oil

- Pour everything except the oils into a bowl.
- Using a hand-blender, mix everything together and slowly pour in the oils – the order doesn't matter – in a gentle steady stream with the hand-blender running.
- The mayo will thicken up quite quickly as the oil incorporates; this is what you want. Continue until you've added all the oil.
- If it gets thicker than the mayo you're used to, add a little warm water to thin it out and carry on adding the oils.
- Store in a glass jar in the fridge; it will last for at least 2 weeks.

_____

MAYO TIPS:

For curry mayo
Add 1 teaspoon curry powder, ½ a teaspoon ground turmeric, 1 teaspoon ground coriander, a little honey to taste and a dash of lemon juice. It's also great with some freshly chopped coriander stirred through it.

For tartar sauce
Add some chopped capers, gherkin, spring onion, parsley and a squeeze of lemon.

For lime mayo
Add the zest and juice of 1 juicy lime, and perhaps a bit of chopped chilli.

_____

BASIL PESTO (not pictured) .... Makes a small bowl

Homemade basil pesto doesn't have the seed oils of storebought pestos – plus it just tastes better.

50g pine nuts or blanched almonds
100g parmesan, grated
50g fresh basil leaves (no stalks)
2 cloves garlic
½ cup (125ml) extra virgin olive oil
salt and pepper, to taste

- Lightly toast the nuts in a pan until golden.
- Using a hand-blender or food processor, blitz all ingredients to a paste.
- For younger children consider using cheddar instead of parmesan; it's milder and more affordable.
- Play around with the ingredients: you can try rocket and walnut, parsley and mint or coriander and almond.

"THE LOWER LIMIT OF **DIETARY CARBOHYDRATE COMPATIBLE WITH LIFE APPARENTLY IS ZERO,** PROVIDED **ADEQUATE AMOUNTS OF PROTEIN AND FAT ARE CONSUMED.** "

– Institute of Medicine of the
United States National Academies

"AS WITH OTHER ADDICTIVE SUBSTANCES, **EXPOSURE** IS THE KEY TO SETTING UP [THE] ADDICTION FOOD CYCLE. THUS IF YOU WANT TO GET HUMANS **ADDICTED TO HIGHLY PROCESSED FOOD,** YOU NEED TO **EXPOSE THEM TO IT AT THE YOUNGEST POSSIBLE AGE.** "

– Dr Bill Wilson, US obesity specialist

THE KIDS' NUTRITION REVOLUTION
BY PROF TIM NOAKES
A SCIENTIFIC REVIEW OF CHILDREN'S NUTRITION TODAY

The idea that launched *Super Food for Superchildren* was a simple one: let's take our critical learnings from *The Real Meal Revolution* and apply them to a book on nutritional advice and recipes for children. But just as that book caused consternation because it challenged the accepted dietary dogma of the past 50 years, so too will *Super Food for Superchildren* attract official ire because it also challenges some of the current dietary guidelines for children, especially those that promote high-carb industrial diets almost from birth.

The three fundamental pillars of advice on which this book rests are the following:
- eliminate (or drastically reduce) sugar from your child's diet;
- eliminate (or drastically reduce) refined carbohydrates from your child's diet;
- include real, non-processed whole foods rather than non-nutritious, unhealthy processed foods in your child's diet.

In preparing my contribution to this book I wanted to investigate the bigger picture of children's nutrition, a process informed by my personal dietary and health history – as described in the Prologue – and my experience and training in studying, analysing and reporting the scientific literature in order to expose the bedrock truth. I had an open agenda and no specific expectations.

My questions were broad. What does the science tell us about children's nutrition today? How has the commercial food industry affected, perhaps directed, the way we feed our babies and children? If we've managed to be so wrong in so much of our general nutritional advice (for example by promoting low-fat, high-carb eating), where else have we made mistakes? What other advice, besides the three fundamentals described above, should we be highlighting?

The art in science is always to begin with the most important question. So to start, I asked the question that logically follows the Prologue: if my generation grew up lean, what happened to subsequent generations? When and why did it all go wrong?

THE KEY DRIVER OF THE MODERN OBESITY EPIDEMIC

There is now clear evidence that the global obesity epidemic began in 1980 (Figure 1), three years after the promotion of the 1977

United States Dietary Goals for Americans (USDGA) and about a decade before global diabetes rates also took off (Figure 2). This change occurred consequent to an increase in the consumption of carbohydrates, including sugar and high fructose corn syrup, as well as vegetable oils, including margarine, with a corresponding reduction in eggs, butter, full-cream dairy and red meat intake – precisely as the guidelines had advised us.

Thus there is a close relationship between the adoption of these novel dietary guidelines in 1977 and the subsequent increase in global rates of both these conditions. But surely, you would ask, there could be important social and other factors to explain why this has happened? That is indeed the case, but our innate human biology predicts which factors are the most likely drivers of these twin epidemics.

Lack of exercise is not the most important reason why we have become fat and diabetic. The problem is appestat malfunction

Everyone knows that to become fat we must eat more calories than we need. That insight does not require a university education. But this knowledge has not helped either prevent or reverse the obesity epidemic. And the reason is simple. This theory explains *how* we became fat; it does not help us understand *why* so many adults across the world have accumulated so much fat in such a short time.

For 3 million years, our pre-historic ancestors and our modern genus *Homo sapiens* have always been lean (as are most animal species living in the wild where they continue to eat the foods with which they co-evolved). Humans have remained lean over the millennia because, even without knowing how or why (or being told how and why), we have eaten exactly the correct number of calories to match our needs. We have done this not as a result of conscious science-based decisions about when to eat and how much, but rather because of internal subconscious controls in our brains that direct our actions with exquisite accuracy. We call the site in the brain that is responsible for this control the *appestat*.

When functioning properly, the appestat directs us to eat the exactly correct number of calories to balance our daily expenditure – not a single calorie more, or less. Indeed it is

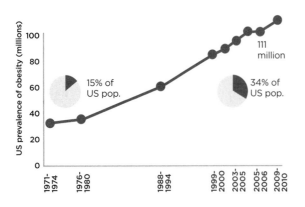

Figure 1. The prevalence of obesity in the US began to rise immediately after the adoption of the 1977 USDGA. [1]

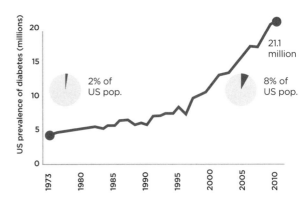

Figure 2. The prevalence of Type 2 diabetes in the US began to rise dramatically 20 years after the adoption of the 1977 USDGA. This is known as the 20-year rule – the time between an increase in sugar and carbohydrate intake and a rise in the prevalence of Type 2 diabetes. [2]

calculated that if the appestat is off by as little as 21 kilocalories a day – the number of calories found in about 4g of potato chips – the result will be a progressive weight gain of 2kg per year or 20kg per decade. Given how precise the action of the appestat must be, the miracle is not perhaps that so many humans gain weight during their lives but rather that there is even a single lean person on the planet.

The appestat must also accommodate for changes in how much exercise we do or fail to do each day, and it does this so successfully that when humans (eating the correct foods) exercise more or less than usual, they don't lose or gain weight. Instead they simply eat appropriately – either more or less – remaining lean as a result.

Although the appestat will impel us to take in more calories if we do more exercise, it is not designed to force us to exercise more (to burn off excess calories) if we eat too much – perhaps because these mechanisms evolved when the chance to overeat didn't exist. The problem thus begins when humans consume more calories than they require because they are eating "addictively" and no longer in response to valid biological drives. The body responds to overfeeding by producing the hormone insulin, which converts those excess calories into stored fat. Perversely, the more calories we have stored and the heavier we become, the less inclined we are to exercise. Or to eat less. Some argue that obesity is in this way not caused by physical inactivity and overeating; rather, obesity begets sloth and gluttony, perpetuating further weight gain (Figure 3).

The manner in which the healthy appestat functions explains why the obesity epidemic cannot be the result of an epidemic outbreak of mass global laziness and couch potato-ness. For if reduced daily physical activity is the sole factor that has changed in our environment since 1977,

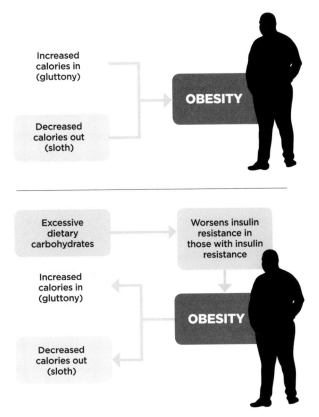

Figure 3. *Top:* The Calories In, Calories Out "You're to blame" model of obesity. According to this model, obesity is a personal choice since it results from gluttony and sloth. *Bottom:* The Carbohydrate (Insulin) model of obesity. In this model an excessive carbohydrate intake worsens an underlying insulin resistance in those with the genetic predisposition. This leads to abnormal appestat function causing progressive weight gain and eventually obesity as a result of the excessive calorie consumption. Obesity then causes hunger and overeating (gluttony) and physical inactivity (sloth) – not the other way around. [3]

we would not detect this as a sudden increase in global obesity rates. Instead, we would notice only that the world's people are eating less, while remaining the same weight. Simple.

In other words, even if humans are exercising less in 2015 than they were in 1977, this cannot explain why more humans are fatter now than they were in 1977.

Rather, the sudden onset of the global obesity epidemic after 1977 proves that the human appestat, so effective for 3 million years, has been damaged by something that has changed in our environment only very, very recently. In my opinion, that factor is very likely the change in the nature of the foods that we began to eat after the introduction of the USDGA in 1977.

These foods contain more carbohydrates and more sugar; they are more processed and have been designed specifically to be irresistible (addictive). In short, these novel foods contain carefully engineered combinations of fat, salt and sugar that make them addictive[4] and so tamper with the proper regulatory functioning of the appestat[5]. This is why we are perpetually hungry and overeat as a result.

According to this explanation, at its core, obesity is a brain disorder caused by a malfunctioning appestat, which has been hijacked by the novel, highly addictive foods that have been introduced into the food chain in recent decades.

As we will reveal, the groundwork for this change was inadvertently laid by the progenitor of the industrial diet: the processed baby foods introduced into the US in the late 1920s by the company that became Gerber's Baby Food.

Understanding that obesity is a (subconscious) brain disorder helps explain why advising patients to eat less and exercise more cannot prevent or reverse obesity (because the role of the brain is ignored). For example, a recent study from University College London has shown that genetic markers for obesity predict satiety responses to feeding.[6] Thus those with genetic markers for obesity are less likely to be satiated when eating. As a result, they must eat more to feel full, and thus develop obesity. This is also compatible with other evidence showing that "obesity risk genes influence adiposity via the appetite regulatory mechanisms" and prospective studies from the same group showing that "a larger appetite rating, greater enjoyment of food, greater food responsiveness, faster eating speed, and lower satiety responsiveness were all related to higher weights and faster weight gains over 6- and 12-month periods during infancy".[7]

So the appestats of those who will become obese are different genetically and less easily satiated by feeding. This is important information because it suggests that the only way to prevent and treat this condition of the brain is to better understand the true cause of the problem – and to act decisively on that information. Until we do, we will have failed yet more generations.

Addictive, sugar-rich processed foods are a key driver of appestat malfunction

In *The Real Meal Revolution* we presented the evidence that the key effect of the 1977 USDGA was to demonise real foods, especially dietary fat from animal sources. In their place we were advised to eat more carbohydrates, especially in the form of grains. Initially this change posed a major threat to the manufacturers of processed foods, because they soon learnt that removing the fat from foods removes taste along with it. But in time they appreciated that this provided a fantastic opportunity with a greater potential for profit than they could ever have imagined. The solution was to replace the fat in our food with a substance that would drive hunger and, as a result, overeating. That magic ingredient was sugar, and the industry began to replace "unhealthy" fats in the diet with ever-increasing amounts of "healthy" sugar, along with high fructose corn syrup and even artificial sweeteners. All the while, skilful marketing informed us that this substitution would be beneficial to us because our foods no longer contained "dangerous" fats that clogged our arteries.

Hence the idea was born that "low fat" foods were particularly healthy, though we missed the obvious qualification: that low-fat foods must be full of sugar in order of us to eat them. And not only do fat-free foods taste like cardboard; they also fail to satiate. Instead, we now know that these artificial foods drive hunger. Sugar, for example, is a powerfully addictive substance, with similarities to the addictive recreational drugs heroin or cocaine.[8]

Sugar also produces important behavioural effects, stimulating hyperactivity especially in younger brains. And too late we also learned that the fructose in sugar and high fructose corn syrup must be turned into fat in the liver, which leads to fatty liver disease, with important consequences for our health.[9]

But it's not just the sugar. By increasing our intake of carbohydrates, especially in the form of grains, we had inadvertently added other appestat dysregulators that promote sensations of continual hunger and the further overconsumption of ever more calories.

Carbohydrates have one other undesirable characteristic: they promote the secretion of insulin which, as also described in *The Real Meal Revolution*, causes blood-insulin concentrations to be continuously elevated (Figure 4) – and insulin is the "natural" fat-building hormone, turning excess carbohydrates into fat. Even worse, the continuous secretion of insulin each time we eat carbohydrates locks our bodies into the obese state by preventing the use of that stored fat as an energy fuel; instead, we force our bodies to burn those carbohydrates, in preference to fat.

In summary, since 1977 we have systematically removed from our diets the natural ingredient, fat, that best regulates appestat function – and we have replaced it with its polar opposites, sugar and high fructose corn syrup, which drive hunger.

In my opinion, the obesity epidemic that begins after 1977 can best be explained by the commandeering of the normal human appestat function by the modern highly addictive processed foods that have entered our food chain over the past 35 years. [11]

The problem is compounded in two further ways: one, we have also learnt to use these highly palatable foods as a stress-coping mechanism[12], and two, the persistent elevations in blood-insulin concentrations produced by the high-carbohydrate low-fat (HCLF) diet maintain the vicious cycle of obesity (Figure 4).

How do we reverse the obesity/diabetes epidemic?

If these ideas are correct, as we believe, they suggest that the prevention of obesity and diabetes does not necessitate some Nobel Prize-winning discovery. All it requires is that we stop eating addictive, highly palatable foods and that each of us eats only that amount of dietary carbohydrate that our individual bodies are able to tolerate. As our work on *The Real Meal Revolution* has shown, when the formerly obese follow these rules and begin to eat real foods, they can quite easily reverse their "sloth and gluttony", becoming lean and healthy with minimal effort and without ever again having to suffer perpetual hunger. In the process, they prove that obesity is not due to an irreversible character flaw, as some who do not understand this simple biology would have us believe.

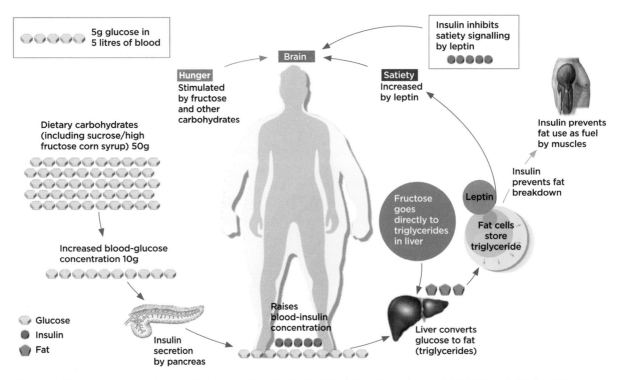

Figure 4. The Carbohydrate Insulin (Abnormal Fat Storage) model of obesity. In this model a high-carb intake causes the blood-glucose concentration to rise, stimulating increased insulin production by the pancreas. The increased blood-insulin concentration produces four key effects: it directs the conversion of glucose into fat (triglyceride) in the liver; it drives the storage of triglyceride in the fat cells; it prevents the breakdown of triglyceride in fat cells for use by the body as an energy fuel; and it inhibits the action of leptin on the brain in promoting feelings of satiety. Note that the bloodstream normally contains only 5g of glucose in 5 litres, yet a high-carb meal can add 50-100g of glucose within minutes. Note also that fructose in sucrose or high fructose corn syrup can only be metabolised to fat (triglyceride) in the liver and that fructose also has a unique action in stimulating hunger. [10]

WHY YOU MUST PREVENT YOUR CHILD FROM BECOMING OBESE

The focus in *The Real Meal Revolution* was on the prevention and reversal of adult obesity. But childhood obesity is increasing at uncontrolled rates that are beyond alarming. A 2014 report of the International Obesity Task Force estimates that worldwide more than 200 million school-age children are already overweight or obese.

Childhood obesity is not simply an aesthetic issue. Children who are obese are more likely to become overweight adults, with all the associated risks: Type 2 diabetes, hypertension, metabolic syndrome, gout, cancer and dementia (as described in *The Real Meal Revolution*).

This probability is especially high if obesity occurs before the age of 10 years. The long-term consequences are dire: their lives will on average be shorter, as childhood obesity is a strong predictor of premature death.

(To give it some personal perspective, when I was in medical training, Type 2 diabetes was known as "adult-onset diabetes". But in the past two decades this term has had to be dropped because so many adolescents now suffer from the condition.)

Equally importantly, and certainly more applicable during childhood, children who have been raised to become overweight or obese may experience fewer opportunities in many fields, particularly in sport and other physical activities, and may be psychologically constricted by lives that are less fulfilling than they would have been had they been raised with normal body weights. The prevention of childhood obesity is thus of critical importance – and it begins before the child is even conceived.

THE ORIGINS OF CHILDHOOD OBESITY

It is now abundantly clear that the beginnings of obesity and metabolic syndrome can be traced in many people to childhood. In fact, the factors determining a baby's birth weight and risk for developing obesity and metabolic syndrome may begin before birth itself, in the mother's own early life nutritional experiences[13] and health status[14]. Remarkably this influence may stretch even further back – to the baby's grandmother's nutrition during *her* early life.

There are two main ways in which the mother's eating choices during pregnancy can influence her unborn child: either because she eats too little or too much. Both alternatives produce predictable outcomes[15], which we know in part from the results of some tragic natural experiments.

Towards the end of the Second World War, during the summer and autumn of 1944, German forces occupying the Netherlands placed an embargo on the supply of food to the western parts of that country. Although the embargo was lifted in November 1944, extreme winter conditions prevented adequate food supplies reaching these deprived Dutch citizens, and their average calorie intake fell from approximately 1,000 calories/day to 400 calories/day at the height of the winter famine.

As a result, many children born in 1945 suffered severe intra-uterine malnutrition. Later, follow-up studies of these and other children affected by foetal malnutrition established that such children are at substantially increased risk for the subsequent development of insulin resistance, Type 2 diabetes and coronary heart disease beginning at a young age. [16, 17]

More recently it has been appreciated that foetal over-nutrition during pregnancy produces babies programmed to be at increased risk for exactly the same conditions.

Thus either malnutrition or over-nutrition during pregnancy produces detrimental long-term effects on the unborn.

It is not, however, just any form of over-nutrition that produces damage. Rather, it is over-nutrition with a high-carbohydrate diet in a mother whose carbohydrate metabolism is compromised because she has (usually unrecognised) insulin resistance that produces this undesirable outcome. Such a mother will expose her unborn child to high blood-glucose concentrations that in turn will require the developing pancreas of the foetus to over-secrete insulin. Since insulin is a stimulator of growth, fat accumulation and, paradoxically, of increased insulin resistance, this produces a larger, fatter, more insulin-resistant baby who is at much greater risk of developing insulin resistance in later life, especially if raised on a high-carb diet. Subsequently I present the theory that insulin resistance may be present in the foetus and may have developed for important survival reasons.

One study found that children of mothers with an abnormal blood-glucose response during the final trimester of pregnancy are at about a two-fold greater risk of developing

Type 2 diabetes in later life, and the offspring of mothers who develop gestational diabetes (diabetes that occurs only during pregnancy) have more adipose tissue at age seven than do those born to mothers whose blood-glucose concentrations remain normal during pregnancy. Yet for the children of mothers with Type 2 diabetes, the risk is much greater; almost half of the children born to such mothers will develop Type 2 diabetes by age 25. [18]

How can risk for Type 2 diabetes transfer so powerfully from mother to infant?

This outcome may result from epigenetic effects; that is, changes in the manner in which the genes express their function (without changes in the genetic material). Epigenetic effects can be produced by any number of influences, most as yet unknown. Logically this effect from mother to child would be produced by the continuously elevated blood-glucose concentrations in mothers with Type 2 diabetes promoting insulin resistance in their infants. Insulin does not cross the placenta so the foetus is protected from high maternal insulin, but not from high glucose concentrations.

Dietary carbohydrates are the macronutrients that most elevate blood-glucose (and insulin) concentrations. Thus high-carb diets are very likely to be an environmental influence producing these epigenetic effects in the unborn.

Other risk factors linked to childhood obesity

The focus in this book and in *The Real Meal Revolution* is on the nutritional risk factors for obesity and diabetes because we believe that *dietary factors are the key drivers of both conditions*. For completeness we should include a study that identified eight of 25 possible risk factors for childhood obesity.[19] These were:

- the presence of parental obesity
- high birth weight
- increased weight at age 8 months
- increased weight gain during the first year
- increased catch-up growth between birth and 2 years
- short sleep duration at age 3 years
- very early elevated body mass index or adiposity rebound (at age 43 months)
- more than 8 hours a week watching television at age 3 years

In reality, the majority of these factors are simply measures of developing obesity – which we would argue are all being driven by nutrient-poor diets high in carbohydrates and other appestat dysregulators.

There is also growing interest in the role of the bacterial content of the intestine – the gut biome – on the risk of developing obesity. The mechanism by which this might occur is still unknown but it seems probable that the future of all medicine lies in understanding the role of the gut biome in health and disease. [20]

The newborn's gut biome begins to be established during its passage through the birth canal when it is exposed for the first time to its mother's bacteria. Recent work suggests that infants born by Caesarean section – and who therefore do not pass through the mother's birth canal – have an increased risk of becoming obese, among other risks. [20]

The gut biome (at all ages) is also altered by the use of antibiotics, and it has been seen that infants of mothers treated with antibiotics during pregnancy are also at a greater risk of obesity.[21] Boys treated with antibiotics during the first year of life were found to be at a greater risk of becoming overweight by age 9, though the same was not found for girls.[22]

Although antibiotics play an important role

in fighting off bacterial infections, their use on infants (and at all ages, in fact) should thus be weighed against this evidence and not advised lightly.

HOW WE GOT HERE: THE ONSLAUGHT OF HIGHLY PROCESSED, HIGHLY ADDICTIVE INDUSTRIAL CHILDREN'S FOODS

If obesity ultimately requires that we take in more calories than we expend, and the cause of this is the appestat malfunction that we have described, then what does this tell us about the foods we should be feeding our children?

Simply, they should be foods that *do not* entrap children's appestats from the moment of conception. Thus a critical responsibility of parents and grandparents everywhere is the protection of our children's and grandchildren's appestats from the onslaught of the addictive, highly processed, high-carbohydrate industrial foods that are designed to do just that. We can do this best by ensuring that our children and grandchildren are raised on a diet of real foods, of the kind we first promoted in *The Real Meal Revolution* and continue to do here – a process that should begin with the mother's food choices.

We'll get to the specifics of those recommendations shortly. First, to appreciate how pervasive and destructive industrial children's foods have become, we need to consider the history of infant formulas and baby foods. These were among the first processed industrial foods that initiated the slide away from our eating real foods and towards the modern industrial diet – with such disastrous consequences. Their introduction in the first half of the 20th century had far-reaching effects.

The falling age of weaning

For countless generations the infants of humans and our ancient predecessors were raised on breast milk for the first 24-28 months of life. This experience suggests that breast milk provides all the nutrients that infants require, perhaps for as long as the first two years of life.

In this era of prolonged breastfeeding, breast milk was provided by the mother or, if she was unable, by so-called "wet" nurses[23] who retained their ability to produce breast milk by continuously suckling (different) infants for months or years. In the absence of other sources of food for infants, the availability of wet nurses in all cultures would have been critical for higher rates of infant survival. Typically infants in those cultures were introduced to whole foods only after 18-24 months, in part because meat was considered damaging and vegetables and fruits were thought to increase risk for infections, even cholera – which was perhaps true but only if these foodstuffs were washed with unclean water contaminated by harmful bacteria.

Only in the past century has the age of human infant weaning decreased dramatically.* How did this come about?

---

* Interestingly humans wean their infants much earlier than do chimpanzee mothers, our nearest relative, who suckle their young for 4-5 years, even though the life expectancy of chimpanzees is less than that of humans. It appears that the early weaning of humans is a direct consequence of our more nutrient-dense diet provided by our carnivorous ways, and earlier weaning allowed humans to breed more rapidly. [24]

Industrial food for babies: where it all began

The key invention in the move away from breastfeeding was a device to make possible a practical alternative delivery method of liquid to an infant: this was the infant-feeding bottle with an effective rubber nipple, perfected in 1912.[23] Once it had been developed, the next key driver of the process was the progressive introduction of infant formulas and processed baby foods to mothers in industrialised countries, especially the United States. This in turn was a result of the development of the food-canning industry in the US after the 1880s, which resulted in canned foods becoming increasingly cheaper and more affordable by the 1920s.

In 1835 an Englishman by the name of William Newton patented a method to develop evaporated cow's milk, and in 1853 the Texan Gale Borden added sugar to evaporated milk, canned the product and named it condensed milk. This became the first infant "food".[23] Similar developments were occurring in the United Kingdom at the same time.[25] In 1862 an Englishman, Ridge, patented an infant food made from cooked flour with added sugar and bicarbonate of potash. Five years later another Englishman, Justus von Liebig, produced a competitor, which he described as "A Food for Infants: A complete substitute for that provided by Nature". Believing that Ridge's product was unhealthy because it contained only carbohydrates, Von Liebig's invention was a mixture of wheat flour, cow's milk and malt-flour with some bicarbonate of potash, first in a liquid form and ultimately in a powdered form to which water or milk was added.[26] Neither of these products was commercially successful.

Around the same time, Swiss pharmacist Henri Nestlé produced the first patented food formula for infants: baked wheat rusks made from hard twice-baked bread crumbled into sweetened condensed milk. The concoction was then dried and sold as brown granules. By the late 1880s there were a number of similar infant foods. One of the most popular in the US continued to be canned condensed cow's milk, which didn't spoil in the hot summer months.

These innovations stimulated the introduction of a large number of similar products over the next 20 years. The effects were not good:

> A large proportion of them [infant formulas] were predominantly farinaceous; that is, they consisted of flour, starch, malted flour and similar materials. They were responsible for an appalling amount of sickness and malnutrition because they were deficient *not only in protein and fat* but in most of the vitamins... The trouble was that children fed on these foods, which were usually, it is true, mixed with a certain amount of milk, grew in a deceptively encouraging manner. *Indeed they usually put on weight too well.* At two or three years they were overweight for their age but pale, fat and flabby. Almost invariably they developed mild rickets, usually undetected, and in later life their teeth were affected. [25] [Italics my emphasis.]

In time it was realised that many of these children were also suffering from mild scurvy, a condition that became known as Barlow's Syndrome after the London physician Sir Thomas Barlow who first described it. Together with another London physician, Walter Butler Cheadle, Barlow was convinced that these infant foods were harmful because they contained too much carbohydrate, especially too much starch. Both believed that infants required a "properly balanced mixture of proteins, fats and carbohydrates". Cheadle's belief was perhaps influenced by the years he had spent traversing the high Canadian Arctic[27], during which time he would have eaten the foods of the Arctic, mainly fat and protein with little carbohydrate.

So it is clear that, beginning at the end of

the 19th century, cereals and sugar were the first foodstuffs onto which infants were weaned. But it is also clear that many considered this a failed experiment – one that we have since forgotten, to the cost of our children.

The first canned baby foods and their influence on breastfeeding and weaning

Before 1900 and the invention of commercial refrigeration, there was a limited capacity to store fruits and vegetables. They were eaten only when in season. As a result, diets in the US "were fairly monotonous regimes of soups, stews, bread, dairy produce, meat (fresh when available, salted, dried, or smoked when not), and fruits and vegetables (fresh in season or preserved through pickling, jams, or preserves, or through drying and some home canning)". [26]

The discovery in 1912 by British scientist Frederick Hopkins that vitamins present in fruit and vegetables play an important role in human health provided the commercial stimulus to provide fruits and vegetables in preserved forms, in cans, all year round. In 1926, the Fremont Canning Company in Fremont, Michigan decided to extend its range of canned fruits and vegetables to include specific baby formulas. It began by producing puréed vegetables and fruits – termed "sieved" or "strained" at the time – and later added cereals, chopped produce and dinner combinations. By 1928 the company was producing strained peas, prunes, carrots, spinach and beef vegetable soups for infants. The commercial success of these baby foods was so great that in time the company changed its name to Gerber's Baby Foods. Its trademark, the Gerber Baby, soon became an iconic symbol for "properly raised and nourished children, signifying the adoption of modern values of progress, efficiency, capitalism, industrialization, and reliance on scientific expert opinion", as described by Amy Bentley in her comprehensive investigation into the baby-food industry, *Inventing Baby Food*, published in 2014. [26]

From the outset the company appreciated that in order to sell its novel products it needed to convince mothers to introduce solid feeding at a younger age than had been the practice. To achieve this, it adopted the thoroughly modern approach of first convincing dieticians of their message by sponsoring advertisements in the *Journal of the American Dietetics Association*, an influential science publication. Next they needed to convince mothers not just of the "wholesomeness of their product but also implicitly to reduce their confidence in their ability to care for their infants... without the help of these experts and their products".[26] Skilful marketing proposed that "scientifically based" formulas with added vitamins must be healthier than breastfeeding.

In this way Gerber successfully medicalised motherhood, changing it from the natural activity that human mothers and their ancestors had practised for millions of years. As Bentley puts it:

> By playing on parents', especially mothers', emotions, presenting medical doctors as the ultimate baby experts, and positioning the uncontested assumption that commercially prepared foods are superior to, or at least far more efficient than, those cooked at home, the new commercial baby food advertising in the 1930s successfully imbued its products with the qualities of exceptional purity and wholesomeness, convenience and modernity and scientific efficiency. [26]

The consequences of these commercial actions are still apparent today. First, through their alliance with dieticians, paediatricians and other child healthcare providers, the industry created the public perception that two industrial products – infant formulas and baby foods – are entirely "natural" products. A century's worth of such systematic programming explains why the threats to our health posed by industrial foods were not anticipated until quite recently (as described in *The Real Meal Revolution*).

Second, the entirely natural process of breastfeeding came to be perceived as inconvenient and even primitive, during a time when American values were sweeping the world. Breastfeeding "was rendered unnatural and deviant... As breastfeeding became aligned with backwardness, commercial baby food became conflated with civilized society, especially in contrast to developing nations, where strong traditions of breastfeeding remained". Whereas before the industrial era 95% of infants were breastfed at birth, by the late 1960s this number had fallen to less than 25%, with only about 5% continuing at six months of age. [26]

Third, modern baby foods have encouraged the introduction of infant formulas and infant weaning to occur at progressively younger ages. By the 1930s most children in industrial countries were being introduced to solid foods by the age of 3 months; two decades later this had fallen to the first month of their lives (Figure 5).

Modern baby foods in a (commercially processed) nutshell

The Second World War became the major driver of the processed food industry in the US,

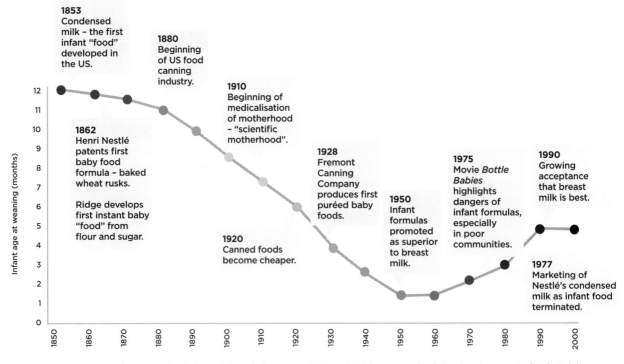

Figure 5: The age of infant weaning fell precipitously between 1870 and 1950 as a result of the development of industrial processed foods that began to replace breast milk. More recently this has been reversed somewhat with campaigns to promote breastfeeding as the healthiest option for all. [28]

as American forces fighting overseas wanted foods of their preference, prepared back home and shipped to the battle front. The final Allied victory produced the Baby Boomer generation and helped launch what became known as the American Century.

Infant formulas captured the essence of the optimism of that era, as Bentley well describes it:

> Commercial baby food was emblematic of midcentury American strength and power, complementing other societal values as modernity and mobility. Its little (bottle) jars of products laden with sugar, salt, and starch were gateway foods to the industrialized American diet that blossomed in the mid-twentieth century. Using them made mothers feel confident and modern, fuelling capitalist enterprise and quelling more "natural" – that is, free and low cost – alternatives, such as breastfeeding and homemade. Commercial baby food made it easier and more convenient for women with small children to enter the paid work force and stay there. [26]

In summary, we can see that infant formulas and baby foods are the original processed foods, the forerunners of the modern industrial diet that really took off with the promotion of the 1977 US Dietary Guidelines. (Indeed, to promote the modern industrial diet in more recent times, the food industry has used precisely the same methods pioneered by Gerber in the 1930s.) At the same time, the targeted undermining of the value of breastfeeding by industry has been a particularly effective strategy, greatly reducing the extent to which breastfeeding is practised globally.[29] Together with the ever-earlier introduction of weaning and changes in methods of weaning, it all raises questions that have profound importance for the future of children's nutrition.

If modernity wants to present itself in a little jar of baby food, what is to become of mother's milk? As breastfeeding has been replaced with processed infant foods at ever younger ages, have we sacrificed our children's health for convenience? Specifically, at what age should babies be weaned onto these convenience foods? And what are the best first foods?

WEANING – WHEN AND WHAT?

The introduction of processed baby foods produced what Bentley describes as the single rule that has remained constant for more than 50 years: infants should begin solid food "one puréed item at a time". There was even a particular order: "usually white rice cereal first, followed by apple-sauce or mashed banana, and progressing on to puréed vegetables and meat. By the post-war period, refined white rice cereal, introduced by Gerber in the 1940s, had become the iconic first food American families fed to their infants." [26]

The critical point is that Gerber introduced this food to infants, not because it was proven to be healthy but because it was good for business.[30] Decades later, when the American (and subsequently Western) diet was overhauled as a result of the 1977 USDGA, it was at least debated openly, even if inconclusive scientific evidence and the power of personality won the day (as described in *The Real Meal Revolution*). But when Gerber effectively invented baby foods in the 1920s and '30s and promoted them as superior to the process that had sustained humans for millennia – breastfeeding, followed by later weaning – it did this without any scientific evidence whatsoever to show that this was the healthiest option. It simply insisted, convincingly, that this was the case.

Bentley argues that white rice cereal became the standard food for infant weaning because it continued a philosophy of feeding thin cereal gruels and beef broths to the elderly, invalids and the very young, largely because this mixture had similarities to breast milk. That it was bland was considered valuable as the alimentary system of children was considered too immature to handle "tasty" foods, the introduction of which needed to be delayed until much later. Thus "white rice cereal became popular not for what it contained but for what it did not...[as] it was regarded as the most benign of the grain cereals".[26]

Corn, rice, wheat, barley and oatmeal were all introduced as alternatives in the 1940s but ultimately white rice cereal was the winner; its smooth bland texture and easy digestibility made it the default first food. In time it was fortified with iron and was considered especially safe because it did not produce allergies.

Thus the introduction of infant foods based on white rice cereal was justified entirely on an unproven, indeed untested, perception of how the gastrointestinal tract of an infant works and without any consideration of what might be the infant's most important nutritional requirements.

But there was another consideration. Baby food manufacturers realised that no mother would feed her infant foods that she herself would not find acceptable. So these foods were formulated to taste good to mothers, and they have been adapted over time to continue to do so. The problem is that mothers' tastes have in recent decades become conditioned to find commercially processed foods palatable. Thus infant formulas have necessarily taken on the taste of the industrialised American diet – high in sugar, salt and refined carbohydrates.

With this background we can begin to address current infant feeding guidelines and where they might be right – or wrong.

The World Health Organization (WHO) dietary guidelines

The WHO guidelines for a healthy diet[31] include advice for infants and children. Much of it is excellent; for example, it acknowledges that the "first 2 years of a child's life are vital as optimal nutrition during this period reduces the risk of dying and of developing (chronic) non-communicable diseases. It also fosters better development and healthy growth and development overall".

Thus the guidelines advise that children should be breastfed exclusively for the first 6 months of life and should continue to be breastfed until 2 years and beyond. From 6 months of age, breast milk should be complemented "with a variety of adequate, safe and *nutrient dense* complementary foods" (my emphasis).

But on further review, the WHO document includes information on what it considers to be a healthy diet that can vary in light of the scientific evidence from unconvincing to outright disastrous.

Fruit and vegetables

Eating at least 5 portions, or 400g, of fruit and vegetables per day reduces the risk of non-communicable diseases, and helps an adequate daily intake of dietary fibre. In order to improve fruit and vegetable consumption, you can: Always include vegetables in your meals. Eat fruit and raw vegetables as snacks. Eat fresh vegetables in season. Vary choices of fruits and vegetables.

We will see subsequently that the evidence that "at least 5 portions" of fruit and vegetables prevents non-communicable diseases is slight at best, and that the nutritional value of fruit and vegetables, though important, has been overplayed.

Fats

Reducing the amount of total fat intake to less than 30% of total energy helps prevent unhealthy weight gain in adult populations... Also the risk of developing non-communicable diseases is lowered by reducing (dietary) saturated fats to less than 10% of total energy, and trans fats to less than 1% of total energy, and replacing them with unsaturated fats contained in vegetable oils... Fats [sic] intake can be reduced by: Changing how you cook – remove the fatty part of meat; instead of butter, use vegetable oil (not animal); and boil, steam or bake rather than fry. Avoid processed foods containing trans fats; limit the consumption of food containing high amounts of saturated fats (e.g. cheese, ice cream, fatty meat).

This advice is simply not supported by the published scientific evidence, as we discussed at length in *The Real Meal Revolution*. It has subsequently also been forensically demolished by Nina Teicholz in her excellent book, *The Big Fat Surprise: Why Butter, Meat and Cheese Belong in a Healthy Diet.* (See p346.) The obesity epidemic after 1980 has occurred precisely as humans, especially in the US and UK, have begun to eat *less* fat and more carbohydrate. It has been known since the 1820s that carbohydrates are uniquely fattening[32], an accepted wisdom that was bulldozed aside by the drafters of the 1977 USDGA who declared (incorrectly) that henceforth fat and not carbohydrate causes weight gain. In so doing, they have brought on the global obesity epidemic, assisted by the likes of the World Health Organization, which has supported their claims without evidence.

The WHO guidelines finish with warnings about consuming too much sugar and salt. While there is no question that eliminating sugar from our diets will produce massive benefits – a fact that forms a pillar of this book – the suggestion that we should reduce our salt intake is not as strongly supported by the evidence. Some studies suggest that an increased salt intake may

reduce mortality in people with Type 2 diabetes.[33] Whether we should be encouraging everyone to reduce salt intake is simply not an established medical fact.[34]

South African and UK dietary guidelines

Both South African guidelines and those put out by the NHS in the UK also promote the introduction of solid foods only after six months of exclusive breastfeeding. But subsequently they offer, or until recently have offered, some suspect advice; for example, when it comes to first foods from 6 months of age.

The 2003 South African guidelines previously suggested that cereals, fruit and vegetables were ideal at this age, but as Bourne et al noted in their review, "it is cause for concern that complementary foods such as chicken, meat and egg yolk, rich in protein, iron and zinc, were seldom mentioned" as important food choices for infants.[35] The guidelines have subsequently come up for revision, and the latest proposals – "still to be tested" as of 2013 – advise parents to provide "diets with adequate fat content". They note that the "eating of foods from animal sources is associated with improved nutrient intake and diet quality which results in better growth outcomes", and thus they specifically recommend that "meat, poultry, fish and eggs should be eaten daily, or as often as possible". They also warn that at "this age, vegetarian diets cannot meet nutrient needs, unless nutritional supplements or fortified products are used." [36]

Acknowledging that such foods may be expensive, the South African authors propose the following: "Examples of relatively inexpensive food from animal sources, containing adequate amounts of protein, iron, zinc and vitamin A include chicken, beef or sheep liver, and eggs.

The regular intake of liver was associated with a favorable vitamin A status in children in the Northern Cape Province." [36]

Meanwhile, the NHS still recommends fruit, vegetables and "baby rice or baby cereal mixed with your baby's usual milk" as first foods from 6 months, before suggesting pasta, noodles, toast and rice in its next foods, along with chicken, fish and eggs, but not red meat. It then goes on to specifically warn as follows: "You should avoid giving your baby certain foods as they may cause food allergies or make your baby ill. These include foods that contain wheat, gluten, nuts, peanuts, peanut products, seeds, liver, eggs, fish, shellfish, cows' milk and soft or unpasteurised cheese." [37]

While the argument can be made that no humans should ever be eating gluten-containing grains (see point 7 below), there is growing evidence that the early introduction of certain foods does not increase but in fact *reduces* the risk for the development of specific allergies to those foods (see point 6 below).

Both South African and UK guidelines also advise that babies should be offered a range of different "healthy" foods and should not be given foods that contain added sugar. The NHS promotes homemade foods as "best" and warns that overreliance on jar or packet foods may "make it harder for your baby to accept more varied textures and to move to family foods as they get older".

Are these guidelines helpful? And if not, why not?

Most of the advice in these and other dietary guidelines for babies and children is supported by solid science and thus, theoretically, should be extremely helpful. There are, however, enough divergences from the most recent accepted evidence to bring their practical usefulness into question. Moreover, the reality is that their promotion has not reversed the epidemics of obesity and diabetes and related conditions in our children. They may actually have caused the problem.

In my opinion a major weakness of many of these guidelines is their failure to recognise that infants with insulin resistance can only remain lean and healthy if they restrict the amount of carbohydrates they eat – from a very young age.

I also believe that grains are nutrient-poor options and have no proven health benefits. On the contrary, they cause dental cavities and a range of debilitating medical conditions known collectively as Non Coeliac Gluten Sensitivity (NCGS).

A key is to identify at the earliest possible opportunity those children who are insulin resistant, and then to ensure that they eat a cereal-and-grain-free diet with restricted carbohydrate content. (See p344.)

Then there is the question of providing sufficient nutrients during the first 24 months of life when the infant brain is growing very rapidly. During this time, infants need nutrient-dense foods including eggs, meat, organs, brains (from animals younger than 1 year), viscera and marrow,[38, 39, 40, 41, 42] which have high concentrations "of iron, calcium, iodine, sodium, zinc as well as vitamins A, B1, niacin, B6, folate, vitamin K and other micronutrients as well as high quality protein and essential fatty acids"[40].

When infants are weaned to meat rather than cereals, they show greater growth in length without any increase in adiposity[43]; they also consume three times as much zinc and show a significantly higher rate of growth of head circumference[44]. Weaning onto eggs improves infant blood DHA (an important omega-3 fatty acid, full name docosahexaenoic acid) and iron levels.[38] In other studies this more rapid brain growth after birth predicts higher intelligence.[45] In evolutionary terms "meat, particularly organ tissues... would provide the ideal weaning food".[46] Even our own South African guidelines now acknowledge as much, or were at least on track to do so, as noted earlier.

Those are the broader points at which I think these guidelines fall down, and there are specific failures elsewhere. But amid this confusion, what advice should a parent be following?

THE SUPERCHILDREN DIETARY GUIDELINES

In analysing the (sound, peer-reviewed) scientific evidence, I advise the following guidelines.

1 **Breastfeeding is nutritionally superior to formula feeding, a point that may not be sufficiently stressed in major feeding guidelines.** Breast milk is truly a miracle food.[47] Thus the health messaging around breastfeeding should be simple: ideally, breastfeed exclusively until weaning begins (at around 6 months), then continue for as long as possible in conjunction with first foods, preferably to 2 years.

As noted earlier in the book, breastfeeding can be painful and even physiologically difficult for new mothers (though we believe rarely impossible with the correct guidance), and is later logistically difficult for many working mothers. These factors must of course be taken into account, as well as the truism that a happy mother makes for a happy child. Nevertheless, the marginalisation, or even demonisation, of breastfeeding in the face of the rising baby-food industry's promotion of infant formulas has undoubtedly harmed our children.[29]

There is now good evidence that breastfed babies have greater intelligence; they spend more time in education and have higher earnings. And the longer the breastfeeding, the greater the benefits. In one major Brazilian study conducted over several decades, babies who were "breastfed for 12 months had an IQ that was four points higher than those breastfed for less than a month, had nearly a year's more schooling and earned around £70 a month more – about a third more than the average income".[48]

The senior author concluded that the "likely mechanism underlying the beneficial effects of breast milk on intelligence is the presence of long-chain saturated fatty acids (DHAs) found in breast milk... Our finding that predominant breastfeeding is positively related to IQ in adulthood also suggests that the amount of [breast] milk consumed plays a role".[48] Long-chain saturated fatty acids are an essential fat necessary for brain development (see point 6 below) and, unless added, are not naturally present in cereal-based processed baby foods.

By contrast, children raised on processed "junk foods" had lower IQ at 8 years of age[49] and lower levels of academic achievement by the eighth grade of schooling[50].

A key benefit of breastfeeding is that it maintains a state of ketosis in the newborn baby for as long as it continues[51], as opposed to formula milks that do not stimulate ketosis to the same extent[52]. The critical importance of ketone bodies to the development of the infant's brain are discussed in point 2.

2 **A high-fat diet is optimal for brain development in newborn infants and babies, while carbohydrates should be considered a non-essential foodstuff.** The current guidelines overemphasise the need for carbohydrates in part because they

fail to appreciate that humans of all ages, but especially newborn infants and babies during the first two years of life, are perfectly adapted to eating low-carb diets.

In *The Real Meal Revolution* we made the point that the human body has no essential requirement for carbohydrate – a fact that has been known for years[53]. Table 1 lists all the nutrients the body cannot manufacture by itself and which must therefore be provided from dietary sources. While there are fats and proteins (amino acids) that are utterly essential – in other words, humans die if their diets lack those ingredients – there is *no essential carbohydrate*.

Humans certainly do require glucose for the functioning of specific organs of the body. But we have a very powerful liver that has all the necessary capacity to convert fat and protein into glucose for use by those glucose-dependant organs, including the brain. The point being: we do not need to eat glucose directly (in the form of carbohydrate) for our bodies to be able to produce all the glucose we need.

This raises an important question: how is it possible that some expert guidelines continue to advise that up to 65% of a child's daily energy requirement come from a nutrient for which humans have no essential requirement? Moreover, do these guidelines not recognise the health dangers of weaning onto a high-carb diet?

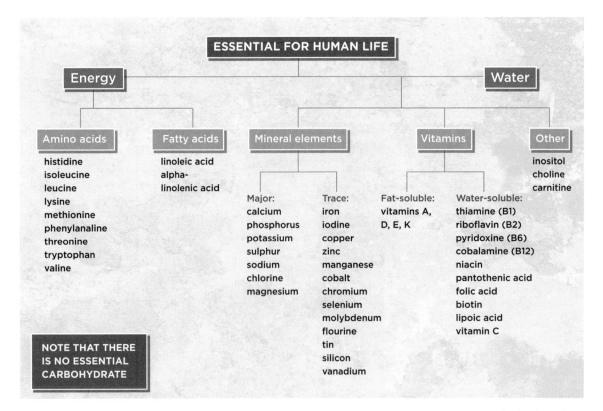

Table 1. The essential nutrients for humans, without which we face malnourishment and ultimately death, include a number of amino acids, fatty acids, mineral elements, vitamins and other compounds – but no carbohydrates. [54]

A high-carb diet will raise blood-glucose concentrations, causing elevated insulin concentrations. In time this will produce obesity and Type 2 diabetes in those with insulin resistance.

A high-carb diet will likely include foods with high concentrations of sugar or high fructose corn syrup that also increase risk for the development of obesity and Type 2 diabetes.

A high-carb diet will likely include nutrient-poor gluten-containing grains that can lead to the leaky gut syndrome that has been implicated as the cause of a variety of auto-immune disease, including Type 1 diabetes and the recently described condition non-coeliac gluten sensitivity (NCGS). (See point 7, below.)

We went to great lengths in *The Real Meal Revolution* to expose the negative health consequences of eating high-carb diets for those with insulin resistance, and the reasons why they will benefit from eating low-carb diets. But at least some of the resistance to the adoption of low-carb diets, especially by mothers during pregnancy and during the weaning of their babies, stems from the nonsensical food-industry-circulated myth that such diets will cause brain damage because a low-carb diet cannot provide the brain with sufficient glucose. In fact, the reason why children are advised to eat high-carb diets has nothing to do with helping their brains to work

better. Rather it is, as we've described before, the result of the industry-driven obsession with the falsehood that a high-fat diet will cause heart disease in adulthood. But we now know this to be incorrect: the evidence is clear that it is carbohydrate intake, not fat intake, that has increased so dramatically in the past four decades (Figure 6) and is thus the most likely cause of the obesity and diabetes epidemics that have emerged in this time (Figures 1 and 2).

Logically the need to reduce the excess carbohydrate intakes of many mothers (who become obese) during pregnancy and of babies and infants (who become obese) should be the first priority in reversing these epidemics. But this is vigorously opposed by an industry stacked with businesses looking to protect the sales of their cheap but highly lucrative carbohydrate foods. Like Gerber in the 1930s, these businesses act through proxy scientific organisations to ensure their message becomes the accepted creed. And, as I have learnt by experience, woe betide anyone who dares to question those dogmas.*

The supposed rationale behind the industry myth that low-carb diets lead to brain damage in young children is that they cause ketoacidosis, which is especially dangerous for the unborn baby because ketones produce birth defects, otherwise known as "teratogenic" effects.

---

* In 1985 my colleagues and I described the first case of a novel medical problem in sport: water intoxication in those who over-drink during prolonged exercise. The then-accepted wisdom that those who don't drink sufficiently during exercise risk dying from "dehydration" was, it turns out, based on incorrect, commercially driven advice. The truth is the opposite: over-drinking, not under-drinking, is the real threat during prolonged exercise. This sparked a 30-year search for the truth, leading to the publication of my book *Waterlogged: The Serious Problem of Overhydration in Endurance Sports*. During those three decades I was ostracised by a sports-drink industry pursuing profit in developing a product ultimately worth more than $2 billion a year in US sales alone. In the end, however, the science won out, and drinking guidelines during exercise are now what I first proposed in 1988 – specifically that we should drink to thirst at all times.

Similarly, I believe we are at the beginning of a sea-change from the recent dietary dogma of low-fat high-carb eating to the high-fat low-carb lifestyle on which the Real Meal Revolution is based. But before we get there we will have to endure a backlash from the food industry protecting its commercial interests, just as the sports-drink industry reacted when its dogma was challenged.

But the science suggests a quite opposite interpretation: that maternal ketone production during pregnancy is utterly essential for the survival of the foetus.

In the first place, no teratogenic effects have been shown experimentally at the blood ketone concentrations found in normal pregnancies (4mmol/L).[56]

Second, adequate ketone production during the first two years of life is crucial for the growth of the baby's brain. This is because "ketones are a key source of carbon for the brain to synthesize the cholesterol and fatty acids that it needs in the membranes of the billions of developing nerve connections... Ketones are the preferred carbon source for brain lipid synthesis and they come from fatty acids recently consumed or stored in body fat. This means that, in infants, brain cholesterol and fatty acid synthesis are indirectly tied to the mobilization and catabolism of fatty acids stored in body fat"[39, 41, 51] Thus "mildly elevated blood ketones are *essential* for normal brain development, at least in humans"[41] (my emphasis).

In addition, maternal ketone body production protects the foetal brain during times of food scarcity when the mother's blood-glucose concentrations must fall; the foetal brain uses ketones instead of maternal glucose to cover its energy requirements.[39]

In fact, pregnancy induces a state of maternal (and perhaps foetal – see later) insulin resistance,[57] the goal of which is to ensure that glucose use by the mother's body is not wasteful but is "spared" and transferred to the foetus via the placenta. Part of this adaptation

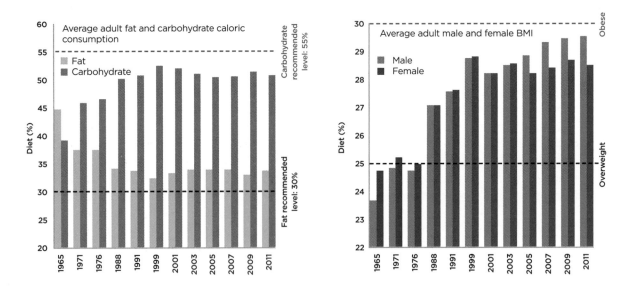

Figure 6. *Left panel:* Changes in % calories from dietary fat and carbohydrates since adoption of the 1977 USDGA that promoted increased dietary carbohydrate and reduced fat intake. Note the dramatic changes between 1965 and 1999. *Right panel:* There has been a progressive increase in US average Body Mass Index (BMI) since the adoption of the 1977 USDGA. The logical assumption, argued here, is that the increased carbohydrate consumption (left panel) increased BMI (right panel). [55]

is an increased production of maternal ketones for use as a fuel in place of glucose by both the mother and, it turns out, the foetus. Thus pregnant mothers show increased blood ketone rises in response to both short-term (overnight)[58] and prolonged (days) starvation.[59]

In addition, during the final trimester of pregnancy, the maternal liver begins to produce ever more triglyceride so that blood-triglyceride concentrations rise markedly.[60] Since maternal blood-borne triglyceride does not cross the placenta, this hypertriglyceridemia cannot be of direct benefit to the foetus. Rather, hypertriglyceridemia increases the mother's capacity to produce even more ketones whenever her carbohydrate intake falls; for example, if she fasts or if she is subject to starvation.

It is highly improbable that this mechanism of enhanced maternal ketone production in response to fasting, starvation or a low-carb diet could have evolved with the goal of harming the brain of the unborn foetus. Instead, it is clearly a mechanism designed to *protect* the foetal brain from potentially dangerous fluctuations in the mother's blood-glucose (and hence placental/foetal-glucose) concentrations whenever her own food intake is reduced.

A key point is that, even during short-term (overnight) fasting, maternal blood-glucose concentrations are very much lower than in non-pregnant women and they can fall further to profoundly low levels (<3mmol/L) after four days of starvation.[59] Since the immature liver of the foetus has a limited capacity to raise the foetal blood-glucose concentration by producing glucose, so the blood-glucose concentration to which the foetus is exposed will mirror the mother's concentration and will be reduced to potentially dangerous levels whenever the mother does not eat for more than about six hours.[58] If the foetus did not have the capacity to use fuels other than glucose for its brain function, it is probable that foetal brain damage would occur every time a mother fasted for more than six hours. Since humans evolved in an environment of food insecurity for millions of years, absence of such a mechanism would have led rapidly to our extinction, as all our children would invariably have been stillborn or born with brain damage.

The solution that evolution provided was to allow the foetal brain to use ketone bodies in place of glucose when maternal (and therefore placental) blood-glucose concentrations fell. It has been known since 1967 that in starvation the brain's glucose requirement can fall by 75%, to be replaced by the use of ketones[61] without any impairment in brain function. In those studies blood ketone levels rose to >6mmol/L, higher than values measured in pregnant mothers during prolonged starvation (4mmol/L), but only about 10% of values measured in diabetic ketoacidosis (>50mmol/L).

Evidence for the importance of ketones to infant metabolism is substantial: it has been found that 30% of the foetal brain's energy requirements are provided by ketones[62]; the use of ketones is continued by the newborn at delivery[63, 64]; there is a further up-regulation after birth of enzymes in the brain that direct the use of ketones; and blood-ketone levels in infants are elevated during the suckling period[65] so that the brains of infants have a "greater uptake of ketone bodies than has been reported in adults"[66] with the result that "as much as 25% of the neonate's basal energy requirements in the first several days of life" come from the use of ketones[67]. In fact, ketone uptake by the brain is five times faster in older infants compared to adults.[45] Even more convincing is the finding that the foetus has the capacity to produce its own ketones, independent of those its mother provides.[68]

None of these adaptations would ever have occurred if blood ketones endangered the brain health of the foetus. Instead these adaptations are clearly designed to shield the brain and bodies of the unborn and newborn from starvation. Thus: "During maternal starvation, ketone bodies may maximize chances for survival both in utero and during neonatal life by restricting cell replication and sustaining lipid and protein and lipid stores in foetal tissues."[69] Or, in the words of colleagues who taught me at the University of Cape Town Medical School, "Since ketone bodies can be used by the brain (including foetal brain) as natural fuel, and there is evidence that the synthesis of essential cerebral lipids occurs from these substances, it is inconceivable that the blood levels reached during calorie-restricted diets could cause harm."[70]

On the other hand, it is clear that the diabetic ketoacidosis that develops in mothers with Type 1 diabetes who fail to use insulin correctly *can* be associated with foetal damage. But whether this is a direct effect of the 10-fold higher maternal and foetal blood-ketone concentrations or is due to other metabolic consequences of diabetic ketoacidosis, including hyperglycaemia, is not yet established.

In review, it is clear that the baby food industry and its proxy scientific and medical bodies have done all of us a massive disservice by spreading the false message that any form of ketosis – whether the mild form in nutritional ketosis (in those eating low-carb diets) or the severe and potentially fatal form in diabetic ketoacidosis – are equally dangerous to the health of the unborn or the newly born.

Few understand that at birth the newborn undergoes "an abrupt change from a high-carbohydrate and a low-fat diet to a high-fat and low-carbohydrate diet".[71] That high-fat diet provided by the mother's breast milk and the ketosis that it induces in the newborn is critical for the subsequent growth of the infant's brain.[41]

Since rapid brain growth continues for the first two years of the infant's life, it is logical that the foods onto which he or she is weaned should be those that will continue to provide the fuel needed for building the brain. And that, it turns out, is ketones. As a result, some specialists have convincingly argued that "weaning onto a ketogenic diet would be healthier than weaning onto a high-carb diet".[72]

The final word on this point belongs to Lily Nichols, author of *Real Foods for Gestational Diabetes.* She notes a strange irony. Many women with polycystic ovary syndrome, a condition associated with insulin resistance, become pregnant only after they increase their dietary fat intakes by adopting a low-carb high-fat diet. Yet once this form of therapy allows them to fall pregnant they are advised to revert to the same high-carb diet that prevented them from becoming pregnant in the first place. That makes no sense. She advises as follows:

> Many women do just fine eating a more moderate level of carbohydrates in pregnancy, so I do not believe *everyone* needs to go low carb. But if you have medical conditions that are tied to blood-sugar issues, such as gestational diabetes, preeclampsia, or you simply want to prevent excess weight gain, you should know it's safe to eat a lower-carbohydrate diet while pregnant. [73]

3 **Though there is uncertainty about the correct timing of the introduction of foods to babies, both premature weaning and the late introduction of potentially allergenic foods are best avoided.**

As outlined above, the age of introduction of first foods dropped quite markedly in the US during the 20th century and particularly after the success of commercial baby foods from the 1920s – to the point that weaning typically began as early as a month after birth in some populations. There was even that set order of foods: "white cereal rice first, followed by apple-sauce or mashed banana, and progressing on to puréed vegetables and meat".[26] This rigid American approach was and is not followed universally, however, indicating a lack of consensus on the matter. Today advice on "complementary feeding" can vary greatly between countries.

The need for weaning to solid foods is the result of the rapid growth of the infant, and especially of its brain, so that after about 6 months of age it becomes increasingly impossible for mother's milk alone to provide all the energy and nutrients required to ensure optimum growth. Six months is thus generally accepted as the reasonable upper limit by which time complementary foods should be added to mother's milk. Early weaning is, however, not recommended, as the infant's renal and gastrointestinal functions need to mature for it to be able to metabolise non-milk foods. Considering this, a 2008 position paper by the the European Society for Paediatric Gastroenterology, Hepatology and Nutrition suggests four months as the earliest age at which weaning should begin.[74] Thus 4-6 months seems the best-considered weaning window. As outlined in the Wonder Weaning chapter (see p68), we suggest waiting a little longer if possible so that your baby might be able to better handle more complex, nutrient-dense foods (animal proteins rather than vegetable purées, for example), but his or her physical needs and interest in non-milk foods will likely be the deciding factor. (Note that the type of weaning food is likely more important than the time of weaning – see point 4.)

A related matter of timing has to do with the avoidance of allergies. By the early 2000s there was clear evidence for the rising incidence of specific food allergies; for example, the prevalence of peanut allergy in the US quadrupled in the 13 years between 1997 and 2010. As a result the American Academy of Allergy, Asthma and Immunology has suggested that new foods be introduced to the infant one at a time for a period and only continued if there was no evidence for any allergic reactions. Other authorities have suggested delaying the introduction of potentially allergenic foods. Following these proposals, the introduction of the infant to more solid foods could take many months.

More recently, however, the thinking has again changed, as it has become apparent that the late introduction of foods may actually *increase* the likelihood that an allergy to that foodstuff will develop[75], while the early introduction of eggs[76] and peanuts[77, 78] may *reduce* the risk that an allergy to that foodstuff will develop. The landmark Learning Early about Peanut Allergy (LEAP) study, led by South African-trained scientist Dr George du Toit in London, found that the early introduction of peanuts reduced the risk that the infant would develop a peanut allergy by 70-80%![77] As a result the suggestion is now that infants should be introduced to peanuts between 4 and 8 months under controlled conditions. Following the LEAP study, there will likely be an increasing interest in the possible role of the earlier introduction of potentially allergenic foods to prevent future food allergies.

4 Wean onto real foods. Not onto non-foods such as white rice cereal or porridge, as some guidelines – and commercial food companies – will have you do.

The traditional weaning of infants onto white (or even brown) rice cereal is not based on some magical nutritional value exclusive to rice cereals without which infants will not thrive. Rather, it is because that is what Gerber decided was good for babies some eight decades ago. The reality is that rice cereal is a nutritionally deficient foodstuff that contains little other than cheap non-essential carbohydrates. Its popularity has been sustained because of the perception that it is a safe foodstuff that is unlikely to produce allergies, and because it is easily digestible (and thus more suitable for premature weaning). More recently, it has the added perceived benefit of being low in fat, which supposedly causes heart disease. The fact that this has been thoroughly refuted, in *The Real Meal Revolution* and elsewhere, is further enforced by the very specific nutritional requirements of babies during the first two years of life; if ever a high-fat diet is required it is during this critical growth stage.

Consider a 100g serving of typical dry brown rice cereal instant baby food: it packs a solid 75g of carbohydrate with 7.5g of protein and only 2.5g of fat, and it comes with a mere fraction of the vitamins and minerals that are present in liver, sardines and eggs (Table 2). The same applies to white rice, only more so.

Research in the past decade has shown that infants raised on bland-tasting, colourless, textureless meals develop a preference for these "beige foods". Thus children raised on diets containing rusks, processed cereals and milk were found to be more likely to prefer white bread, plain pasta, potato chips and milk as they aged. In part this is because infants learn that these processed foods are "food", while "other more colourful foods seem foreign, and even 'non-food like'"[26]. In contrast, infants fed a wider range of colourful, textured foods were more likely to show an interest and preference for these foods in their adolescence.

More discomforting evidence has come from the 2002 and 2008 Feeding of Infants and Toddlers Study (FITS).[80, 81, 82] This study of the feeding behaviours of 3,000 babies in the US found that by seven months of age some babies had already adopted the industrial American diet low in vegetables and fruits, with the result that by 15 months French fries were the most common "vegetable" consumed. By 8 months nearly 50% of infants consumed some type of dessert, sweet or sweetened beverage; by 24 months 62% consumed a baked dessert, 20% candy and 44% a sweetened beverage.[80] By age 2-3 years, these numbers had only worsened so that 85% of infants between those ages consumed some type of sweetened beverage, dessert, sweet or salty snack in a day. The incidence of obesity in these infants was double that of children three decades earlier.[81] Importantly, *nearly all* of these children ate commercially processed white rice cereal (98%) and jarred baby foods (99%).[83]

Though they have uncovered some startling results, in my opinion the FITS authors and others[84] have failed to understand fully the implications of their studies. Their dietary advice is in essence that infants need to eat more fruits and vegetables ("with emphasis on dark green, leafy, and deep yellow vegetables and colourful fruits"[80]), more iron-rich infant cereal, more iron-fortified grains, more low-fat dairy products, more meat and more "healthier" fats, and "limit consumption of low-nutrient, energy-dense foods and beverages".[81, 83]

These authors fail to grasp the point that it is a nutrient-poor high-carb low-fat diet of highly processed non-foods that is causing the obesity epidemic amongst these US children. Advising these children to eat high-carb fruits, cereals, grains and porridge, even if iron-fortified, and to limit their fat intake, while not warning of the real dangers of sugar and perhaps wheat addiction (see point 7), is in my opinion the gateway to adult obesity.

And it's one that can be traced back to Gerber's introduction of industrial infant foods in the 1920s.

Amy Bentley concurs: "Feeding infants food such as bland, highly processed rice cereal, its critics argue, puts them on the pathway to a lifetime of consumption of highly processed unhealthy calories, which is one cause of the rising rates of overweight, obesity, and related diseases such as diabetes."[26]

(All per 100g of product)	SELECTED NUTRIENT-RICH FOODS			INFANT CEREALS	
	Chicken liver	Sardines	Eggs	White rice	Brown rice
Essential fats – omega 3 (mg)	6	**1,480**	74	13	40
Essential fats – omega 6 (mg)	486	**3,544**	1,148	62	900
Protein quality (100+ = complete protein)	**149**	148	136	-	-
Vitamins					
A Retinol (900 mcg)	**3,290**	32	139	0	0
A Carotene (assumed retinol equivalent)	**6**	0	1	3	0
B1 (Thiamin) (1.2 mg)	**0.3**	0.1	0.1	0.2	0
B2 (Riboflavin) (1.3 mg)	**1.8**	0.2	0.5	0	0
B3 (Niacin) (16 mg)	9.7	5.2	0.1	1.5	**15**
B5 (Pantothenic acid) (5 mg) (AI)	**6.2**	0.6	1.4	0.4	0
B6 (1.7 mg)	**0.9**	0.2	0.1	0.1	0
Folate (400 mcg)	**588**	12	47	58	12.5
B12 (2.4 mcg)	**16.6**	8.9	1.3	0	0
C (90 mg)	**17.9**	0	0	0	0
D (600 IU) (AI) (*)	Neg	**272**	35	0	0
E (15 mg)	0.7	**2**	1	0	0
K (120 mcg) (AI)	0	**2.6**	0.3	0	0
Minerals (M)					
Calcium (1,000 mg) (AI)	8	**382**	53	10	48
Magnesium (420 mg)	19	39	12	12	**43***
Phosphorus (700 mg)	297	**490**	191	43	238
Minerals (T)					
Copper (0.9 mg)	**0.5**	0.2	0.1	0.1	0
Iron (18 mg)	**9.0**	2.9	1.8	1.2	**43***
Manganese (2.3 mg) (AI)	0.3	0.1	0.0	**0.4**	0
Selenium (55 mcg)	**54.6**	52.7	31.7	7.5	20
Zinc (11 mg)	**2.7**	1.3	1.1	0.5	0

Table 2. The nutrient composition of three nutrient-rich foods – chicken liver, sardines and eggs – compared to white and brown rice in infant rice cereals. The foodstuff providing the most of each particular nutrient is shown in **bold**. [79]

* Note that magnesium and iron absorption from meat and fish are much greater than from fortified cereals.

The movement against white rice cereal as the staple infant food in the US has been led by a clinical professor of paediatrics at Stanford, Dr Alan Greene, who has labelled it "junk food". Greene argues that white rice cereal is a nutritionally deficient food that programmes the infant to seek foods that are equally highly processed and nutritionally incomplete, and usually high in sugar and refined carbohydrates.

Dr Greene believes that "white rice cereal can predispose to obesity", and he expands on this without equivocation in a way to grab the attention of those who recognise the dangers of sugar:

"In fact I think [white rice cereal] is the tap root of the child obesity epidemic. The problem is that it is basically like feeding kids a spoonful of sugar."

He further clarifies this thought by comparing white rice cereal to drinking sugary fizzy drinks: "I'm saying you might as well be putting soda in a bottle as feeding the white rice cereal. It would be soda with added vitamins [and] added iron. But yeah, that's what you are doing".

Gerber, now owned by Nestlé, disagrees; they are, they say, "not aware of any scientific studies that support the theory that white rice cereal contributes to childhood obesity, and welcome the opportunity to review any relevant data". [85]

Perhaps, at this point, it is important to remember that there are no essential carbohydrates and that there are only three uses for carbohydrates in the human body. They can be stored as glycogen – the human equivalent of starch – in the liver and muscles; or they can be used as an energy fuel; or they must be turned into fat. There are no other alternatives.

A growing baby cannot build muscles and bones from carbohydrates. Nor, for that matter, brains.

5 **Optimum nutrition in the first 24 months of life is critical, and it's absolutely essential to focus on the foods and nutrients that assist brain development in this time, especially fats, vitamins, iron, iodine, copper, zinc and selenium.**

The emphasis of the Feeding of Infants and Toddlers Study authors is to encourage infants to eat more carbohydrates in grains and some "healthier fats", while drinking low-fat milk. In fact, the focus of early infant nutrition should, in my opinion, be on restricting carbohydrates and emphasising the essential fats, proteins, vitamins and minerals provided by nutrient-dense real foods, especially for the proper development of the brain and circulatory system.

In *The Real Meal Revolution* we repeatedly made the point, as we do here, that carbohydrates are not an essential human foodstuff (Table 1). There are, rather, essential proteins and fats; the latter include the omega-3 and omega-6 polyunsaturated fats, alpha-linolenic acid (ALA) and linoleic acid (LA) or their products, docosahexaenoic acid (DHA) and arachidonic acid (AA). Remember, however, that the modern diet is generally excessive in LA and omega-6 fats (found in vegetable oils and margarines, for example) and deficient in omega-3 fats (found in oily fish and dairy from grass-fed cows), which we'll look in to further below.

Fifty to 60% of the structural matter of the brain and retina comprises DHA, the majority of which is laid down during the period of maximum brain growth that begins at 26 weeks of conception and continues until about 2 years, with 80% occurring between weeks 26 and 40 after conception. During this period of rapid growth, as much as 70% of the baby's energy is partitioned for brain growth. Many believe that a key driver of human evolution and the development of our large brain occurred when we added foods rich in omega-3 oils and the other brain specific nutrients[40,41,86], perhaps as recently as 200,000 years ago. In *The Real Meal Revolution*, we provided evidence that this defining event may have occurred along the southern Cape coast near Mossel Bay.

The developing brain has an elevated demand for DHA, AA, ALA and LA and other brain-specific nutrients during this critical period of accelerated growth.[87] While adult humans have some capacity to convert ALA and LA to DHA and AA, the foetus does not. Instead, the maternal placenta actively extracts DHA and AA from the mother's circulation to provide these critical nutrients for the developing foetus's brain.[88] A deficient maternal dietary DHA and AA intake may lead to both brain and circulatory complications in the newborn[89] and could contribute to the development of insulin resistance in child and adulthood, especially in those exposed to high sugar and carbohydrate intakes from a young age.

To ensure optimum brain development, we need to ensure that newborns and infants are provided with an abundance of DHA and AA. They will not find this in an industrial diet based on grains and from which animal foods, dairy and especially fish and shellfish are excluded, nor in a vegetarian-type diet.

As one commentator put it, "Fetus brains are not made from romaine lettuce and low-cholesterol omega-6 soybean oil salad dressings. Fetus brains are not made from rice milk. Fetus brains are not made from organic fruit or fruit juices. Fetus brains are not made from carbohydrates, starches or fibre." [90]

Indeed, as we've emphasised, carbohydrates are not essential for human survival, and can, in fact, be harmful. Meanwhile, a healthy foetus brain *is* made from saturated fats, omega-3 fatty acids, amino acids from proteins and essential vitamins and minerals, all of which must be found in abundance in the pregnant mother's blood supply. The best way to achieve this is to remove omega-6-rich industrial seed oils from the mother's diet – particularly corn, soybean, canola, sunflower, safflower and grapeseed oils – and to encourage consumption of fishes that are rich in DHA and AA. Excellent sources are fatty fish like salmon and tuna, with well-cooked crab, prawns and eggs also good options. (If you're pregnant or planning to get pregnant and have been avoiding tuna, remember that current NHS guidelines recommend no more than two 150g tuna steaks or four 140g (when drained) cans of tuna a week.)

And what might be the outcome? One prospective study compared the effects of supplementing the diet of pregnant mothers with either predominantly omega-6 polyunsaturated fat, corn oil, or predominantly omega-3 polyunsaturated fat, cod liver oil, on the mental development of their children. The results showed superior mental performance at four years of the children whose mothers had supplemented with cod liver oil.[91] But other studies have not been as successful.

While associational studies can really only provide material for new hypotheses, it is interesting that the DHA:LA (linoleic acid) content of human milk samples – that is, the (good) omega-3 to (bad) omega-6 breast-milk ratio – from 26 countries was positively associated with the each country's average test

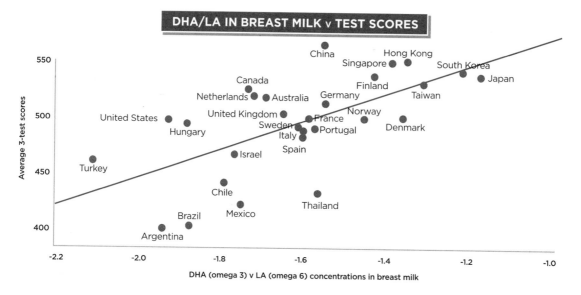

Figure 7. The log of docosahexanoic (omega 3) to linoleic (omega 6) acid concentrations in human milk samples from 28 countries predicts test scores in mathematics, reading and science in those countries. Together, these two human milk fatty acids explained 46% to 48% of the variance in test scores in these countries. Note that lower values (moving to the right on the horizontal axis) indicate more (healthy) omega 3 and less (less healthy) omega 6 in breast milk. [93]

scores in mathematics, reading and science measured from the Program for International Student Assessment[92] (Figure 7). The authors suggest that dietary LA may impair cognition by decreasing brain DHA and AA concentrations. In contrast, dietary DHA, AA and ALA would be expected to increase the brain concentrations of these critical fats.

The remarkable finding of the study was that these two dietary measures explained 46-48% of the variance in these scores with no improvement in predictive power when socioeconomic variables were included. Imagine if a nation's prosperity really is determined by the quality of its mothers' breast milk – a frightening thought!

Then there is the evidence that only a meat-based weaning diet will provide all the zinc, iron and other nutrients required by the rapidly growing brain.[42] In addition, iron absorption from meat is much greater than from iron-fortified cereals, and meat produces a healthier gut bacterial flora (biome) than do cereals[94] (the negative health implications of cereals notwithstanding).

Recently Health Canada, the Canadian Paediatric Society, Dieticians of Canada and the Breastfeeding Committee of Canada have advised that infants "should be served meat, fish, poultry, or meat alternatives daily. The amount of food offered should be guided by the infant's hunger and satiety cues. Breastfeeding continues to provide the main source of nutrition as other foods are introduced."[95] These recommendations tie in closely with those in the revised South African dietary guidelines mentioned earlier.

Just how important is this emphasis on

providing the newborn with the correct amount of brain-specific nutrients? The World Health Organization warns, for example, that, "The brainpower of entire nations is slipping because of a shortage of the right dietary nutrients, including iodine, iron, vitamin A and zinc. The report claimed that inadequate iron intake reduces a child's IQ by five to seven points, while insufficient iodine reduces childhood IQ by 13 points. Iron deficiency is pervasive enough that it is estimated to reduce the gross domestic product of the most affected countries by 2%. So ubiquitous is vitamin and mineral deficiency that it debilitates in some significant degree the energies, intellect and economic prospects of nations." [41]

WHY ARE HUMAN BABIES BORN FAT?

Professor Steven Cunnane of the University of Sherbrooke, Quebec has made the interesting observation that humans are the only land mammals whose neonates are born fat.[39, 41] Since the newborn of our nearest relatives, the chimpanzees, do not contain such body fat, Cunnane has concluded that something has happened in the past 6 million years or so to ensure that human newborns accumulate fat especially in the final three months of gestation. Since the much greater brain mass of humans is the other key difference between land mammals and humans, Cunnane wonders whether these two are linked. What if human babies accumulate body fat in the final trimester of their intra-uterine life in order to fuel the explosive growth in brain size that occurs during the first two years of life?

He argues that the greater human brain size is entirely dependent on the capacity of the foetus to store about 500g of body fat before birth, and on the infant liver's ability to convert those fat stores and the fat in its diet into the ketones needed to grow the brain. In this way fat in the infant's body, fat in its diet and fat (ketones) in its blood explain why humans have such big brains.

The point of all this is to show that for the first two years of life, the infant is a metabolic machine designed to turn its body fat stores and the fat in its diet into ketone bodies to build its brain.

And the more effectively it is able to do this, the cleverer the infant is likely to be as an adult.[45]

Not unsurprisingly, it is mothers with a university education or higher socioeconomic status who raise infants with the largest brains, and hence the greatest future intellectual prospects.[45] Infants raised on diets deficient in the key brain-specific nutrients will carry that disadvantage all their lives.

I have another theory. What if the genes for insulin resistance arose spontaneously in humans in the last million years or so and produced fat babies in the high-carbohydrate environment of their mother's womb? And what if those fat babies were more likely to develop bigger brains during infancy especially when exposed to nutrient-specific brain foods and so to become cleverer than their peers? Since this genetic variant would provide a significant biological advantage, with time the genes for insulin resistance would be conserved and those without those genes would become fewer and fewer, according to the Darwinian principle of survival of those most fitted to the environment.

Unfortunately while insulin resistance might be an advantage during the short period of intra-uterine life, as described in *The Real Meal Revolution*, it becomes a serious disadvantage for those living their entire adult lives eating a high-carbohydrate diet.

6 **The consumption of five or more servings of fruit and vegetables every day has been overplayed by the official guidelines, and should be of secondary nutritional concern compared to nutrient-rich fats and proteins.**

Parents around the world have always struggled to get their kids to eat their fruit and vegetables... But what if they've been getting their priorities wrong? Should they in fact be focusing on other foods? The first inkling that this may be the case comes with the realisation that parents haven't "always" struggled with this problem; the idea that eating a number of servings of fruit and veg each day is healthy is of quite recent origin. Before canning, refrigeration, reliably clean water and the discovery of vitamins, fruits and vegetables were viewed with suspicion since they were often associated with ill health (due to their preparation in bacterially contaminated water).

The reality is that most fruits and vegetables are relatively poor sources of vitamins and minerals compared to some other foods (Tables 2 and 3), and a nutrient-dense diet of the kind promoted in this book and in *The Real Meal Revolution* is more likely to provide optimum vitamin and mineral intakes than is a diet that includes five ("or more") servings of fruits and vegetables per day but excludes nutrient-dense foods. That noted, fruits and vegetables can provide phytochemicals and anti-oxidants, and may alter the gut biome positively. For this reason we promote vegetables and to a lesser extent fruits as a valuable dietary component in the Real Meal Revolution eating plan and thus for children.

Table 3 lists five genuinely nutrient-dense foods – chicken livers, sunflower seeds, sardines, eggs and kale – of which the former two have the highest concentrations of 9 of 24 nutrients and are thus particularly highly recommended. Note that three are animal products and only one, kale, is a vegetable. By comparison, the nutrient density of five popular fruits and vegetables listed in Table 4 – apples, bananas, oranges, carrots, peas – is poor, the sole exception being the high concentration of carotene in carrots.

In debunking the "five-a-day" myth, obesity researcher Zoë Harcombe writes, "The fruit and veg five-a-day has traces of essential fats; no complete protein; no retinol (the form in which the body needs vitamin A – don't assume that carotene can be converted); no B12 and no vitamin D (note also that D3 is only available in animal foods – D2 is the plant version). Not one nutrient RDA/AI [recommended daily allowance/ adequate intake] can be provided by 100g of any of the fruit and veg – not even vitamin C." [96]

She goes on to list the enormous quantities of each of the five fruits or veg needed on a daily basis to satisfy recommended vitamin and mineral requirements; for example, 2.1kg of carrots for vitamin E – carrots being the best source of vitamin E in Table 4.

Of more concern, however, is the "significant sugar content in fruit and veg". While a meal of 100g of each of the five foods in Table 3 would contain just 3 grams of sugar – less

(All per 100g of product)	Chicken liver	Sardines	Eggs	Sunflower seeds	Kale
Essential fats – omega 3 (mg)	6	**1,480**	74	74	180
Essential fats – omega 6 (mg)	486	3,544	1,148	**23,048**	138
Protein quality (100+ = complete protein)	**149**	148	136	88	92
Vitamins					
A Retinol (900 mcg)	**3,290**	32	139	0	0
A Carotene (assumed retinol equivalent)	6	0	1	3	**769**
B1 (Thiamin) (1.2 mg)	0.3	0.1	0.1	**1.5**	0.1
B2 (Riboflavin) (1.3 mg)	**1.8**	0.2	0.5	0.4	0.1
B3 (Niacin) (16 mg)	**9.7**	5.2	0.1	8.3	1
B5 (Pantothenic acid) (5 mg) (AI)	**6.2**	0.6	1.4	1.1	0.1
B6 (1.7 mg)	0.9	0.2	0.1	**1.3**	0.3
Folate (400 mcg)	**588**	12	47	227	29
B12 (2.4 mcg)	**16.6**	8.9	1.3	0	0
C (90 mg)	17.9	0	0	1.4	**120**
D (600 IU) (AI)	neg	**272**	35	0	0
E (15 mg)	0.7	2	1	**33.2**	0
K (120 mcg) (AI)	0	2.6	0.3	0	**817**
Minerals (M)					
Calcium (1,000 mg) (AI)	8	**382**	53	78	135
Magnesium (420 mg)	19	39	12	**325**	34
Phosphorus (700 mg)	297	490	191	**660**	56
Minerals (T)					
Copper (0.9 mg)	0.5	0.2	0.1	**1.8**	0.3
Iron (18 mg)	**9.0**	2.9	1.8	5.2	1.7
Manganese (2.3 mg) (AI)	0.3	0.1	0.0	**1.9**	0.8
Selenium (55 mcg)	**54.6**	52.7	31.7	53.0	0.9
Zinc (11 mg)	2.7	1.3	1.1	**5.0**	0.4

Table 3. The nutrient composition of five nutrient-rich foods: chicken liver, sardines, eggs, sunflower seeds and kale. The foodstuff providing the most of each particular nutrient is shown in **bold**. [96]

than a teaspoon, all of which comes from the sunflower seeds – a similar meal of 100g of each of the fruit and veg in Table 4 would contain 41 grams, or more than 10 teaspoons, of sugar.

To make her point that fruit and veg have been promoted without sufficient evidence and to the detriment of far more nutritious foods, Harcombe has calculated that adult human RDAs for all nutrients can be achieved by eating just five foods in these amounts each day: 500g

(All per 100g of product)	Apple	Banana	Orange	Carrots	Peas
Essential fats – omega 3 (mg)	9	27	9	2	**35**
Essential fats – omega 6 (mg)	43	46	23	115	**152**
Protein quality (100+ = complete protein)	31	62	58	-	**84**
Vitamins					
A Retinol (900 mcg)	0	0	0	0	0
A Carotene (assumed retinol equivalent)	3	3	12	**835**	38
B1 (Thiamin) (1.2 mg)	0	0	0.1	0.1	**0.3**
B2 (Riboflavin) (1.3 mg)	0	0.1	0.1	0.1	**0.1**
B3 (Niacin) (16 mg)	0.1	0.7	0.4	1	**2.1**
B5 (Pantothenic acid) (5 mg) (AI)	0.1	0.3	0.3	**0.3**	0.1
B6 (1.7 mg)	0	**0.4**	0.1	0.1	0.2
Folate (400 mcg)	3	20	34	19	**65**
B12 (2.4 mcg)	0	0	0	0	0
C (90 mg)	4.6	8.7	**59.1**	5.9	40
D (600 IU) (AI) (*)	0	0	0	0	0
E (15 mg)	0.2	0.1	0.2	**0.7**	0.1
K (120 mcg) (AI)	2.2	0.5	0	13.2	**24.8**
Minerals (M)					
Calcium (1,000 mg) (AI)	6	5	**43**	33	25
Magnesium (420 mg)	5	27	11	12	**33**
Phosphorus (700 mg)	11	22	23	35	**108**
Minerals (T)					
Copper (0.9 mg)	0	0.1	0	0	**0.2**
Iron (18 mg)	0.1	0.3	0.1	0.3	**1.5**
Manganese (2.3 mg) (AI)	0	0.3	0	0.1	**0.4**
Selenium (55 mcg)	0	1.0	0	0.1	**1.8**
Zinc (11 mg)	0	0.2	0.1	0.2	**1.2**

Table 4. The nutrient composition of five popular fruits and vegetables. The foodstuff providing the most of each particular nutrient is shown in **bold**. Note how poorly these figures rate in comparison to the nutrient rich foods in Table 3, previous page. [96]

whole milk, 450g (10 medium-sized) eggs, 300g spinach, 250g raw mushrooms, and 50g sunflower seeds. She suggests that a simple diet that contains the following nine foods would ensure optimum nutritional balance: liver, sardines, eggs, whole milk, sunflower seeds, oats, cocoa, spinach and broccoli.[96, 97] In contrast, strict vegetarians who eschew milk and eggs will have great difficulty achieving their vitamin A (retinol), vitamin D3, vitamin K2 and vitamin B12 requirements especially, since all these vitamins exist naturally only in animal foods (meat, fish, eggs and dairy produce).

As an aside, there is a spurious counter to the suggestion that liver is a super food (Table 3): the claim is that anyone eating liver risks developing vitamin A toxicity. The reality is that vitamin A toxicity has been documented in Arctic explorers forced to eat either dog or polar bear livers in order to survive[98, 99] and in those consuming *synthetic* vitamin A at doses of 300,000 IU. Since 100g of liver contains 11,000 IU of retinol, an individual would need to eat 3kg of liver in one sitting to reach a toxic dose. Usual intakes are less than 60g. In contrast to this suggestion, eating liver has been seen to improve the vitamin A status of low-income children in South Africa's Northern Cape.[100]

Similarly, though a high fruit-and-veg intake has been promoted as a means to prevent cancers, a major cross-sectional study published in 2010 found that there was no difference in the risk of developing cancer in those eating the least or the most fruit and vegetables per day.[101] The conclusion from this and other work is: "The possibility that fruit and vegetables may help to reduce the risk of cancer has been studied for more than 30 years, but no protective effects have been firmly established."[97]

Thus we see that the WHO guideline that we should each eat "at least 5 portions, or 400g, of fruit and vegetables per day" is not evidence-based. While children with normal carbohydrate metabolism – that is, children without any signs of weight problems (let alone diabetes) – might be able to follow this advice with some beneficial effects, for those with insulin resistance, pre-diabetes or Type 2 diabetes, the high-carb load present in fruits especially will harm long-term health. In general, we see no reason why anyone should ever eat more than 200g of carbohydrate per day.

Interestingly, between 1991 and 1998 fruit and vegetable intake in the US increased by nearly 20%. But in the same time obesity rates increased 50%. While no-one can claim that the one caused the other, it is clear that "five-a-day" advice has not had a measurably positive impact on obesity rates. By increasing the carbohydrate load in those with insulin resistance, the emphasis on "healthy" fruits especially will likely have contributed to the obesity and diabetes epidemics – for in obesity, increased fruit consumption is simply another (delicious) way of ingesting more unnecessary carbohydrates.

In summary, there can be no denying that there are certain nutritional and health benefits to be had from fruit and in particular vegetables, and we still recommend vegetables and lower-sugar fruits for children, as can be seen in the recipes throughout this book. The point is that their nutritional importance has been overplayed to the detriment of more vital nutrient-dense foods.

7 There is increasing evidence, often overlooked in the dietary guidelines, that the consumption of gluten-containing grains, including wheat, barley and rye, can cause a variety of health problems, especially in the genetically-predisposed.

There is a growing concern that gluten-containing grains like wheat, barley and rye directly cause long-term ill health. The concern was perhaps first popularised by US cardiologist Dr William Davis[102], followed by his countryman Dr David Perlmutter[103], a neurologist. More recently, the champion of this cause has become Dr Alessio Fasano of the Harvard Medical School.[104, 105]

Dr Fasano is a potential future Nobel Laureate for his discovery of the manner in which gluten in wheat causes the auto-immune disease coeliac disease, and perhaps other auto-immune conditions.[106] On purely scientific grounds, Dr Fasano will become an increasingly irresistible candidate as his ideas become increasingly mainstream.

In a series of the remarkable studies, Dr Fasano has shown that gliadin, a breakdown product of gluten in wheat, rye and barley, induces the production of the protein zonulin within the gut. Zonulin then binds with the intestinal cells, opening the tight junctions between these cells. Once these tight junctions are compromised, large molecules can enter the bloodstream, potentially setting the stage for a range of auto-immune and other diseases in those at specific genetic risk (Table 5). This has been termed "leaky gut syndrome".

Importantly for those with a family history of Type 1 (insulin deficient) diabetes mellitus, Dr Fasano has presented evidence that this form of diabetes may be an auto-immune disease initiated by this "leaky gut" mechanism in response to the consumption of gluten.[106, 108]

Perhaps of equal interest is the growing realisation that while the diseases listed in Table 5 are relatively less common, a much more common cause of human ill health is the condition known as non-coeliac gluten sensitivity (NCGS). [105] I became interested in this condition as a result of my personal conversion to the low-carb high-fat diet, in which I removed all gluten from my diet. Miraculously, a large number of minor medical irritations – weekly migraines, irritable bowel syndrome (IBS), gastric reflux and recurrent bronchitis with occasional exercise-induced asthma, amongst others – suddenly disappeared and have not returned in four years. I have to conclude that all these conditions are related to foods that I no longer eat, with wheat as the most probable culprit.

The "classical" presentation of NCGS is considered to be the following:

Autoimmune diseases	Diseases of the nervous system	Cancers
Ankylosing spondylitis	Chronic inflammatory demyelinating polyneuropathy	Brain cancers (gliomas)
Coeliac disease	Multiple sclerosis	Breast cancer
Inflammatory bowel disease (Crohn's disease)	Schizophrenia	Lung adenocarcinoma
Rheumatoid arthritis		Ovarian cancer
Systemic lupus erythematosus		Pancreatic cancer
Type 1 diabetes mellitus		

Table 5. Diseases that may be linked to the "leaky gut syndrome" produced by gliadin-induced zonulin released in the intestine. [107]

A combination of IBS-like symptoms including abdominal pain, bloating, bowel habit abnormalities (either diarrhoea or constipation), and systemic manifestation such as "foggy mind", headache, fatigue, joint and muscle pain, leg or arm numbness, dermatitis (eczema or skin rash), depression and anaemia...many NCGS patients already report the causal relationship between the ingestion of gluten-containing foods and worsening of symptoms. In children, NCGS manifests with typical gastrointestinal symptoms, such as abdominal pain and chronic diarrhoea, while the extra-intestinal manifestations seem to be less frequent, the most common extra-intestinal symptom being tiredness. [109]

More recently, these groups of authors have shown that all humans develop "leaky gut" when exposed to gliadin, the digestion product of gluten.[110] Dr Simon Murch of Warwick University in the United Kingdom has advanced the hypothesis that gliadin is part of the plant's defence mechanism that prevents predation by inducing an immune response in most creatures that eat it. He notes, for example, that the only insects that eat wheat are those producing enzymes that breakdown gliadin. But all humans lack those enzymes.

Thus Dr Fasano believes that no humans should eat wheat, as we are not designed fully to digest gluten/gliadin. This opinion is unlikely ever to be popular in his adopted country, the US, which grows more than 58 million tons of wheat annually, of which 50% is exported at a value of $9 billion.

Interestingly, despite the advice that humans should eat "healthy whole grains" for long-term health, there are no long-term randomised controlled trials showing benefits from such "health foods". Instead, all the published studies have failed to show any benefits of this dietary change.[111-118] Nor is there evidence that an increased fibre intake alters short-term (2-4 years) risk of developing colon cancer.[119]

It is surprising how effectively this science has been hidden and instead the (unproven) health benefits of grains continue to be touted by those marketed as the world's leading nutritional scientists.[120]

8 **To avoid major dental problems, feed your child a cereal-free diet full of vitamin D, fats and calcium provided by real foods – in contrast to some older guidelines that are effectively the ideal dietary prescription for the promotion of dental cavities.**

Before the agricultural revolution and the introduction of grains into the human diet, humans did not suffer widely from dental cavities (except for one group of North Americans eating acorns), a perhaps obvious realisation, since without easy access to dentists those with cavities must live painful lives and will likely die from dental abscesses.

Dental cavities, or caries, are thus a modern disease caused by carbohydrate-containing foods, as observed by McCollum writing in 1941: "Caries of teeth is restricted to people and animals who eat liberally of carbohydrate containing foods. Carnivorous man and animals do not suffer from this disease."[121]

Dr Weston Price was the person who first observed that peoples eating their traditional diets do not suffer from dental cavities until exposed to the modern industrial diet.[122] He concluded that there were four dietary factors that cause dental cavities:

- Lack of the minerals calcium, magnesium and phosphorus in the diet;
- Lack of soluble vitamins A, D, E and K with special emphasis on vitamin D;
- Excessive consumption of foods containing phytic acid (found in grains, nuts, seeds

and beans that have not been sprouted or fermented before consumption);
- Excessive sugar consumption.

That Dr Price was correct was essentially proven by a series of classic studies published in 1932, which established that a cereal-free (that is, phytic-acid-free) diet supplemented with vitamin D in abundance (in cod liver oil, irradiated ergosterol, pasture-raised eggs, raw milk and/or butter) had "greater inhibitory and curative effects on dental caries than any previously tested... The hardening of carious areas, which indicates the diminution in activity of the carious process and ultimate arrest, was one of the characteristic changes brought about by the diets used. It will be observed that the removal of cereals from the diet also increased the amount of arrest of caries as compared with that produced by the diets containing this food." [123] (Figure 8.)

The authors also wrote that "Experimental work on dogs and other animals has shown that for the normal development of the teeth the diet should include abundant vitamin D and calcium, and not be overweighted with cereals."

Subjects in the study replaced dietary cereals – bread, oatmeal, rice and tapioca, for example – with "an increased intake of potatoes and other vegetables, milk, fat, meat and eggs". Interestingly the beneficial effects of removing phytic-acid-containing foods occurred even though subjects were allowed to continue eating their usual amounts of sugar (around 60g a day) in the form of sugar, jam and syrup.

Sadly these studies and others coming to essentially the same conclusions[125] have simply been ignored[126]. Instead, the current advice of the American Dental Association (ADA) is that tooth decay occurs when "foods containing carbohydrates (sugar and starches) such as milk, pop, raisins, cakes or candy are frequently

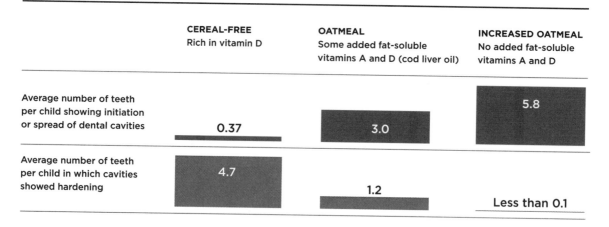

Figure 8. The effects of three different diets on the progression of dental cavities in children. Note that children eating the cereal-free diet rich in vitamin D showed the least increase in cavities and the greatest increase in dental hardening during the trial. By contrast, children eating diets high in cereals and low in fat-soluble vitamins had the opposite results. [124]

left in the mouth. Bacteria that live in the mouth thrive on these foods, producing acids as a result. Over a period of time, these acids destroy tooth enamel, resulting in tooth decay."

Thus the ADA has failed to advertise the proven role of vitamin D supplementation, raw milk, a high-fat diet and the removal of phytic acid in the prevention of dental cavities. I would suggest that the organisation could do better by warning us all that the perfect prescription that will cause dental cavities is the breakfast favoured by the USDGA: phytic-acid-loaded cereals topped with vitamin-D-deficient skimmed milk (and inevitably added sugar) plus phytic-acid-loaded bread with further added sugar (in the form of jams and other spreads). They could then advise widely that dental cavities can be prevented by eating real foods and by putting the fat back into our diets.

This unstated advice in the face of clear evidence certainly does raise awkward questions. Is the ADA, along with other organisations, unaware of the advice because their experts have not read the literature? Or is it because they have significant conflicts of interest in a nation in which grains are king?

A more important question for now, however, is: why is it so important to prevent cavities in children? The obvious answer is to prevent the pain, trauma and cost of the dental work required to fix these problems. But there is a more profound and far-reaching reason.

There is a strong body of scientific evidence indicating that dental cavities are the early marker of risk for developing the evil triad of chronic diseases: obesity, diabetes and heart disease.[121, 127] There is even evidence that the bacteria causing dental gum disease may be directly involved in coronary artery narrowing (atherosclerosis).[128] The point is that the same diet that causes dental cavities also causes chronic ill-health.

In other words, the presence of even a single dental cavity should indicate to you that your child is eating the wrong foods.

How then do we protect our children's teeth? Here are the simple rules, as advised by Dr Josh Axe, creator of the Food Is Medicine website.[129]

- **Remove sugar from the diet.**

- **Remove phytic acid from the diet by avoiding grains, beans (unless they have sprouted or been properly soaked before consumption) and soy.**
Phytic acid binds the minerals in grains and beans, including calcium, magnesium, phosphorus, iron and zinc, that are necessary for teeth mineralisation, preventing their absorption. Nuts also contain phytic acid but have other beneficial health effects and so should be eaten in appropriate amounts and not avoided. Phytic acid content is increased in foods grown using high-phosphate fertilisers.

- **Eat raw dairy and nutrient-rich foods.**
Raw dairy contains abundant calcium, vitamin K2, vitamin D3, magnesium, phosphorus and vitamins A and E. Note, however, that "raw milk" is unpasteurised, and so may contain organisms harmful to health. (Raw milk and dairy products made from raw milk must be clearly labelled as such.) As a result, we suggest eating organic cheeses and butter.

- **Emphasise foods that are rich in fat-soluble vitamins and minerals.**
In other words, eat the foods promoted in this book and *The Real Meal Revolution*, and remember that Dr Axe emphasises that there must be "NO processed food, packaged food or fast food".

BABY-LED WEANING: BYPASSING THE CONVENTIONAL PURÉED BABY FOOD STAGE

Just as the Banting revolution that we re-launched with *The Real Meal Revolution* proposed a return to eating real foods, so the latest movement in infant feeding is a return to the eating of real foods. If adult humans were healthier before they ate the modern industrial diet, so the argument goes, surely infant humans would be too? How did infants survive and become strong before the introduction of industrial processed baby foods? Is it not possible that the early weaning of infants onto processed industrial foods was promoted simply for the financial advantage of the manufacturers of commercial baby foods?

Advocates of the ancient approach argue that babies should bypass the purées and spoon-feeding stages of infant feeding. Instead, after the first six months of breastfeeding, they should be offered small chunks of real foods that they can manipulate with their fingers and consume by themselves. The goal is to develop co-ordination, independence and chewing as solid foods are introduced. This weaning bypasses "the baby food mush stage altogether,

a fairly radical proposition given the entrenched nature of puréed baby food in US infant feeding practices".[22]

Like most novelty in science, this is nothing new. In 1928 Clara M Davis, a doctor in Winnetka, Illinois, began a decade-long experiment in what would become known as "infant-led weaning".[130] In a home she established for 15 orphans, she began what has been called the world's longest, most detailed and most ambitious dietary experiment.[131] She wished to test the theory that when it comes to food, a child's body instinctively knows what is best for it – what has since been termed "the wisdom of the body".

To test this theory, at each meal she provided those 15 children with a range of 31 different foods and three drinks (water, sweet milk and sour milk) from which they could choose what they wished to eat and drink. These foods included vegetables, fruits, four cereals, and 10 foods of animal origin (Table 6). All foods were "procured fresh in the market all year round"; there were no processed foods and no sugar or flour or vegetable oils. Perhaps surprisingly, cream, butter and cheese were not included.

The key was that the food choices were left entirely to each child.

Water	Peaches	Spinach	Beef	Kidneys
Sweet milk	Tomatoes	Potatoes	Lamb	Fish (haddock)
Sour (lactic) milk	Beetroot	Lettuce	Bone marrow	
Sea salt	Carrots	Oatmeal	Bone jelly	
Apples	Peas	Wheat	Chicken	
Bananas	Turnips	Corn meal	Sweetbreads	
Orange juice	Cauliflower	Barley	Brains	
Fresh pineapple	Cabbage	Rye crisp bread	Liver	

Table 6. The list of foods provided in the feeding experiment of Clara M Davis. [132]

At each meal a nurse would place before them 6 or 8 servings containing a variety of wholesome unrefined foods. There were vegetables, fruits, eggs, cereals, meats, wholegrain bread, milk, water and fruit juices. The nurse was told, "Don't help the baby till he shows you what he wants". ["The nurses' orders were to sit quietly by, spoon in hand, and make no motion."[130]] The 8-month-old baby would lean forward and dip his fist into a dish of beets and then try to eat it off his hand. Now the nurse was permitted to give him a spoonful of beets. Then she must wait until he showed his choice again. Another spoonful of beets or maybe apple sauce. [133]

The type and amount of food eaten by each child at every meal was carefully logged: "the amount of every single thing eaten or spilled at every single meal over 4½ years of their eating life was assiduously recorded. To this was added records of changes in height and weight, the nature of bowel movements, and regular bone radiographs and blood tests".[131] By the end of the experiment, which was terminated when Davis exhausted her financial reserves, she had collected 36,000-37,000 daily food records.

Davis concluded that her study supported her hypothesis since there were "no failures of infants to manage their own diets; all had hearty appetites; all throve. Constipation was unknown among them and laxatives were never used or needed." A visiting physician noted that these children "were the finest group of specimens from the physical and behaviour standpoint that I have ever seen in children that age". A radiologist was no less enthusiastic: "The beautifully calcified bones in roentgenograms of your group of children stand out so well that I have no trouble in picking them out when seen at a distance."

The children ate precisely the number of calories that were expected so that "after six months [there were] no noticeably fat or thin children but a greater uniformity of build than often obtains among those of the same family". The chosen diets provided on average 17% protein (range from 9-20%), 35% fat and 48% carbohydrate.

Davis was left to conclude that the "successful juggling and balancing of more than 30 nutritional essentials that exist in mixed and different proportions in the foods from which they must be derived suggests at once the existence of some innate, automatic mechanism for its accomplishment" so that "errors that children's appetites must have made [...] were too trivial and too easily compensated for to be of importance or even to be detected".

As a result she proposed that the key to healthy infant feeding is to provide healthy foods and to allow the children to decide how much and what they will eat.

These ideas caught the attention of Dr Benjamin Spock, author of the hugely influential *Baby and Child Care*, first published in 1946. "Dr Davis discovered three important things," wrote Spock.

First, babies who chose their own diet from a variety of natural foods develop very well; none of them got too fat or too thin. Second, every baby, over a period of time, chose what any scientist would agree was a well-balanced diet. Third, from meal to meal and day to day, the appetite varied a lot. Each separate meal wasn't well balanced. For several meals in a row a baby might feed largely on greens. Then he would change and go more heavily for starches. [133]

Spock also noted that children would often "go on a real jag" and eat only one foodstuff at a meal in amounts that grownups would not consider "polite"; or drink "a quart of milk" or eat "6 hard-boiled eggs in addition to a full meal" or "his appetite for beef would begin to increase. He might work up to four times as much beef as we would ordinarily think proper, keep up that rate for several days, and then taper off".

The current status of infant-led weaning

There were two great weaknesses in Dr Davis's experiment.[131] First, it lacked a control group to show what normally happens to children weaned according to the traditional baby food mush phase. Thus Dr Davis could not ever conclude that her method produced superior results. Second, she did not ever report her data; she only ever presented her conclusions from her personal analysis of those data. This was because she was not primarily a scientist, but a busy physician with all the constraints imposed by her need to make a living.

The result was that Dr Davis collected a mountain of data that probably overwhelmed her, especially living in the pre-computer era. By the time the computer age finally came around, all her carefully collected data had tragically been destroyed.

But from her work we can conclude that there were no obvious health risks associated with this method of weaning. She also established that an infant's appetite is not fixed but has the capacity to adjust on a daily/weekly basis to ensure that over time a properly balanced diet is eaten.

The first modern study evaluating aspects of Dr Davis's method was published in 2011.[134] Unlike hers, this was a retrospective study that evaluated the outcomes in infants whose parents stated that their child had been weaned either by the usual baby-mush spoon-feeding method or by baby-led weaning. The nature of the foods provided to the infants, whether natural or industrial, was not reported. The study found that children who directed their own food choices were more likely than spoon-fed infants to eat healthily and to be an appropriate weight as they aged. The key weakness of this study is that there is no record of the foods the infants were offered. And so we must conclude:

Ultimately it is the quality of the food choices that children are offered that will best determine their long-term health, regardless of how that food is presented to them and how they eat it.

Mothers wishing to try this method can find a great resource in Gill Rapley's book *Baby-Led Weaning: Helping Your Child to Love Good Food*[135] although some might argue that the food options include perhaps more carbohydrate than is necessary.

She writes: "No purées, no ice cube trays, no food processor, no potato masher, no baby rice, no weird fruit and veg combos...just you and your child, eating food that you enjoy with you and your family."

Refer back to the relevant advice in the Wonder Weaning chapter (see p72), where we provide information and advice for both baby-led weaning and traditional puréed feeding – and suggest trying a combination of both.

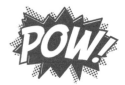

HOW TO FEED YOUR SUPERCHILDREN

My own experience suggests that if you want your children to be lean and healthy for life and not to develop obesity or Type 2 diabetes, as I did, then you need to do what I did *not* do. I thought that tons of exercise would protect me and that I did not need to worry about what I ate, just as long as I followed the diet that the experts assured me was "healthy". By the time I discerned their lies, it was too late for me to reverse my Type 2 diabetes. So here are the key foundation guidelines for parents on which, in my opinion, a healthy life is based:

Encourage your children to be life-long athletes.

Exercise is excellent for all-round health for a number of reasons. That said, we also need to understand that exercise alone is not enough – you cannot, as we now say, outrun a bad diet. In fact, I now believe that nutrition is a more important determinant of our long-term health than is regular exercise. But the combination is unbeatable.

Understand that obesity is a disorder of the brain, specifically due to appestat malfunction.

The traditional explanation that obesity is due simply to eating too much and exercising too little is unhelpful since it explains *how* but not *why* obesity develops. We overeat when our individual brain appestats controlling how many calories we eat each day are hijacked by the addictive processed foods of the industrial diet that incrementally have become the global norm since the introduction of the 1977 USDGA.

The key to the prevention of obesity and subsequent chronic ill health in our children and grandchildren (as well as us) is to ensure that we do not allow their appestats to be hijacked by addictive processed foods. And the earlier we can attune them to avoiding these foods and eating real foods instead, the better – the prevention of the addiction is better than the cure of it.

Wean your children onto non-commercial real foods.

We have shown in this book that infant foods first produced by the Fremont Canning Company in the 1920s and '30s, which then became Gerber's Baby Foods, were the prototype processed foods – the forerunners of the modern industrial diet. So if we are to ensure that our children do not become hooked on processed foods, we need to wean them onto real foods, not the types of food that are the descendants of those Gerber creations.

Especially in their crucial younger years, our children need to eat foods that are designed to maximise their health, not processed foods based on cheap carbohydrates that are designed to maximise the commercial health of the companies producing them.

Realise that current national feeding guidelines for babies and children are often not perfect. And sometimes they are quite far from perfect. Following them to the letter will not ensure the future health of your children. Instead, brave parents need to be aware that the guidelines can be wrong in a number of the principles they profess.

They fail to stress the importance of continuing breastfeeding beyond six months.

They overemphasise the need to eat a non-essential foodstuff, carbohydrate, at any age, in part because they fail to appreciate at all ages, humans (including babies and infants) are perfectly adapted to eating low-carb diets.

They place too much faith in the unproven health benefits of eating five or more servings of fruit and vegetables every day.

There is uncertainty about the correct timing of the first introduction of (real) foods to babies.

Some of these guidelines encourage the weaning of babies onto non-foods like white rice cereal, rather than onto real foods.

The need for key essential nutrients, especially fats but also iron and zinc, during the first 24 months of life is not always sufficiently emphasised.

The guidelines do not warn of growing concerns about the medical consequences of eating gluten-containing cereals including wheat, barley and rye, especially by the genetically predisposed.

The guidelines ignore evidence showing that a cereal-free diet full of vitamin D, fats and calcium provided by real foods can prevent the development of dental cavities.

Consider the value of baby-led weaning to introduce your babies to real foods.

Understand that insulin resistance is perhaps the single most prevalent medical condition across the globe, and one to be responded to decisively if it is apparent in your children. When driven by a high-carb diet, the level of each individual's insulin resistance becomes the greatest determinant of that person's long-term (ill) health, since it determines whether or not they are more likely to develop Type 2 diabetes and heart disease, and perhaps even cancer and dementia, amongst many other conditions.

It is therefore critical to establish whether or not your children have levels of insulin resistance that place them at increased risk for these conditions should they eat a high-carb diet (as I unfortunately did) for too many years.

The good news if they do have a measure of insulin resistance is that treatment is simple: reduce the amount of carbohydrates eaten each day. For those with the most severe degrees of insulin resistance, an intake of 25g carbohydrates per day is appropriate; for those with lesser degrees, carbohydrate intakes of 100-200g per day may still be effective.

SIGNS THAT YOUR CHILD MAY BE INSULIN RESISTANT

The main warning sign for insulin resistance is the presence of Type 2 diabetes in family members, especially parents, grandparents, aunts and uncles. The closer the relation, the greater the probability, and a parental history of Type 2 diabetes increases the risk that a child will also develop the condition up to ten-fold.

The first visible indicator that your child may be insulin resistant to some degree is a spell of progressive weight gain without significant growth. A key indicator is the progressive accumulation of an "insulin roll" – a roll of subcutaneous fat around his or her waist at the height of the belly button. Should this occur you could then consult your paediatrician for testing.

The first blood-test indicator for insulin resistance in the young is a rising blood-insulin concentration measured after an overnight fast. Next, the blood-insulin concentration becomes elevated after meals. As the condition progresses the blood-glucose concentration becomes elevated after meals, then after an overnight fast, and finally at all times both day and night.

The glycated haemoglobin value measures the average 24-hour blood-glucose concentration and becomes of concern when it rises above 5.5%; a value of 6.5% is high enough to support a diagnosis of Type 2 diabetes.

Finally, as the insulin resistance progresses, other markers of metabolic disturbance develop, including elevated blood triglyceride and small LDL particle numbers and lowered HDL-cholesterol concentrations.

Together all these measures give an indication of an individual's degree of insulin resistance. The key point is that the more abnormal the results, the greater the urgency to do something effective. And the first step, as we promoted in *The Real Meal Revolution*, and to a slightly lesser extent here, is to start reducing carbohydrate intake.

IN SUMMARY, IF THE PARENTS OF NEWBORNS AND YOUNGSTERS WERE ALL TO FOLLOW THE ADVICE IN THIS BOOK WE WOULD REVOLUTIONISE THE LONG-TERM HEALTH OF EVERYONE. AND THAT CONTINUES TO BE THE GOAL OF OUR EATING REVOLUTION.

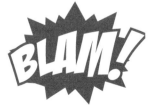

REFERENCES, NOTES & BIBLIOGRAPHY

The science and history of high-fat low-carb versus low-fat high-carb eating have been covered in great detail in three books that serve as a general reference for *Super Food for Superchildren*, and which we recommend. The first, unsurprisingly, is our own:

- *The Real Meal Revolution* by Tim Noakes, Jonno Proudfoot, David Grier and Sally-Ann Creed; Cape Town: Quiver Tree, 2013
The other two are:
- *Good Calories, Bad Calories* by Gary Taubes; New York: Anchor Books; 2007 – published in South Africa and elsewhere as *The Diet Delusion*
- *The Big Fat Surprise* by Nina Teicholz; New York: Simon and Schuster; 2014

PART I

Introduction: How To Raise Superchildren

1. World Health Organization. Health, history and hard choices: Funding dilemmas in a fast-changing world (2006), and Life expectancy (2013); www.who.int
2. World Health Organization. The top 10 causes of death. Fact sheet 310; www.who.int; 2014
3. World Health Organization. Obesity and overweight. Fact sheet 311; www.who.int; 2015
4. United States Department of Health and Services and Department of Agriculture. Scientific Report of the 2015 Dietary Guidelines Advisory Committee; www.health.gov; 2015
5. The short summary of *The Real Meal Revolution* here is broad and sweeping. We have used that book, as well as Taubes and Teicholz for much of the detail.
6. This information was compiled by in-house researchers in London, and was correct as of December 2015. We have used the standard conversion of 4g sugar = 1 teaspoon sugar
7. This information was compiled by in-house researchers in London, and was correct as of December 2015. We have used the standard conversion of 4g sugar = 1 teaspoon sugar
8. This information was compiled by in-house researchers in London, and was correct as of December 2015. We have used the standard conversion of 4g sugar = 1 teaspoon sugar

PART II

Marvellous Mums

1. Y Kelly, et al. "Light drinking versus abstinence in pregnancy – behavioural and cognitive outcomes in 7-year-old children: A longitudinal cohort study"; *BJOG: An International Journal of Obstetrics & Gynaecology*; 2013; 120 (11): 1340-1347
2. KD Setchell, et al. "Exposure of infants to phyto-oestrogens from soy-based infant formula"; *The Lancet*; 1997; 350 (9070): 23-27
3. A joint statement of Health Canada, Canadian Paediatric Society, Dietitians of Canada, and Breastfeeding Committee for Canada: www.hc-sc.gc.ca

Wonder Weaning

1. C Agostoni, et al. "Complementary feeding: A commentary by the ESPGHAN Committee on Nutrition"; *Journal of Pediatric Gastroenterology and Nutrition*; 2008; 46: 99-110
2. Practice-based Evidence in Nutrition. Infant nutrition complementary feeding: Evidence summary; www.pennutrition.com; 2014
3. D de Silva, et al. "Primary prevention of food allergy in children and adults: Systematic review"; *European Journal of Allergy and Clinical Immunology*; 2014; 69 (5): 581-589
4. S Cameron, et al. "How feasible is baby-led weaning as an approach to infant feeding? A review of the evidence"; *Nutrients*; 2012; 4 (11): 1575-1609

Terrific Toddlers

1. JC McCann and BN Ames. "Is docosahexaenoic acid, an n-3 long-chain polyunsaturated fatty acid, required for development of normal brain function? An overview of evidence from cognitive and behavioral tests in humans and animals"; *The American Journal of Clinical Nutrition*; 2005; 82 (2): 281-295
2. SN Young. "The effect of raising and lowering tryptophan levels on human mood and social behaviour"; *Philosophical Transactions of the Royal Society*; 2013; 368 (1615)
3. MW Louwman, et al. "Signs of impaired cognitive function in adolescents with marginal cobalamin status"; *The American Journal of Clinical Nutrition*; 2000; 72 (3): 762-769
4. M Singh and RR Das. "Zinc for the common cold"; *Cochrane Database of Systematic Reviews*; 2011; 16 (2): 1364

General resource for this chapter: Pan American Health Organization, as recommended by World Health Organization. Guiding principles for complementary feeding of the breastfed child. www.who.int; 2003

Incredible Kids

1. S Qamar, et al. "Vitamin D levels in children with growing pains"; *Journal of the College of Physicians and Surgeons Pakistan*; 2011; 21 (5): 284-287
2. M Viuda-Martos, et al. "Functional properties of honey, propolis, and royal jelly"; *Journal of Food Science*; 2008; 73 (9): R117-R124
3. R Lemus-Mondaca, et al. *"Stevia rebaudiana* Bertoni, source of a high-potency natural sweetener: A comprehensive review on the biochemical, nutritional and functional aspects"; *Food Chemistry*; 2012; 132 (30): 1121–1132
4. AJ Lanou, et al. "Calcium, dairy products, and bone health in children and young adults: A reevaluation of the evidence"; *Pediatrics*; 2005; 115 (3): 736-743

General resource for this chapter: JM Tanner. *Fetus Into Man: Physical growth from conception to maturity.* Cambridge, MA: Harvard University Press; 1989

Tremendous Teens:

1. RP Kelch and IZ Beitins. "Adolescent sexual development." In: MS Kappy, et al, eds. *The Diagnosis and Treatment of Endocrine Disorders in Childhood and Adolescence*, 4th ed. Springfield, Illinois: Charles C Thomas; 1994
2. RN Smith, et al. "A low-glycemic-load diet improves symptoms in acne vulgaris patients: A randomized controlled trial"; *The American Journal of Clinical Nutrition*; 2007; 86: 107-115
3. K Steventon and F Cowdell. "Acne and diet: A review of the latest evidence"; *Dermatological Nursing*; 2013; 12(2): 28-34
4. P Ozuguz, et al. "Evaluation of serum vitamins A and E and zinc levels according to the severity of acne vulgaris"; *Cutaneous and Ocular Toxicology*; 2014; 33 (2): 99-102
5. British Dietetic Association. Food and Mood Fact Sheet; www.bda.uk.com; 2014
6. JL Beard. "Iron requirements in adolescent females"; *Journal of Nutrition*; 2000; 130 (2S Suppl): 440S-442S

PART III

The Children's Food Revolution

1. Figure 1: reproduced from G Taubes. Why we get fat: The diet/weight

relationship, an alternative hypothesis; www.youtube.com; 2014

2. Figure 2: reproduced from G Taubes. Why we get fat: The diet/weight relationship, an alternative hypothesis; www.youtube.com; 2014

3. Figure 3: T Noakes

4. M Moss. *Salt Sugar Fat: How the food giants hooked us.* New York: Random House; 2013

5. DA Kessler. *The End of Overeating.* London: Penguin Books; 2009

6. CH Llewellyn, et al. "Satiety mechanisms in genetic risk of obesity"; *JAMA Pediatrics*; 2014; 168 (4): 338-344

7. CH van Jaarsveld, et al. "Prospective associations between appetitive traits and weight gain in infancy"; *American Journal of Clinical Nutrition*; 2011; 94 (6): 1562-1567

8. NM Avena, et al. "Evidence for sugar addiction: behavioral and neurochemical effects of intermittent, excessive sugar intake"; *Neuroscience & Biobehavioral Reviews*; 2008; 32: 20-39

9. X Ouyang, et al. "Fructose consumption as a risk factor for non-alcoholic fatty liver disease"; *Journal of Hepatology*; 2008; 48: 993-999

10. Figure 4: T Noakes

11. K Coveleskie, et al. "Altered functional connectivity within the central reward network in overweight and obese women"; *Nutrition & Diabetes*; 2015; 5: e148.

12. MM Boggiano, et al. "Eating tasty food to cope: Longitudinal association with BMI"; *Appetite*; 2015; 14 (87C) 365-370

13. GC Chung and CW Kuzawa. "Intergenerational effects of early life nutrition: Maternal leg length predicts offspring placental weight and birth weight among women in rural Luzon, Philippines"; *American Journal of Human Biology*; 2014; 26 (5): 652-659

14. CM Boney, et al. "Metabolic syndrome in childhood: Association with birth weight, maternal obesity, and gestational diabetes mellitus"; *Pediatrics*; 2005; 115 (3): e290-e296

15. AC Estampador and PW Franks. "Genetic and epigenetic catalysts in early-life programming of adult cardiometabolic disorders"; *Diabetes, Metabolic Syndrome and Obesity: Targets and Therapy*; 2014; 7: 575-586

16. M Hanson and P Gluckman. "Developmental origins of noncommunicable disease: Population and public health implications"; *American Journal of Clinical Nutrition*; 2011; 94 (6 Suppl): 1754S-1758S

17. SA Norris, et al. "Size at birth, weight gain in infancy and childhood, and adult diabetes risk in five low- or middle-income country birth cohorts"; *Diabetes Care*; 2012; 35 (1): 72-79

18. PW Franks, et al. "Gestational glucose tolerance and risk of type 2 diabetes in young Pima Indian offspring"; *Diabetes*; 2006; 55 (2): 460-465

19. JJ Reilly, et al. "Early life risk factors for obesity in childhood: Cohort study"; *BMJ*; 2005; 330 (7504): 1357

20. D Perlmuter and K Loberg. *Brain Maker.* New York: Little, Brown and Company; 2015

21. NT Mueller, et al. "Prenatal exposure to antibiotics, cesarean section and risk of childhood obesity"; *International Journal of Obesity*; 2015; 39 (4): 665-670

22. MB Azad, et al. "Infant antibiotic exposure and the development of childhood overweight and central adiposity"; *International Journal of Obesity*; 2014; 38 (10): 1290-1298

23. EE Stevens, et al. "A history of infant feeding"; *The Journal of Perinatal Education*; 2009; 18 (2): 32-39

24. E Psouni, et al. "Impact of carnivory on human development and evolution revealed by a new unifying model of weaning in mammals"; *PLOS ONE*; 2012; 7 (4): e32452

25. JC Drummond and A Wilbraham. *The Englishman's Food.* London: Pimlico; 1991

26. A Bentley. *Inventing Baby Food.* Oakland, California: University of California Press; 2014

27. WF Milton and WB Cheadle. *The North-West Passage by Land*, 2nd edition. London: Cassell, Petter, and Galpin; 1865

28. Figure 5: based on information from Bentley (26) and collated by T Noakes

29. G Palmer. *The Politics of Breastfeeding: When breasts are bad for business.* London: Pinter and Martin Ltd; 2009

30. G Palmer. *Complementary Feeding: Nutrition, Culture and Politics.* London: Pinter and Martin Ltd; 2011

31. World Health Organization. Healthy diet. Fact sheet 394; www.who.int; 2014

32. G Taubes. *Good Calories, Bad Calories*; New York: Anchor Books; 2007

33. EI Ekinci, et al. "Dietary salt intake and mortality in patients with type 2 diabetes"; *Diabetes Care*; 2011; 34 (3): 703-709

34. AP Kalogeropoulos, et al. "Dietary sodium content, mortality, and risk for cardiovascular events in older adults: The health, aging, and body composition (Health ABC) study"; *JAMA Internal Medicine*; 2015; 175 (3): 410-419

35. LT Bourne, et al. "The process followed in the development of the paediatric food-based dietary guidelines for South Africa"; *Maternal & Child Nutrition*; 2007; 3 (4): 239-250

36. LM du Plessis, et al. "Complementary feeding: A critical window of opportunity from six months onwards"; *South African Journal of Clinical Nutrition*; 2013; 26: S129-S140

37. NHS. Your baby's first solid foods; www.nhs.uk; 2015

38. M Makrides, et al. "Nutritional effect of including egg yolk in the weaning diet of breast-fed and formula-fed infants: A randomized controlled trial"; *American Journal of Clinical Nutrition*; 2002; 75 (6): 1084-1092

39. SC Cunnane and MA Crawford. "Survival of the fattest: Fat babies were the key to evolution of the large human brain"; *Comparative Biochemistry and Physiology Part A: Molecular & Integrative Physiology*; 2003; 136 (1): 17-26

40. K Milton. "The critical role played by animal source foods in human (Homo) evolution"; *The Journal of Nutrition*; 2003; 133 (11 Suppl 2): 3886S-3892S

41. SC Cunnane. *Survival of the fattest: The key to human brain evolution*; Singapore: World Scientific Publishing Co; 2005

42. KM Hambidge and NF Krebs. "Zinc deficiency: A special challenge"; *The Journal of Nutrition*; 2007; 137 (4): 1101-5

43. M Tang and NF Krebs. "High protein intake from meat as complementary food increases growth but not adiposity in breastfed infants: A randomized trial"; *The American Journal of Clinical Nutrition*; 2014; 100 (5): 1322-1328

44. NF Krebs, et al. "Meat as a first complementary food for breastfed infants: Feasibility and impact on zinc intake and status"; *Journal of Pediatric Gastroenterology and Nutrition*; 2006; 42 (2): 207-214

45. CR Gale, et al. "Critical periods of brain growth and cognitive function in children"; *Brain*; 2004; 127 (Pt 2): 321-329

46. GE Kennedy. "From the ape's dilemma to the weanling's dilemma: Early weaning and its evolutionary context"; *Journal of Human Evolution*; 2005; 48 (2): 123-145

47. O Ballard and AL Morrow. "Human milk composition: Nutrients and bioactive factors"; *Pediatric Clinics of North America*; 2013; 60 (1): 49-74

48. S Boseley. "The longer babies breastfeed, the more they achieve in life - major study"; *The Guardian*; 2015

49. K Northstone, et al. "Are dietary patterns in childhood associated with IQ at 8 years of age? A population-based cohort study." *Journal of Epidemiology and Community Health*; 2012; 66 (7): 624-628

50. KM Purtell and ET Gershoff. "Fast food consumption and academic growth in late childhood"; *Clinical Pediatrics*; 2014; Epub

51. JM Medina and A Tabernero. "Lactate utilization by brain cells and its role in CNS development"; *Journal of Neuroscience Research*; 2005; 79 (1-2): 2-10

52. L De Rooy and J Hawdon. "Nutritional factors that affect the postnatal metabolic adaptation of full-term small- and large-for-gestational-age infants"; *Pediatrics*; 2002; 109 (3): E42

53. EC Westman. "Is dietary carbohydrate essential for human nutrition?" *The American Journal of Clinical Nutrition*; 2002; 75 (5): 951-953

54. Table 1: AE Harper. "Defining the Essential of Nutrients". In: ME Shills, et al, eds. *Modern Nutrition in Health and Disease*, 9th edition. Baltimore: Lippincott, Williams & Wilkins; 1999

55. Figure 6: Redrawn from E Cohen, et al. "Statistical review of US macronutrient consumption data, 1965-2011"; *Nutrition*; 2015; 31: 727-732

56. N Freinkel, et al. The 1986 McCollum award lecture: "Fuel-mediated teratogenesis during early organogenesis: The effects of increased concentrations of glucose, ketones, or somatomedin inhibitor during rat embryo culture"; *The American Journal of Clinical Nutrition*; 1986; 44 (6): 986-995

57. A Martin, et al. "Glucose tolerance tests and 'in vivo' response to intravenous insulin in the unanaesthetized late pregnant rat and their consequences to the fetus"; *Diabetes & Metabolism*; 1986; 12 (6): 302-307

58. BE Metzger, et al. "'Accelerated starvation' and the skipped breakfast in late normal pregnancy"; *The Lancet*; 1982; 1 (8272): 588-592

59. P Felig. "Maternal and fetal fuel homeostasis in human pregnancy"; *The American Journal of Clinical Nutrition*; 1973; 26 (9): 998-1005

60. E Herrera. "Metabolic adaptations in pregnancy and their implications for the availability of substrates to the fetus"; *European Journal of Clinical Nutrition*; 2000; 54 Suppl 1: S47-S51

61. OE Owen, et al. "Brain metabolism during fasting"; *The Journal of Clinical Investigation*; 1967; 46 (10): 1589-1595

62. PA Adam, et al. "Oxidation of glucose and D-B-OH-butyrate by the early human fetal brain"; *Acta Paediatrica Scandinavica*; 1975; 64 (1): 17-24

63. V Sabata, et al. "The role of free fatty acids, glycerol, ketone bodies and glucose in the energy metabolism of the mother and fetus during delivery"; *Biology of the Neonate*; 1968; 13 (1): 7-17

64. B Persson and R Tunell. "Influence of environmental temperature and acidosis on lipid mobilization in the human infant during the first two hours after birth"; *Acta Paediatrica Scandinavica*; 1971; 60 (4): 385-398

65. MA Page, et al. "Activities of enzymes of ketone-body utilization in brain and other tissues of suckling rats"; *Biochemical Journal*; 1971; 121 (1): 49-53

66. G Settergren, et al. "Cerebral blood flow and exchange of oxygen, glucose, ketone bodies, lactate, pyruvate and amino acids in infants"; *Acta Paediatrica Scandinavica*; 1976; 65 (3): 343-353

67. PF Bougneres, et al. "Ketone body transport in the human neonate and infant"; *The Journal of Clinical Investigation*; 1986; 77 (1): 42-48

68. C Bon, et al. "Feto-maternal metabolism in human normal pregnancies: Study of 73 cases"; *Annales de Biologie Clinique*; 2007; 65 (6): 609-619

69. GE Shambaugh, III. "Ketone body metabolism in the mother and fetus"; *Federation Proceedings*; 1985; 44 (7): 2347-2351

70. EJ Coetzee, et al. "Ketonuria in pregnancy – with special reference to calorie-restricted food intake in obese diabetics"; *Diabetes*; 1980; 29 (3): 177-181

71. J Girard. "Gluconeogenesis in late fetal and early neonatal life"; *Biology of the Neonate*; 1986; 50 (5): 237-258

72. The Ketogenic Diet for Health. Babies thrive under a ketogenic metabolism; www.ketotic.org; 2014

73. L Nichols. *Real Food for Gestational Diabetes*. USA: Lilly Nichols; 2015

74. C Agostoni, et al. "Complementary feeding: A commentary by the ESPGHAN Committee on Nutrition"; *Journal of Pediatric Gastroenterology and Nutrition*; 2008, 46: 99–110

75. BI Nwaru, et al. "Age at the introduction of solid foods during the first year and allergic sensitization at age 5 years"; *Pediatrics*; 2010; 125 (1): 50-59

76. JJ Koplin, et al. "Can early introduction of egg prevent egg allergy in infants? A population-based study"; *Journal of Allergy and Clinical Immunology*; 2010; 126 (4): 807-813

77. G Du Toit, et al. "Randomized trial of peanut consumption in infants at risk for peanut allergy"; *The New England Journal of Medicine*; 2015; 372 (9): 803-813

78. RS Gruchalla and HA Sampson. "Preventing peanut allergy through early consumption – ready for prime time?"; *The New England Journal of Medicine*; 2015; 372 (9): 875-877

79. Table 2: reproduced from Z Harcombe. The perfect five-a-day? www.zoeharcombe.com; 2014, with additional material on brown and white rice from Self Nutrition Data. Babyfood, cereal, brown rice, dry, instant; nutritiondata.self.com; 2015, and Self Nutrition Data. Rice, white, long-grain, regular, cooked. nutritiondata.self.com; 2015

80. MK Fox, et al. "Feeding infants and toddlers study: What foods are infants and toddlers eating?"; *Journal of the American Dietetic Association*; 2004; 104 (1 Suppl 1): s22-s30

81. MK Fox, et al. "Food consumption patterns of young preschoolers: Are they starting off on the right path?"; *Journal of the American Dietetic Association*; 2010; 110 (12 Suppl): S52-S59

82. JT Dwyer, et al. "FITS: New insights and lessons learned"; *Journal of the American Dietetic Association*; 2004; 104 (1 Suppl 1): s5-s7

83. RR Briefel, et al. "Feeding infants and toddlers study: Improvements needed in meeting infant feeding recommendations"; *Journal of the American Dietetic Association*; 2004; 104 (1 Suppl 1): s31-s37

84. L Johnson, et al. "Energy-dense, low-fiber, high-fat dietary pattern is associated with increased fatness in childhood"; *The American Journal of Clinical Nutrition*; 2008; 87 (4): 846-854

85. J Chang and L Salahi. Rice cereal controversy: Does it make kids fat? ABC News; abcnews.go.com; 2011

86. J Bradbury. "Docosahexaenoic acid (DHA): An ancient nutrient for the modern human brain"; *Nutrients*; 2011; 3 (5): 529-554

87. SM Innis. "Dietary (n-3) fatty acids and brain development"; *Journal of Nutrition*; 2007; 137 (4): 855-859

88. M Crawford. "Placental delivery of arachidonic and docosahexaenoic acids: Implications for the lipid nutrition of preterm infants"; *The American Journal of Clinical Nutrition*; 2000; 71 (1 Suppl): 275S-84S

89. MA Crawford, et al. "Are deficits of arachidonic and docosahexaenoic acids responsible for the neural and vascular complications of preterm babies?"; *The American Journal of Clinical Nutrition*; 1997; 66 (4 Suppl): 1032S-1041S

90. Bible Life Ministries. Mommy goes shopping for baby food. Diet and nutrition for infant health; www.biblelife.org; 2015

91. IB Helland, et al. "Maternal supplementation with very-long-chain n-3

fatty acids during pregnancy and lactation augments children's IQ at 4 years of age"; *Pediatrics*; 2003; 111 (1): e39-e44

92. WD Lassek and SJ Gaulin. "Linoleic and docosahexaenoic acids in human milk have opposite relationships with cognitive test performance in a sample of 28 countries"; *Prostaglandins, Leukotrienes and Essential Fatty Acids*; 2014; 91 (5): 195-201

93. Figure 7: Reproduced from WD Lassek and SJ Gaulin. "Linoleic and docosahexaenoic acids in human milk have opposite relationships with cognitive test performance in a sample of 28 countries"; *Prostaglandins Leukotrienes and Essential Fatty Acid*s; 2014; 91 (5): 195-201

94. NF Krebs, et al. "Effects of different complementary feeding regimens on iron status and enteric microbiota in breastfed infants"; *The Journal of Pediatrics*; 2013; 163 (2): 416-423

95. Health Canada. Infant Feeding Joint Working Group. Nutrition for healthy term infants: Recommendations from birth to six months; www.hc-sc.gc.ca; 2015

96. Table 3 and Table 4: reproduced from Z Harcombe. The perfect five-a-day? www.zoeharcombe.com; 2014

97. Z Harcombe. Five a day: The truth; www.zoeharcombe.com; 2012

98. D Mawson. *The Home of the Blizzard*. New York: St Martin's Press; 1998

99. L Bickel. *Mawson's Will: The greatest Polar survival story ever written*. Vermont: Steerforth Press; 2000

100. ME van Stuijvenberg, et al. "Serum retinol in 1-6-year-old children from a low socio-economic South African community with a high intake of liver: Implication for blanket vitamin A supplementation"; *Public Health Nutrition*; 2012; 15: 716-724

101. P Boffetta, et al. "Fruit and vegetable intake and overall cancer risk in the European Prospective Investigation into Cancer and Nutrition (EPIC)"; *Journal of the National Cancer Institute*; 2010; 102 (8): 529-537

102. W Davis. *Wheat Belly*. New York: Rodale; 2011

103. D Perlmutter. *Grain Brain*. New York: Little, Brown and Company; 2013

104. A Fasano. *Gluten Freedom: The nation's leading expert offers the essential guide to a healthy, gluten-free lifestyle*. Bognor Regis, UK: Wiley; 2014

105. A Fasano. *A Clinical Guide to Gluten-related Disorders*. Philadelphia: Lippincott, Williams & Wilkins; 2014

106. A Fasano. "Zonulin and its regulation of intestinal barrier function: The biological door to inflammation, autoimmunity, and cancer"; *Physiological Reviews*; 2011; 91 (1): 151-175

107. Table 5: reproduced from A Fasano. "Zonulin and its regulation of intestinal barrier function: The biological door to inflammation, autoimmunity, and cancer"; *Physiological Reviews*; 2011; 91 (1): 151-175

108. JC Antvorskov, et al. "Dietary gluten and the development of type 1 diabetes"; *Diabetologia*; 2014; 57 (9): 1770-1780

109. C Catassi, et al. "Non-Celiac Gluten sensitivity: The new frontier of gluten related disorders"; *Nutrients*; 2013; 5 (10): 3839-3853

110. J Hollon, et al. "Effect of gliadin on permeability of intestinal biopsy explants from celiac disease patients and patients with non-celiac gluten sensitivity"; *Nutrients*; 2015; 7 (3): 1565-1576

111. ML Burr, et al. "Effects of changes in fat, fish, and fibre intakes on death and myocardial reinfarction: Diet and reinfarction trial (DART)"; *The Lancet*; 1989; 2 (8666): 757-761

112. DJ Jenkins, et al. "Effect of wheat bran on glycemic control and risk factors for cardiovascular disease in type 2 diabetes"; *Diabetes Care*; 2002; 25 (9): 1522-1528

113. AR Ness, et al. "The long-term effect of dietary advice in men with coronary disease: Follow-up of the Diet and Reinfarction trial (DART); *European Journal of Clinical Nutrition*; 2002; 56 (6): 512-518

114. A Andersson, et al. "Whole-grain foods do not affect insulin sensitivity or markers of lipid peroxidation and inflammation in healthy, moderately overweight subjects"; *Journal of Nutrition*; 2007; 137 (6): 1401-1407

115. IA Brownlee, et al. "Markers of cardiovascular risk are not changed by increased whole-grain intake: The WHOLEheart study, a randomised, controlled dietary intervention"; *British Journal of Nutrition*; 2010; 104 (1): 125-134

116. L Enright and J Slavin. "No effect of 14 day consumption of whole grain diet compared to refined grain diet on antioxidant measures in healthy, young subjects: A pilot study"; *Nutrition Journal*; 2010; 9: 12

117. R Giacco, et al. "Effects of rye and whole wheat versus refined cereal foods on metabolic risk factors: A randomised controlled two-centre intervention study"; *Clinical Nutrition*; 2013; 32 (6): 941-949

118. A Colpo. *Whole Grains, Empty Promises*. Kentucky, USA: Lulu Publishing; 2014

119. T Asano and RS McLeod. "Dietary fibre for the prevention of colorectal adenomas and carcinomas"; *Cochrane Database of Systematic Reviews*; 2002; (2): CD003430

120. WC Willett. *Eat, Drink and Be Healthy*. New York: Free Press; 2005

121. P Hujoel. "Dietary carbohydrates and dental-systemic diseases"; *Journal of Dental Research*; 2009; 88 (6): 490-502

122. W Price. *Nutrition and Physical Degeneration*. Oxford: Benediction Classics; 2010

123. M Mellanby and CL Pattison. "Remarks on the influence of a cereal-free diet rich in vitamin D and calcium on dental caries in children"; *British Medical Journal*; 1932; 1 (3715): 507-510

124. Figure 8: reproduced from data in M Mellanby and CL Pattison. "Remarks on the influence of a cereal-free diet rich in vitamin D and calcium on dental caries in children"; *British Medical Journal*; 1932; 1 (3715): 507-510

125. EC McBeath and TF Zucker. "The role of vitamin D in the control of dental caries in children"; *Journal of Nutrition*; 1937; 15 (6): 547-564

126. R Nagel. *Cure Tooth Deay: Heal and prevent cavities with nutrition*, 2nd edition. Oregon: Golden Child Publishing; 2010

127. KJ Mattila, et al. "Association between dental health and acute myocardial infarction"; *BMJ*; 1989; 298 (6676): 779-781

128. A Pucar, et al. "Correlation between atherosclerosis and periodontal putative pathogenic bacterial infections in coronary and internal mammary arteries"; *Journal of Periodontology*; 2007; 78 (4): 677-682

129. Dr Axe: Food is Medicine. How to heal your cavities naturally; draxe.com; 2015

130. CM Davis. "Results of the self-selection of diets by young children"; *Canadian Medical Association Journal*; 1939; 41 (3): 257-261

131. S Strauss and M Clara. "Davis and the wisdom of letting children choose their own diets; *CMAJ*; 2006; 175 (10): 1199

132. Table 6: reproduced from CM Davis. "Results of the self-selection of diets by young children"; *Canadian Medical Association Journal*; 1939; 41 (3): 257-261

133. B Spock. *Baby and Child Care*, 17th edition. New York: Pocket Books; 1972

134. E Townsend and NJ Pitchford. "Baby knows best? The impact of weaning style on food preferences and body mass index in early childhood in a case-controlled sample"; *BMJ Open*; 2012; 2 (1): e000298

135. G Rapley and T Murkett. *Baby-led Weaning: Helping your baby to love good food*. London: Vermilion; 2008

GENERAL INDEX

Page references in italics indicate tables or figures.

RECIPE INDEX

ACKNOWLEDGEMENTS

PROF TIM NOAKES

Challenging conventional eating ideas is, I have learned, not a simple journey. The support of my family and most especially my wife Marilyn Anne has been critical in helping me through the tougher moments. To her and to my children, I am forever deeply grateful. I thank also Jonno Proudfoot and his team for the opportunity to be part of this adventure. And to Sigal Chives, as always, sincere thanks for the perfect diagrams; and to Megan Lofthouse, thank you for helping with the manuscript and, as ever, managing my schedule.

JONNO PROUDFOOT

Thank you to my beautiful and talented wife, Kate George – and my inspiration, baby Imogen. And to Bridget Surtees for bringing her expertise and calming nature to our epic creation. And Steve, Hagen, Spiro and James of Lima Bean. Also to Ann Childers, for Canadian stats and Canadian charm; Karen Thomson, for her vast network and tenaciousness; Caro Gardner, for being an absolute rock star; Toby Murphy, for taking the best food photos in the world; Emily Maguire, for her wealth of knowledge and enthusiasm; John Briffa, for his time and wisdom; Adam Pike, Nick Pemberton and Wendy Hoffman, our legal team. A big thank you to Tim Richman, Fran Beighton and the team at Burnet Media for their hard work in putting it all together. And, finally, a heartfelt thank you to Prof for once again joining us for the ride, and for allowing us access to his wonderful, energetic world and his incredible mind; it's an honour and privilege to work with you.

TIM RICHMAN

My great thanks go to Prof Noakes, Jonno, Kate and Bridget, for being a blast to work with and (most of all) for being brilliant. And to the extended publishing team: Fran Beighton and Bron MacGregor; Simon Richardson and Gary Maverick; Ania Rokita, Lynda Ingham-Brown and Mary Lennox; Bridget Impey, Shay Heydenrych, Kerrie Barlow and Janine Daniel at Jacana; Arlene Gippert at Craft. And, of course, to Jules Richman, my amazing wife, publishing adviser and future-superchild raiser.

ROBINSON

•

First published in South African in 2015 by The Real Meal Revolution

•

First published in Great Britain in 2016 by Robinson

•

A CIP catalogue record for this book is available from the British Library.

•

ISBN: 978-1-47213-726-5 (paperback)
ISBN: 978-1-47213-727-2 (ebook)

•

Typeset in South Africa by Burnet Media
Printed in China

•

Robinson
is an imprint of
Little, Brown Book Group
Carmelite House
50 Victoria Embankment
London EC4Y 0DZ

•

An Hachette UK Company
www.hachette.co.uk

•

www.littlebrown.co.uk

•

The recommendations given in this book are solely intended as education
and should not be taken as medical advice.

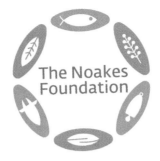

The Noakes Foundation

For decades we have been fed misinformation about nutrition, but following this advice has left us with enormous challenges, such as rising rates of obesity, diabetes and autoimmune diseases.

Having been left frustrated by a decline in his own health, Professor Tim Noakes has made it his mission to reverse this global trend. The Noakes Foundation is the catalyst for this change. It seeks to reveal what genuine healthy nutrition looks like and, in doing so, make a difference in the lives of millions of people, by supporting healthier-eating research, funding independent studies and addressing the research gap into low-carb nutrition.

To tackle this challenge, The Noakes Foundation addresses three key questions.

1 What does the optimal diet look like?

2 How can nutrition reverse the effects of diabetes and other autoimmune diseases?

3 What are the fundamental problems with our current eating habits?

In answering these, the Foundation hopes to take great steps forward in the battle against Type 2 diabetes, obesity and insulin resistance.

Visit www.thenoakesfoundation.org to learn more

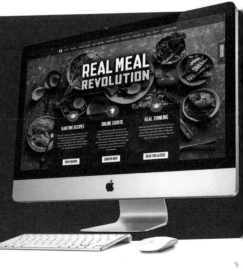

CONVERSION CHARTS

Oven temperatures

°C	Fan °C	°F	Gas	Description
110	90	225	¼	Very cool
120	100	250	½	Very cool
140	120	275	1	Cool
150	130	300	2	Cool
160	140	325	3	Warm
180	160	350	4	Moderate
190	170	375	5	Moderately hot
200	180	400	6	Fairly hot
220	200	425	7	Hot
230	210	450	8	Very hot
240	220	475	8	Very hot

Weights for dry ingredients

Metric	Imperial	Metric	Imperial
7g	¼ oz	400g	14oz
15g	½ oz	425g	15oz
20g	¾ oz	450g	1lb
25g	1 oz	500g	1lb 2oz
40g	1½oz	550g	1¼lb
50g	2oz	600g	1lb 5oz
60g	2½oz	650g	1lb 7oz
75g	3oz	675g	1½lb
100g	3½oz	700g	1lb 9oz
125g	4oz	750g	1lb 11oz
140g	4½oz	800g	1¾lb
150g	5oz	900g	2lb
165g	5½oz	1kg	2¼lb
175g	6oz	1.1kg	2½lb
200g	7oz	1.25kg	2¾lb
225g	8oz	1.35kg	3lb
250g	9oz	1.5kg	3lb 6oz
275g	10oz	1.8kg	4lb
300g	11oz	2kg	4½lb
350g	12oz	2.25kg	5lb
375g	13oz	2.5kg	5½lb
		2.75kg	6lb

Liquid measures

Metric	Imperial	Aus	US
25ml	1fl oz		
50ml	2fl oz	¼ cup	¼ cup
75ml	3fl oz		
100ml	3½fl oz		
120ml	4fl oz	½ cup	½ cup
150ml	5fl oz		
175ml	6fl oz	¾ cup	¾ cup
200ml	7fl oz		
250ml	8fl oz	1 cup	1 cup
300ml	10fl oz/½ pint	½ pint	1¼ cups
360ml	12fl oz		
400ml	14fl oz		
450ml	15fl oz	2 cups	2 cups/1 pint
600ml	1 pint	1 pint	2½ cups
750ml	1¼ pints		
900ml	1½ pints		
1 litre	1¾ pints	1¾ pints	1 quart
1.2 litres	2 pints		
1.4 litres	2½ pints		
1.5 litres	2½ pints		
1.7 litres	3 pints		
2 litres	3½ pints		
3 litres	5¼ pints		

UK-Australian tablespoon conversions
1 x UK or Australian teaspoon is 5ml
1 x UK tablespoon is 3 teaspoons/15ml
1 Australian tablespoon is 4 teaspoons/20ml